VETERINARY DENTISTRY

A TEAM APPROACH

VETERINARY DENTISTRY

A TEAM APPROACH

Third Edition

Steven E. Holmstrom, DVM, Dipl. AVDC
San Pedro, California

ELSEVIER

ELSEVIER

3251 Riverport Lane
St. Louis, Missouri 63043

VETERINARY DENTISTRY: A TEAM APPROACH   ISBN: 978-0-3234-8527-2

Notices

Library of Congress Control Number: 2018943477

Content Strategist: Brandi Graham
Content Development Manager: Lisa Newton
Senior Content Development Specialist: Danielle M. Frazier
Publishing Services Manager: Deepthi Unni
Book Production Specialist: Srividhya Vidhyashankar
Design Direction: Patrick C. Ferguson

Printed in China
Last digit is the print number: 9   8   7   6   5

I would like to dedicate this edition of Veterinary Dentistry: A Team Approach, to the founders of "modern" veterinary dentistry: Drs. Peter Emily, Donald Ross, and. Keith Grove.

Dr. Emily received his Doctor of Dental Surgery at Creighton University, Omaha, Nebraska, and his Certificate of Periodontology from the University of Pennsylvania in the 1960s. He started working in association with veterinarians on many species of animals shortly thereafter. While I had trained by another group of specialist dentists, I credit Peter with stimulating me to spread my knowledge when he stated over lunch, "You know, you really should start lecturing and writing."

Dr. Ross, began his career in veterinary medicine with the U.S. Air Force in 1967 during the Vietnam War. He was assigned to the Military Working Dog Hospital and performed dental procedures on military dogs for 3 years. He developed his dental skills by working with the base endodontist. Once out of the military, he earned his master's degree in dentistry in 1972 and subsequently started giving lectures in veterinary dentistry. He was always available by telephone and contributed to my knowledge.

Dr. Grove was board certified as both a human and veterinary dentist, having earned his DDS degree from the University of Detroit-Mercy School of Dentistry in 1972 and later achieving diplomate status with both the American Veterinary Dental College (AVDC) and the American Board of Periodontology. He presented me with the idea of having "dental labs" at the Veterinary Dental Forum when I was program chair for the second Veterinary Dental Forum. This has grown to become a very popular source of veterinary dental education.

Of course, there were others in the early stages that joined together to form "critical mass" that I feel I should recognize. It was a group effort to get veterinary dentistry to where it is now. The organizing committee for the AVDC also included Drs. Peter Emily, Donald Ross, Keith Grove,. Gary Beard, Benjamin Colmery, Colin Harvey, Sandy Manfra,. Thomas Mulligan, and Charles Williams. The first 10 presidents of the AVDC were Drs. Charles Williams, Colin Harvey, Keith Grove, Steven Holmstrom, Edward Eisner, Robert Wiggs, Gregg DuPont, Kenneth Capron, Barbara Stapleton, and Michael Peak.

Without these dedicated veterinary dentists, our profession would be nowhere near where it is today.

CONTRIBUTORS

Ana C. Castejon-Gonzalez, DVM, PhD, Dipl. AVDC, Dipl. EVDC
Lecturer of Dentistry and Oral Surgery
Department of Clinical Sciences and Advanced
  Medicine
University of Pennsylvania School of Veterinary
  Medicine
Philadelphia, Pennsylvania

Laurie A. Holmstrom, RDH
San Pedro, California

Steven E. Holmstrom, DVM, Dipl. AVDC
San Pedro, California

Alexander M. Reiter, Dipl. Tzt., Dr. med. vet., Dipl. AVDC, Dipl. EVDC
Professor of Dentistry and Oral Surgery
Department of Clinical Sciences and Advanced
  Medicine
University of Pennsylvania School of Veterinary
  Medicine
Philadelphia, Pennsylvania

PREFACE

Veterinary Dentistry: A Team Approach was written with the entire general veterinary practice in mind. It is comprehensive, bringing a practical, working knowledge in veterinary dentistry to the student, veterinary assistant, receptionist, technician, and veterinarian. The collaboration of the team is vital to the expansion of services and the completion of many dental-related tasks, resulting in increasing related productivity of the laboratory, anesthesia, radiology, dentistry, hospitalization, pharmacy, and retail departments.

This edition includes an outline at the beginning of each chapter to give the reader an overview of the chapter contents. Key points and key terms are listed and should be reviewed before and after reading the chapter to ensure that the chapter is understood. Worksheets are provided at the end of each chapter to help the reader retain key information and improve skill competency. The worksheet answers appear in a section at the back of the text. The reader will also find an appendix con-

taining a list of abbreviations. Although this list was current when the text was published, the American Veterinary Dental College (AVDC) Nomenclature Committee is continuing to revise this list. Those studying for Board examinations are urged to visit the AVDC's website (www.avdc.org) for the most current list. There is also an appendix that includes lists of various veterinary dental equipment and one with AVDC-approved definitions. The reader will also find a bibliography and a glossary.

I would like to thank all of the technicians with whom I have had the pleasure to work with in my veterinary dental practice: Jan Yarslov, Gina Gros de Mange, Karen Thomson, Loretto Jaca, Melinda Pyle, Lilian Brown, and Lee Figard, as well as practice manager Stacey Neubert. Thanks to Danielle Frazier at Elsevier for her contributions to making this a useful text.

Steven E. Holmstrom, DVM, Dipl. AVDC

CONTENTS

Introduction to Veterinary Dentistry

LEARNING OBJECTIVES

When you have completed this chapter, you will be able to:
- Differentiate between the terms mesaticephalic, brachycephalic, and dolichocephalic.
- Identify the anatomic components that comprise the mandible and maxilla.
- Describe the structure of the teeth and supporting tissues.
- List the dental formulas for dogs and cats.
- Identify the terms used to designate position and direction in the oral cavity.
- Describe the anatomic and Triadan numbering systems.
- Describe the method for recording pathology on a dental chart.

KEY TERMS

Alveolar mucosa
Alveolus
Ameloblasts
Anatomic numbering system
Apical
Brachycephalic
Buccal
Canine tooth
Cementum
Coronal
Distal

Dolichocephalic
Furcation
Gingiva
Incisors
Interproximal area
Labial
Lateral palatine fold
Mandible
Maxilla
Mesaticephalic
Mesial

Molars
Mucogingival line
Occlusion
Odontoblasts
Palatal
Premolars
Rugae palatinae
Sublingual
Sulcus
Temporomandibular joint
Triadan numbering system

WHY VETERINARY DENTISTRY?

Just as humans need dental care, animals require veterinary dental care to maintain overall health. In addition to the discomfort caused by dental disease, the associated disease processes may cause systemic problems.

The American Veterinary Dental College defines veterinary dentistry as a discipline within the scope of veterinary practice that involves the professional consultation, evaluation, diagnosis, prevention, treatment (nonsurgical, surgical or related procedures) of conditions, diseases, and disorders of the oral cavity and maxillofacial area and their adjacent and associated structures; it is provided by a licensed veterinarian, within the scope of his/her education, training, and experience, in accordance with the ethics of the profession and applicable law. (http://www.avdc.org/Nomenclature/Nomen-Intro.html)

DENTAL ANATOMY AND DENTAL TERMINOLOGY

Communication in veterinary dentistry is as important as communication in veterinary medicine. Medical records and charts must be annotated. Dental terminology differs from that of veterinary medicine because the focus is on the teeth and their relationship to each other and the mouth.

GENERAL ANATOMY

To be able to recognize oral disease, technicians and veterinarians must first understand oral health. After establishing this baseline, technicians and veterinarians can recognize the changes that occur as oral disease progresses. Another reason that understanding normal anatomy is so important is that it helps veterinarians and technicians select the appropriate technique to use to prevent and treat disease. For example, without knowing the number of roots that a tooth has, the practitioner could not extract the tooth.

Types of Heads

Three types of skulls are common: mesaticephalic, brachycephalic, and dolichocephalic. These words have a common root, *cephalic,* which means head.

Mesaticephalic

Mesatic means medium. Mesaticephalic is the most common head type. Poodles, corgis, German shepherds, Labrador retrievers, and domestic shorthair cats are typical examples (Fig. 1.1).

Brachycephalic

Brachy means short. Brachycephalic animals have short, wide heads. This characteristic commonly results in crowded and rotated premolar teeth, a condition that may lead to periodontal disease. Boxers, pugs, bulldogs, and Persian cats are common examples of the brachycephalic type (Fig. 1.2).

Dolichocephalic

Dolicho means long. Dolichocephalic animals have long, narrow heads. Collies, greyhounds, borzois, and seal

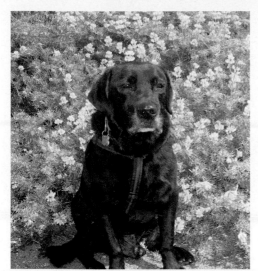

Fig. 1.1 The Labrador is an example of a mesaticephalic head type.

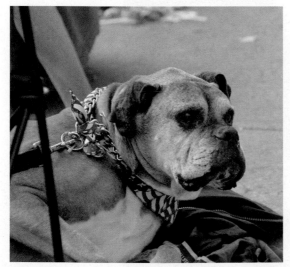

Fig. 1.2 The boxer is an example of a brachycephalic head type.

point Siamese cats are common examples of this type (Fig. 1.3).

Maxilla

The upper jaw, called the *maxilla,* is made up of many bones (Fig. 1.4). The incisal and maxillary bones hold the teeth. The roof of the mouth is composed of the hard and soft palates. The hard palate is the portion of the roof of the mouth that consists of hard bone. The hard palate is covered with a mucous membrane that has irregular ridges, called the *rugae palatinae.* The incisive papilla lies behind the central incisors. The nasopalatine ducts exit on each side of the incisive papilla. The naso-palatine ducts communicate with the vomeronasal organ), which connects to the dog's amygdala, the part of the brain that plays a big role in emotional reactions. This allows dogs to respond emotionally to molecules such as pheromones which travel up the incisive canal. The soft palate is the posterior portion of the roof of the mouth, which does not have underlying bone. This portion separates the oral cavity from the pharynx, which leads to the nasal cavity. Close observation reveals that the teeth are surrounded by the gingiva. The area in which the two jaws join in the back of the oral cavity is known as the *lateral palatine fold.*

Mandible

The lower jaw is known as the *mandible* (Fig. 1.5). It is connected to the maxilla by a hinge joint called the *temporomandibular joint* (TMJ). The two mandibles are fused together at the mandibular symphysis. The symphysis is a synarthrosis, which is a union of the left and right mandible joined together by fibrocartilagenous tissue. So, between the rostral ends of the two mandibles, there is a plate of tissue. This tissue is radiolucent, so radiographs of the rostral mandible in dogs and cats will always show a lucent line running down the mid line. The tongue is a fleshy muscular organ in the mouth used for tasting, licking, swallowing, articulating, and thermoregulation. The tongue lies between the two mandibles; the structures and surfaces beneath the tongue are referred to as *sublingual.* The mandible is covered ventrally by muscle and skin. The oral cavity is covered with a mucous membrane, which becomes the gingiva at the mucogingival line. It is not unusual for dogs and cats to have slightly mobile mandibular symphysis.

Cheeks and Lips

The mucous membrane, or oral mucosa, is the tissue that forms the lining of most of the oral cavity outside the mucogingival line. The oral mucosa ends at the lips. The vestibule of the oral cavity is the part between the cheeks or lips and the alveolar ridge (Fig. 1.6).

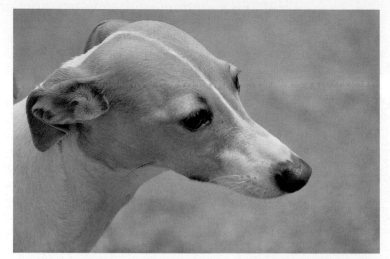

Fig. 1.3 The whippet is an example of a dolichocephalic head type.

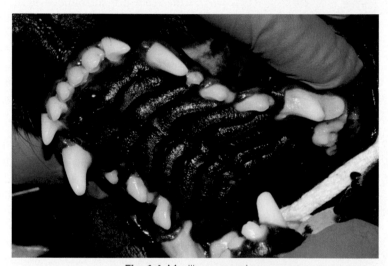

Fig. 1.4 Maxilla or upper jaw.

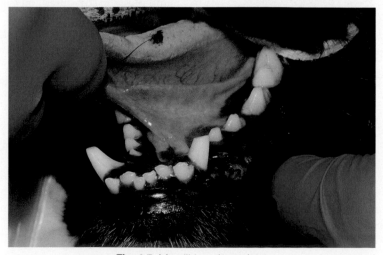

Fig. 1.5 Mandible or lower jaw.

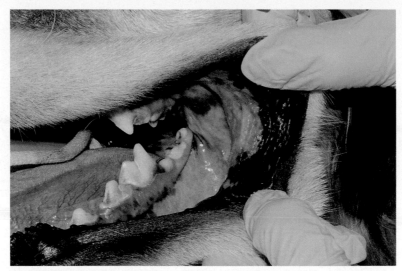

Fig. 1.6 The vestibule is the area between the teeth/gingiva and cheek.

TOOTH ANATOMY

The puppy has 28 teeth, whereas the adult dog has 42 teeth. The kitten has 26 teeth, whereas the adult cat has 30 teeth.

External Tooth

The tooth may be divided into the crown, neck, and root (Fig. 1.7). The **clinical crown (CR/CC)** is that part of a tooth that is coronal to the gingival margin where the **anatomic crown (CR/AC)** is that part of a tooth that is coronal to the cementoenamel junction (or anatomic root). The tip of the crown is known as the *cusp*. The crown is covered with enamel (E), the hardest substance in the body. It will survive normal use and even some abuse without problems. However, it may fracture in patients who chew bones and other hard substances. Normally, enamel is present only above the gumline. Enamel is produced by cells called *ameloblasts* as the tooth is developing. Where the enamel thins close to the gumline, many teeth have a slight indentation. This indentation is known as the *neck* or cementoenamel junction, which is the area of a tooth where cementum and enamel meet. Underneath the gumline is the root. The **anatomic root (RO/AR)** is that part of a tooth that is apical to the cementoenamel junction (or anatomic crown). The **clinical root (RO/CR)** is the part of a tooth that is apical to the gingival margin. The deepest part of

the root is known as the *apex*. At the apex, blood vessels and nerves enter the tooth through a series of small channels known as the *apical delta* or through larger canals known as the *apical foramen*. The cusp is the tip or pointed prominence on the occlusal surface of the crown.

Internal Tooth

The bulk of the tooth consists of dentine or dentin. Both spellings are correct and synonymous. Dentine is produced by odontoblasts, which are cells that line the pulp chamber. Throughout the life of the tooth the odontoblast continues to produce dentine. The innermost portion of the tooth is the pulp, which is further divided into the pulp chamber and root canal. Pulp chamber is the space within the crown of a tooth and the root canal is the space within the root of a tooth. As previously mentioned, the pulp chamber is lined by odontoblasts. The remainder of the pulp chamber consists of nerves, blood vessels, and a variety of different types of cells and fibrous tissue. The root canal is the portion of the pulp chamber below the gumline. The apex of the tooth is the portion deepest in the socket (or alveolus). The apex contains small channels through which blood vessels and nerves enter and exit.

Gingiva

Attached gingiva is made up of epithelial tissue that is harder and more tightly attached to supportive

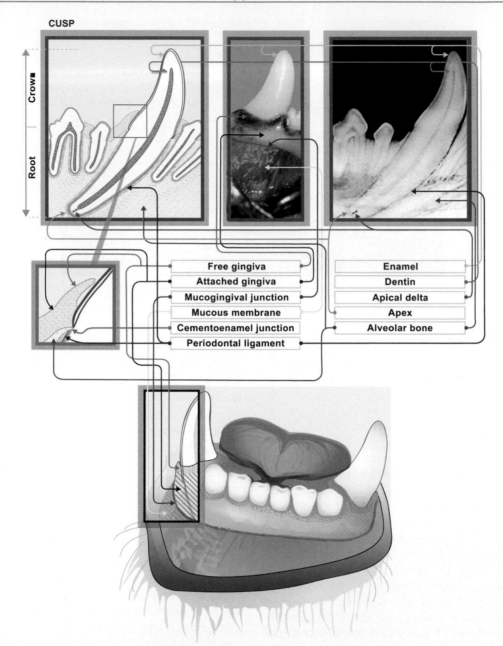

Fig. 1.7 Tooth anatomy. (Courtesy Veterinary Information Network [VIN].)

structures than other tissue in the oral cavity. Gingiva is therefore able to withstand the forces of chewing. This hardening is known as *keratinization*. Free gingiva is the portion of the gingiva that is not directly attached to the tooth or supporting structure. A slight groove exists between the free and attached gingiva, which is known as the free gingival groove. The area between the free gingiva and the tooth is known as the *sulcus* when healthy and without a space. A space between the gingiva and tooth is called a *pocket*. Pockets are considered diseased tissue when periodontal disease is present.

Alveolar Mucosa

The alveolar mucosa is the less densely keratinized gingival tissue covering the bone. Its decreased keratinization increases the susceptibility of the tissue to trauma caused by chewing.

Attachment Apparatus

The attachment apparatus is composed of the structures that support the tooth. The tooth is held in place in the alveolus, or socket, by the periodontal ligament. Cementum, a material that can repair itself if damaged, attaches the periodontal ligament to the tooth. The periodontal ligament is a fibrous structure attached to the tooth/cementum and bone by Sharpey's fibers. These fibers are interlaced in cementum and bone. The alveolar bone is the bone of the upper jaw (maxilla) or lower jaw (mandible) in which the tooth rests.

DENTAL FORMULA FOR THE PUPPY

The deciduous dentition period is that period during which only deciduous (primary or baby) teeth are present. The permanent dentition period is that period during which only permanent (adult or secondary) teeth are present. The mixed dentition period is that period during which both deciduous and permanent teeth are present.

The puppy is born without teeth. Deciduous (primary or "baby") canine dentition consists of 28 teeth. The primary incisors normally erupt at approximately 3 to 4 weeks of age, the canines at 3 weeks, and the primary premolars from 4 to 12 weeks of age. The age at which the teeth erupt varies among breed lines. On each side, upper and lower, the adult dog has three incisors, one canine, and three premolars. Puppies do not have primary molars. The dental formula for the puppy is as follows:

$$2 \times (3/3i, \ 1/1c, \ 3/3p) = 28$$

Generally, primary teeth fall out (exfoliate) 1 to 2 weeks before the eruption of adult teeth. What triggers a tooth to exfoliate is not fully understood. One theory is that as the adult tooth develops, it puts pressure on the primary tooth, stimulating a resorptive process. Once the tooth root is resorbed, the crown loosens from the gingival attachment and falls off.

The approximate ages in which deciduous and adult teeth erupt are listed in Table 1.1.

TABLE 1.1 Approximate Ages (in weeks) When Teeth Erupt in Dogs and Cats

Teeth	DECIDUOUS (PRIMARY)		PERMANENT (ADULT)	
	Puppy	Kitten	Dog	Cat
Incisors	4–6	3–4	12–16	11–16
Canines	3–5	3–4	12–16	12–20
Premolars	5–6	5–6	16–20	16–20
Molars	–	–	16–24	20–24

DENTAL FORMULA FOR THE ADULT DOG

The secondary (adult) canine dental formula on each side of the mouth, upper and lower, consists of three incisors, one canine, and four premolars. On each side, the upper jaw has two molars and the lower jaw has three molars. The incisors are used for gnawing and grooming. The canine teeth are used for holding and tearing. The arrangement of the premolars, which are used for cutting and breaking up food, resembles pinking shears. The molars are used for grinding. The adult incisor teeth erupt at 3 to 5 months of age, the canine and premolar teeth at 4 to 6 months, and the molars at 5 to 7 months. The dental formula for the adult dog is as follows:

$$2 \times (3/3I, \ 1/1C, \ 4/4P, \ 2/3M) = 42$$

DENTAL FORMULA FOR THE KITTEN

The kitten's dentition is similar to that of the puppy except that two, rather than three, deciduous premolars are present in the lower jaw. The kitten's deciduous teeth erupt earlier than those of the puppy. The incisors erupt at 2 to 3 weeks of age. The deciduous canines erupt at 3 to 4 weeks of age, and the deciduous premolars at 3 to 6 weeks of age. The dental formula for a kitten is as follows:

$$2 \times (3/3i, \ 1/1c, \ 3/2p) = 26$$

DENTAL FORMULA FOR THE ADULT CAT

On each side of the mouth, upper and lower, the adult cat has three incisors, one canine, and one molar. On each side the cat has three premolars on the upper jaw and two premolars on the lower jaw. The adult incisors erupt at 3 to 4 months of age, the canines at 4 to 5 months of age, premolars at 4 to 6 months of age, and molars at 4 to 5 months of age. The dental formula for the adult cat is as follows:

$$2 \times (3/3I, \; 1/1C, \; 3/2P, \; 1/1M) - 30$$

ROOT STRUCTURE OF THE ADULT DOG

An understanding of root structure is important. When extracting teeth (with a few exceptions discussed later), all roots should be removed to prevent further complications. To remove all the roots, the practitioner must know the number of roots and understand the anatomy. In the dog the incisors, canines, first premolar, and mandibular third molar have one root each. The maxillary second and third premolars; the mandibular second, third, and fourth premolars; and the mandibular first and second molars have two roots. The maxillary fourth premolar, first molar, and second molar have three roots each. One key to remembering the number of roots is to recall that the mandible does not have any three-rooted teeth (Figs. 1.8 and 1.9).

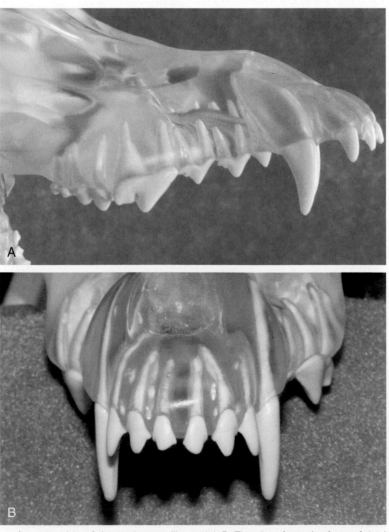

Fig. 1.8 A, View from the side of the canine maxilla model. B, The view from the front of the incisors in the canine model.

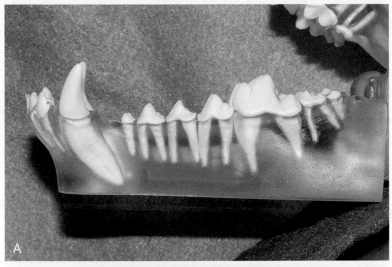

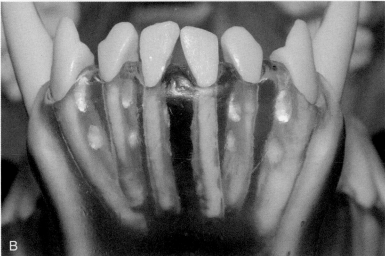

Fig. 1.9 A, Vew from the side of the canine mandible model. B, The view from the front of the canine mandible model.

ROOT STRUCTURE OF THE ADULT CAT

In the cat the incisors, canines, and maxillary second premolar have one root each. The maxillary third premolars, mandibular third and fourth premolars, and mandibular first molar have two roots. The maxillary fourth premolar has three roots. The number of roots in the maxillary first molar varies from one to three roots, which are usually fused together (Figs. 1.10 and 1.11).

FURCATION

The furcation is the area in which the roots join the crown. In two-rooted teeth, it is known as a bifurcation; in three-rooted teeth, a trifurcation.

NOMENCLATURE

The term *nomenclature* is derived from the words "name" and "to call."

POSITIONAL TERMINOLOGY

The reference point for anatomic terms in the mouth is the teeth. The term vestibule *(labial)* indicates the direction toward the outside of the teeth, usually toward the lips. Similarly, vestibule or buccal indicates the direction toward the outside of the teeth, usually toward the cheeks. Palatal and lingual refer to the direction toward the middle of the mouth—palatal for the maxillary and lingual for the mandibular. Although these terms are

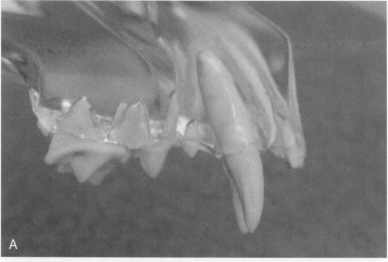

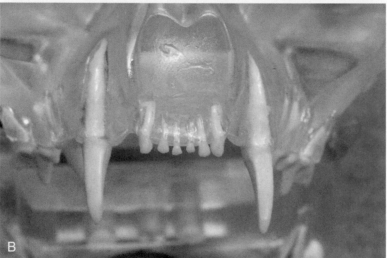

Fig. 1.10 A, View from the side of the feline maxilla tooth model showing all of the teeth. B, The view from the front of the feline maxilla model showing the incisors and canines.

often used interchangeably, they are properly used specifically for upper and lower dentition, respectively. If a line is drawn along the dental arch and a mark is placed representing the center of the line between the first incisors, mesial is the side of the tooth closest to the center of the line and distal is the portion farthest from the center of the line (Fig. 1.12).

Line Angles

Line angles represent the "corners" of the tooth. The mesial buccal line angle is the area in which the mesial and buccal surfaces join. Likewise, the buccal distal line angle joins the distal and buccal walls. The distal lingual

and lingual mesial serve as similar reference points. Line angles and walls are important in describing fractures and tooth defects.

Coronal-Apical Directions

Coronal refers to the direction toward the crown, and *apical* means toward the root of the tooth. For example, a fracture at the tip of the crown could also be described as a fracture in the coronal third of the tooth.

Between Teeth

The area in between two teeth is known as the *interproximal area*.

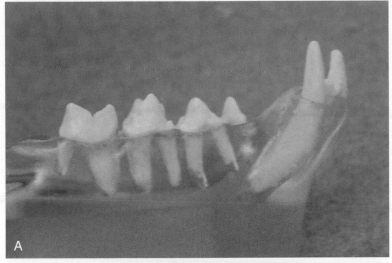

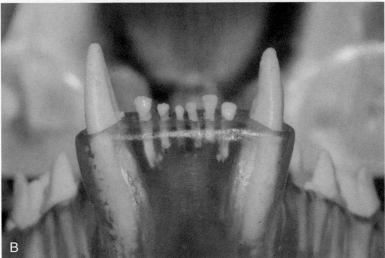

Fig. 1.11 A, Feline mandible. B, Feline mandible incisal.

OCCLUSION

Occlusion refers to the way the teeth fit together. Humans have true occlusal surfaces in which the premolars and molars directly oppose each other. Chewing takes place on a flat surface. Dogs and cats have sectorial occlusion, whereby chewing occurs on the sides of the teeth.

ANATOMIC AND TRIADAN NUMBERING SYSTEMS

In human dentistry the universal nomenclature system is standard. In the nomenclature system the numbering starts with the upper right third molar (#1) and proceeds around the arch to #16. The lower left third molar is #17, and counting proceeds around the arch to the lower right third molar, #32.

Because the veterinary profession treats a variety of species with different numbers of teeth, use of the universal system is impractical and would result in the same tooth being identified by a different number, depending on the animal. For that reason the veterinary profession has adopted the anatomic and Triadan numbering systems. By using the anatomic or Triadan system, veterinary staff members can easily annotate medical records. Currently, both the anatomic and Triadan systems are acceptable. Each system has advantages and disadvantages.

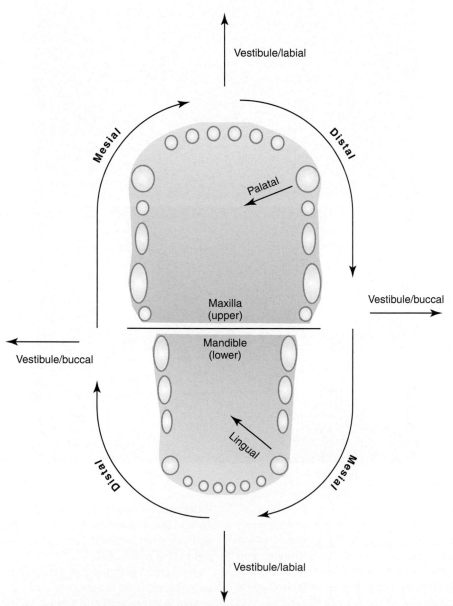

Fig. 1.12 Positional terminology: The oral road map.

Anatomic Numbering System

The first thing to know with the anatomic numbering system is tooth type. The beginning of this chapter contained a review of the types and functions of teeth. The first letter of the tooth is used to identify the tooth type. The correct anatomic names of teeth written out are right or left; maxillary or mandibular; first, second, third, or fourth; and incisor, canine, premolar, or molar, as applicable, written out in full or abbreviated. An example of written out names would be *left maxillary first incisor* or *right mandibular fourth premolar*.

Abbreviations for the tooth types are *I* for incisors, *C* for canines, *P* for premolars, and *M* for molars. To indicate the side of the mouth where the tooth is, a number representing the tooth is written on the left side of the letter for the left side of the patient's mouth or on the right side of the letter for the right side of the patient's mouth. A helpful way to remember this convention is as follows: left side of patient, left side of letter; right side of patient, right side of letter.

The maxillary (upper) teeth are indicated as a superscript number. The mandibular teeth are indicated as a subscript number.

Incisors = I

The incisors are identified by the capital letter *I*. When writing the tooth type on ruled paper, the veterinary staff member should generally write the letter on the line. A lowercase letter *i* should be used in reference to a primary tooth. The incisor located closest to the center of the mouth is incisor #1, incisor #2 is the intermediate incisor, and incisor #3 is the lateral incisor. The central right maxillary incisor is I^1. The central left mandibular incisor is $_1I$.

Canines = C

The adult canine teeth are identified by the capital letter *C*. The primary canine tooth is indicated by the lowercase letter *c*. A quadrant is one quarter, and the mouth has four quadrants: upper right, upper left, lower left, and lower right. Because only one canine tooth is present in each quadrant, only the number *1* is used. The left mandibular canine is known as $_1C$. The right maxillary canine tooth is known as C^1.

Premolars = P

The premolars are represented by the capital letter *P*. Primary premolar teeth are represented by a lowercase *p*.

In the dog the premolars are numbered sequentially beginning with *1* and moving back in the mouth. Because the cat does not have a first premolar in the maxilla (upper jaw) or a first or second premolar in the mandible (lower jaw), premolar numbering starts with *2* in the maxilla and *3* in the mandible. The left maxillary fourth premolar is called ^4P, and the right mandibular fourth premolar is called P_4. The cat does not have ^1P, P^1, $_1P$, $_2P$, P_1, or P_2.

Molars = M

The molars are indicated by the letter *M*. Remember that no primary molars exist. The first molar is indicated by *1*, and successive molars by *2* and *3* if present. The right maxillary first molar is M^1. The left mandibular first molar is $_1M$.

Primary (Deciduous) Teeth

The primary teeth are indicated by lowercase letters. A lowercase *i* indicates a primary incisor, *c* a canine, and *p* a premolar.

Shortcut

A shortcut in the notation of multiple teeth is to indicate the tooth numbers as a chain. For example, $^{321}I^{123}$ indicates all the maxillary incisors.

Modification for Alphanumeric Computers

The use of computers in veterinary medicine is increasing. For the purposes of estimating and invoicing, codes can be created to indicate various types of treatment of individual teeth. The letter *U* is used for upper teeth, and *L* is used for lower teeth. For example, one code might be RCULC (*Root Canal Upper Left Canine*) to indicate a root canal performed on the upper left canine tooth. Similarly, DXLP4 (*Dental eXtraction Lower Premolar*) might indicate an extraction of the lower right fourth premolar.

Advantages

The primary advantage of the anatomic system is that it is easy to remember because it uses anatomic terms that most people already know. Also, by using the previously described shortcut, veterinary staff members can refer to many teeth at once.

Disadvantages

One disadvantage of this system is that it is more time consuming than the Triadan system, which is discussed next. Although shorter than "left maxillary canine," the words "one superscript C" still take more time to say than the numbers of the Triadan system. Moreover, not all computers are alphanumeric. Some computer systems accept only numbers. Because the creation of codes would be difficult with this type of computer, the Triadan system is particularly useful.

Triadan Numbering System

The many numbers in the Triadan numbering system make it seem confusing at first (Table 1.2). Despite its appearance, the Triadan system is quite simple once the code is memorized. The Triadan system uses three numbers. The first number identifies the quadrant (remember that there are four) of the mouth. The second and third numbers identify the tooth, which is always represented by two numbers.

Quadrant

The quadrants are identified as *1xx* for right maxillary, *2xx* for left maxillary, *3xx* for left mandibular, and *4xx* for right mandibular. The quadrant is indicated by the first of three numbers (Fig. 1.13).

Tooth

Numbering of the teeth begins in the front of the mouth. The central incisor is identified as *tooth 01,* the intermediate incisor as *02,* the lateral (or corner) incisor as *03,* the canine as *04,* the first premolar as *05,* and the first molar as *09.* Remember, in the Triadan system the type of tooth is always identified by two numbers. Combined with the quadrant, there are three numbers. For example, the left

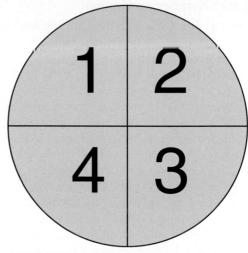

Fig. 1.13 Quadrants used in the Triadan numbering system.

maxillary canine tooth is identified as *204.* The right maxillary fourth premolar is identified as *108,* the left mandibular first molar as *309,* and the right mandibular central incisor as *401* (Figs. 1.14 and 1.15).

Rule of 4 and 9

For species that have fewer teeth, the rule of 4 and 9 has been developed. This rule states that the canine tooth is always designated by *04* and the first molar by *09.* Teeth are counted from 01 to 05. The first molar is counted as 09, and then the count goes backward, with the fourth premolar being 08 and the third premolar being 07, as it is in the dog. This convention allows identical teeth to have identical numbers in different species and decreases confusion.

Deciduous (Primary) Teeth

In the young patient, deciduous teeth are identified as being in quadrants 5 for the right maxillary (upper), 6 for the left maxillary (upper), 7 for the left mandibular (lower), and 8 for the right mandibular (lower).

Advantages

The primary advantage of the Triadan system is that it can be used with nonalphanumeric computers. Secondly, referring to the tooth type as "one-o-one" for the right maxillary first incisor or "three eleven" for the left mandibular third molar is convenient.

Disadvantage

The disadvantage of the Triadan system is that it is not intuitive. The technician must know the code to

TABLE 1.2 Anatomic Numbering System vs. Triadan Numbering System		
	Anatomic	**Triadan**
Computers	Will not work with nonalphanumeric types	Works with both types
Shortcut	Can identify many teeth of the same type	Identifies each tooth separately
Ease of use	Familiar terms, easy to remember	Not intuitive, must be memorized

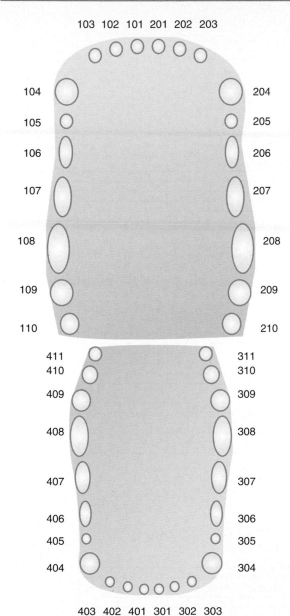

Fig. 1.14 Triadan numbering system in the dog.

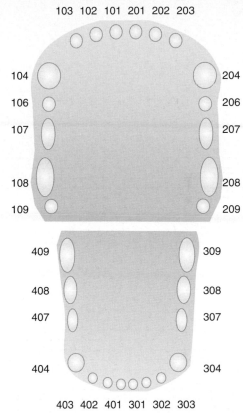

Fig. 1.15 Triadan numbering system in the cat.

understand which tooth is being identified. However, once learned, it is easy to use and therefore its popularity has increased.

DENTAL CHART FOR THE DOG

A dental chart may be used to keep a visual record of the patient's oral health status (Fig. 1.16). The teeth are

oriented to the viewer, who is facing the patient. The patient's right side is indicated on the left side of the chart, and the patient's left side is on the right side of the chart. The first row of teeth represents the labial/buccal (outside) of the maxillary (upper) teeth. The second row of teeth represents the palatal (inside) of the maxillary teeth. The third row of teeth represents the lingual (inside) of the mandibular (lower) teeth. The lowest row of teeth represents the labial/buccal (outside) of the mandibular (lower) teeth. The boxes indicate the depth of the sulcus, or pocket, at the time of successive dental procedures. The first charted depth is indicated in the row closest to the tooth (date #1). Successive procedures are noted in the next rows.

DENTAL CHART FOR THE CAT

Except for the number of teeth, the dental chart for the cat is identical to that for the dog (Fig. 1.17).

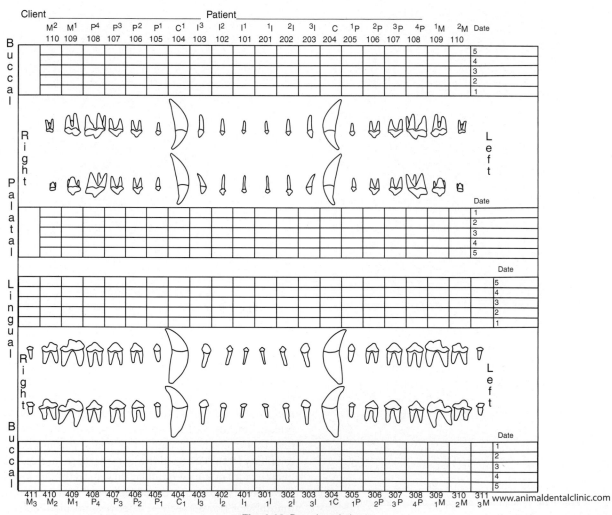

Fig. 1.16 Dog dental chart.

Client _____ Patient _____

www.animaldentalclinic.com

Client _____ Patient_____

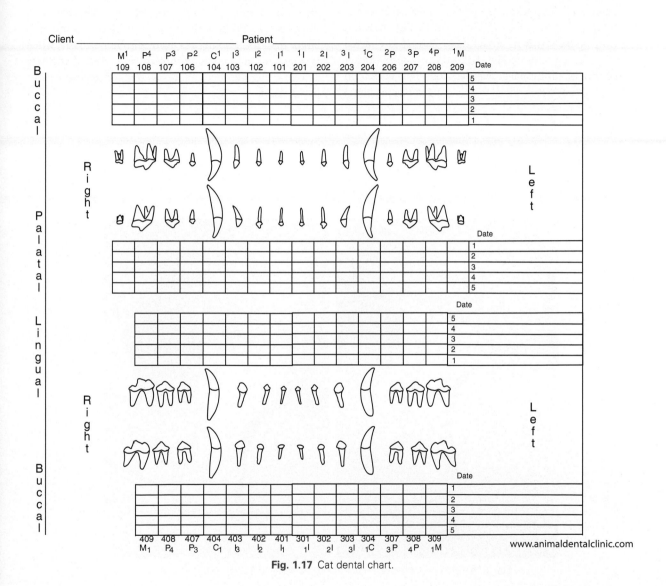

Fig. 1.17 Cat dental chart.

www.animaldentalclinic.com

DENTAL CHARTING

The charts provided allow for multiple visits. Each time the patient is charged, the date is recorded and the pathology is noted. The first number that is written in the square is the pocket depth, the second number is the total attachment loss. The patient in Fig. 1.18 has a 3-mm pocket with no attachment loss. It is charted as 3/0. The patient in Fig. 1.19 has a 3-mm pocket with 2 mm of additional attachment loss. This is charted as 3/5. The patient in Fig. 1.20 has gingival hyperplasia

that is approximately 8-mm deep. The sulcular depth is approximately 2 mm. The 8 mm of pseudopocket and 2 mm of sulcular depth are added together for the first number (pocket depth) of 10, whereas the second number is normally the attachment loss; however, in this case, the 8 mm of pseudopocket is indicated, and thus 10/2 would be written. When the first number is larger than the second, it is a site with hyperplasia; when it is smaller, it is a site with recession; and when there is only one number, there is neither recession nor hyperplasia.

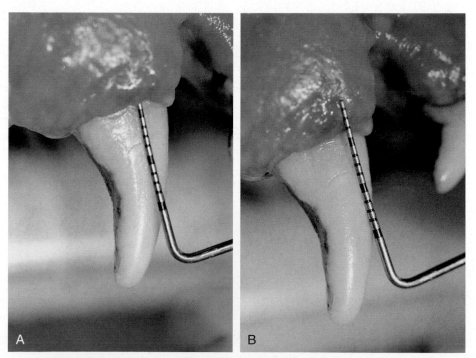

Fig. 1.18 A 3-mm pocket with no attachment loss. A, Probe in. B, Probe out.

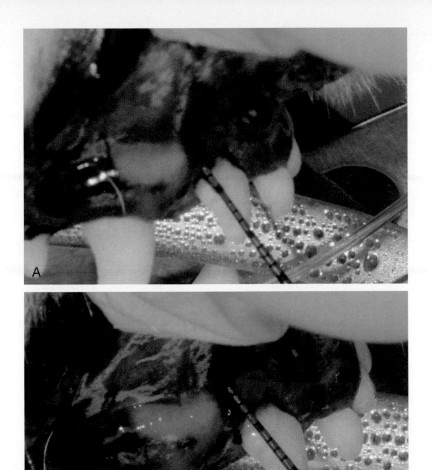

Fig. 1.19 Attachment loss with pocket. A, Probe in. B, Probe out.

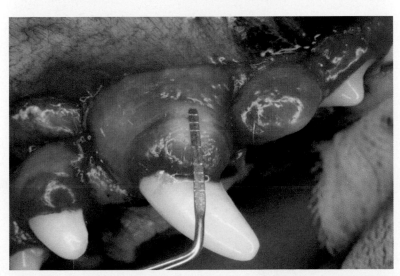

Fig. 1.20 Gingival hyperplasia with probe out of pocket, over hyperplastic area.

CHAPTER 1 WORKSHEET

1. The most common condition in cats over 7 years of age is _____

2. Dental terminology differs from veterinary medical terminology in that the focus is on the teeth themselves and the relationship of the _____ to other teeth.

3. For example, practitioners could not extract a tooth without knowing the number of _____ that the tooth has.

4. The area where the two jaws join in the oral cavity is known as the _____.

5. The puppy has _____ teeth, whereas the adult dog has _____ teeth.

6. _____ is the hardest substance in the body and is fairly resistant to stains.

7. Dentine is produced by _____, which are cells that line the pulp chamber.

8. The area between the free gingiva and the tooth is known as the _____ in healthy animals when there is no space between the gingiva and tooth and a _____ when there is space.

9. The tooth is held in place in the alveolus, or socket, by the _____.

10. The dental formula for the adult dog is: _____.

11. The dental formula for the adult cat is: _____.

12. The following maxillary teeth have one root in the dog (use Triadan or anatomic system): _____.

13. The following mandibular teeth have two roots in the dog (use Triadan or anatomic system): _____.

14. The following maxillary teeth have three roots in the dog (use Triadan or anatomic system): _____.

15. The following maxillary teeth have three roots in the cat (use Triadan or anatomic system): _____.

16. The primary teeth are indicated by _____ letters.

17. In the Triadan system, adult quadrants are identified as _____ for right maxillary, _____ for left maxillary, _____ for left mandibular, and _____ for right mandibular. The quadrant is indicated as the first of three numbers.

18. The central incisor is identified as tooth _____, the intermediate incisor is identified as tooth _____, the lateral (or corner) incisor is identified as tooth _____, the canine as _____, and first premolar as _____.

19. The rule of 4 and 9 states that 04 is always the _____ tooth and the _____ _____ is always tooth 09.

20. The left maxillary first premolar in the dog would be listed as tooth #_____, whereas the right mandibular third premolar in the cat would be listed as tooth #_____.

The Oral Examination and Disease Recognition

OUTLINE

LEARNING OBJECTIVES

When you have completed this chapter, you will be able to:

- Describe the normal occlusion seen in dogs and cats.
- Differentiate between pedodontics, orthodontics, periodontics, prosthodontics, and endodontics.
- Define anodontia and list possible conditions with which it is associated.
- Describe the three classes of malocclusion and discuss the various clinical presentations seen with these conditions.

- List and describe the classifications of oropharyngeal inflammation.
- Describe possible abnormal conditions of the tooth surface, including abnormalities in enamel formation.
- List and describe the various fracture classification schemes that apply to veterinary dentistry.
- List and describe common oral medical diseases, including neoplastic conditions of the oral cavity.

KEY TERMS

Acanthomatous ameloblastoma
Alveolar mucositis
Amelogenesis imperfecta
Anodontia
Attrition
Avulsion
Buccoversion
Canine oral viral oral papillomatosis
Caries
Caudal crossbite
Caudal mucositis
Cheilitis
Cingulum
Class I malocclusion
Class II occlusion
Class III occlusion
Contact mucositis (also contact mucosal ulceration)
Cranial mandibular osteodystrophy
Crossbite
Dentigerous cyst
Dentinogenesis imperfecta
Dilacerated roots
Distoversion

Enamel hypomineralization
Enamel hypoplasia
Endodontics
Fibrosarcoma
Fusion
Gemini tooth
Gingival hyperplasia
Gingivitis
Glossitis
Granuloma
Interceptive orthodontics
Labial/buccal mucositis
Labioversion
Linguoversion
Luxation
Malignant melanoma
Mandibular periostitis ossificans
Mandibular prognathism
Maxillary brachygnathism
Maxillary-mandibular asymmetry
Mesioversion
Nonneoplastic bone
Odontoma
Oral medicine
Oral neoplasia
Oronasal fistula

Orthodontics
Osteomyelitis
Palatitis
Pericoronitis
Pedodontics
Peg teeth
Periodontics
Periodontitis
Peripheral odontogenic fibroma
Persistent primary teeth
Pharyngitis
Prosthodontics
Rostral crossbite
Scissors bite
Slab fracture
Spearing canines
Squamous cell carcinoma
Stomatitis
Sublingual mucositis
Supernumerary teeth
Tonsillitis
Tooth resorption
Ulcerative eosinophilic stomatitis
Uremic ulceration

This chapter is devoted to an overview of the oral examination and the recognition of veterinary dental disease. Because it is an overview, it does not provide in-depth coverage of specific aspects of treatment. The treatment of veterinary dental conditions is covered in subsequent chapters.

All of the members of the veterinary office staff play important roles in health care. Although the diagnosis of disease should be left to the veterinarian, the technician and other staff members can assist the veterinarian by recognizing conditions that appear abnormal and alerting the veterinarian to them. This chapter discusses various disease conditions that staff members might observe.

The wide variety of genetics in the dog (and to a lesser degree the cat) gives rise to a wide variety of size and developmental abnormalities. Fig. 2.1 illustrates this variety in the difference in size between a Chihuahua and Saint Bernard.

ORAL EXAMINATION

The duties of veterinarians and their staff are described in the practice acts of each state. Because state law varies, veterinary staff members should refer to the specific practice acts of the state in which they are employed. However, some generalities apply. The oral examination should always be conducted in a systematic manner. In many states, it is legal for the registered veterinary technician to induce anesthesia under orders of a licensed veterinarian. The placement of the endotracheal tube is a good opportunity for visualization of the pharynx, tonsils, and tongue (Fig. 2.2). While scaling and polishing the teeth, the technician can closely observe the tooth surface and gingiva. The technician should always note any abnormalities and report them to the doctor.

NORMAL OCCLUSION

Normal occlusion in dogs and cats is a scissors bite, in which the mandibular (lower) teeth come into contact with the palatal side (inside) of the maxillary (upper) teeth (Figs. 2.3 and 2.4). Normally, the cusp of the mandibular incisors rests on a ledge on the palatal side of the maxillary incisors known as the *cingulum.* The mandibular canines fit in the diastema (space) between the lateral incisor and maxillary canines. The cusp of the mandibular first premolar fits midway between the maxillary canine and first premolar. The remainder of the premolars are intermeshed in a similar fashion. The lower teeth are approximately one-half a tooth in front of their maxillary counterparts. The maxillary premolar teeth do not contact the mandibular premolar teeth. The crown cusps of the mandibular premolar teeth are positioned lingual to the arch of the maxillary premolar teeth.

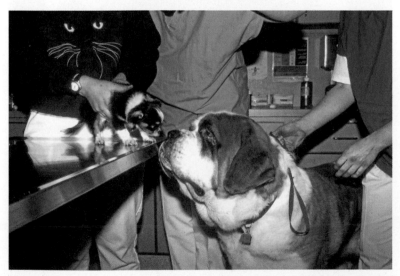

Fig. 2.1 The differences in the canine size expressed by looking at a chihuahua and a St Bernard.

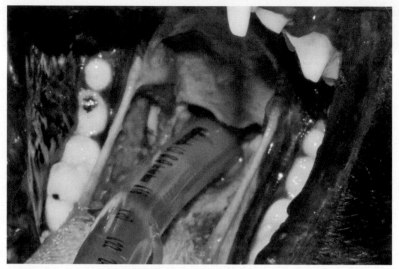

Fig. 2.2 Intubation often allows the first chance for complete visualization of the oral cavity.

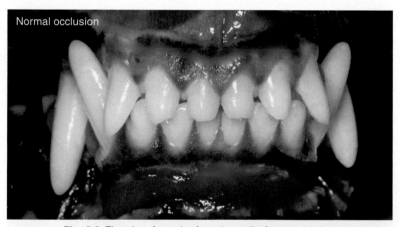

Normal occlusion

Fig. 2.3 The view from the front (rostral) of a normal dog.

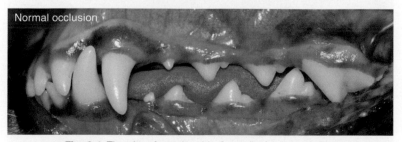

Normal occlusion

Fig. 2.4 The view from the side (buccal) of a normal dog.

SPECIALTIES OF DENTISTRY

In the past, veterinarians were expected to treat all animals for any conditions they might have. Veterinary medicine has since become more sophisticated; with the advancement of knowledge, no veterinarian can perform all facets of veterinary medicine. Consequently, the field is now increasingly specialized. In fact, human dentistry is subdivided into specialties (Table 2.1), a phenomenon that is becoming increasingly common in veterinary dentistry as well. The more a practitioner performs a particular skill, the better the practitioner becomes. Therefore, treatment of advanced periodontal disease, fractured teeth, and orthodontic conditions may not be in the patient's best interest when the practitioner performs these procedures only occasionally. Furthermore, preparing the practice for the occasional specialized procedure requires considerable expense, training, and time. In this case, the "win-win" solution is referral.

TABLE 2.1	Dental Disciplines
Branch of Dentistry	**Area of Specialization**
Endodontics	Treatment of diseases that affect the tooth pulp and apical periodontal tissues
Exodontics	Extraction of teeth and related procedures
Oral surgery	Surgery of the oral cavity
Orthodontics	Guidance and correction of malocclusion of the juvenile teeth and adult tooth positioning
Periodontics	Study and treatment of diseases of the tooth-supporting tissues
Prosthodontics	Construction of appliances designed to replace missing teeth and/or other adjacent structures
Restorative/ operative dentistry	Restoration of form and function of teeth

From Wiggs RB, Lobprise HP: *Veterinary Dentistry: Principles and Practice*, Philadelphia, 1997, Lippincott-Raven; and Holmstrom SE, Frost P, Eisner ER: *Veterinary Dental Techniques*, Philadelphia, 1998, WB Saunders.

ORAL DISEASES AND DENTAL SPECIALTIES

Because of the variety of disease conditions, a variety of dental specialties exists. Pedodontics is the treatment of dental disease in the puppy and kitten. Orthodontics is the treatment of disease related to the way the teeth fit together. Periodontics is the treatment of conditions in the surrounding tooth structure (*perio* means around, and *dontics* means tooth). Prosthodontics involves the process of restoring the tooth to normal health. Endodontics means "inside the tooth." Oral medicine deals with the effects of cancer and other medical conditions on the mouth.

Pedodontics

Puppies and kittens exhibit a variety of dental conditions, both genetic (inherited) and acquired.

Missing Teeth

Anodontia, the absence of teeth, can occur in dogs or cats. Teeth may be missing because they never developed in the first place, are slow to erupt, or were present and fell out. Dental radiographs must be taken to evaluate the area of the missing tooth. In dental charts a circle around the tooth indicates that it is missing. A radiograph should be taken to evaluate the oral structure for missing teeth (see Chapter 11 for technique). The radiograph indicates whether the root is missing or retained. The absence of the root may be inherited or the result of trauma.

Some breeds, notably the boxer, pug, and dachshund, are likely to retain their teeth in the bone subgingivally. This may lead to the formation of a dentigerous or follicular cyst. The cyst is lined by epithelial cells derived from the enamel epithelium of the tooth-forming organ; they are known as "dentigerous cysts." Dentigerous cysts can occur in a variety of breeds, but brachycephalic dog breeds have a greater frequency than those with other skull types. Fig. 2.5 shows a radiograph of a cyst in a 5-year-old boxer.

Persistent Primary Teeth

Persistent primary (also called *retained, deciduous,* or *baby*) teeth may cause orthodontic and periodontic abnormalities. Extraction of these teeth may help

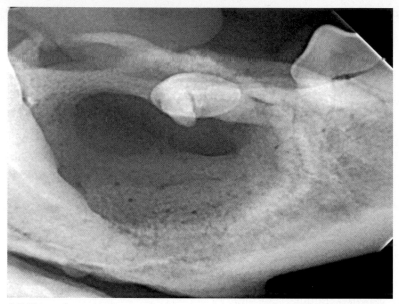

Fig. 2.5 This radiograph shows a dentigerous cyst as a result of a tooth that did not erupt.

prevent such complications. In the patient shown in Fig. 2.6, the primary tooth is displacing the maxillary canine. In addition to causing the possible displacement of the adult canine, the abnormal periodontal border may cause periodontal disease resulting from plaque being trapped between the primary and adult teeth. The general rule applies: There is no room for two teeth of the same type in the same mouth at the same time. Unless they are extremely loose, retained primary teeth should be extracted as soon as possible after the adult tooth starts to erupt. The patient in Fig. 2.6 has a persistent left maxillary canine (^{1}c, 604), which should be extracted. The patient in Fig. 2.7 has a persistent left maxillary lateral incisor (^{3}i, 603). The important question to answer for this patient is: "Where is the adult lateral incisor?" Intraoral radiographs are indicated to see if the adult tooth never formed or if it is impacted and potentially causing a dentigerous cyst.

The term *interceptive orthodontics* describes the process of extracting primary teeth to prevent orthodontic malocclusions. Extraction of these teeth does not cause the jaw to grow correctly or longer. Rather, it removes any possible obstruction to the full development of the jaw. Normally, the primary mandibular (lower) canine occludes mesial to the primary maxillary (upper) canine. In this case the mandibular primary canine is "trapped"

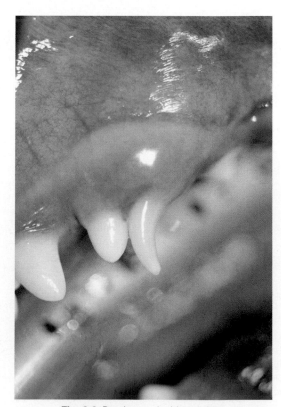

Fig. 2.6 Persistent deciduous 604.

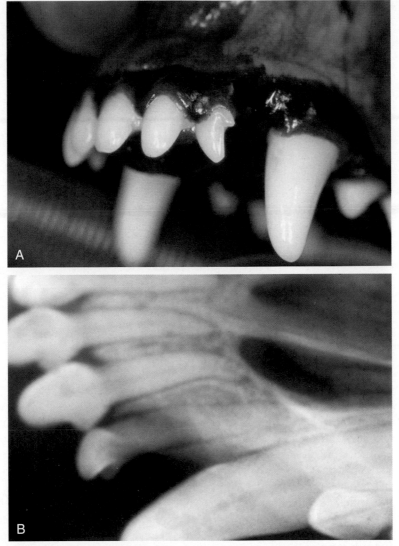

Fig. 2.7 A, A persistent deciduous lateral incisor. B, Radiograph showing that the adult tooth never formed.

by the maxillary primary canine. Further forward growth of the mandible cannot occur. To be effective, this type of interceptive orthodontic treatment should be performed before the patient reaches 12 weeks of age, preferably much earlier. Additional reasons for interceptive orthodontics are discussed in Chapter 13.

Dentinogenesis Imperfecta

Dentinogenesis imperfecta is caused by mutations of a specific protein called dentin sialophosphoprotein (DPP), which is necessary for initiation of mineralization of dentin. Without DPP, the teeth become brittle. Patients with this condition have discolored teeth that are susceptible to fracture (Fig. 2.8).

Pericoronitis/Operculitis

The soft tissue covering a partially erupted tooth crown is called the *operculum*; it is an area that is difficult to access for oral hygiene. An accumulation of oral debris bacteria beneath this tissue or biting the operculum with

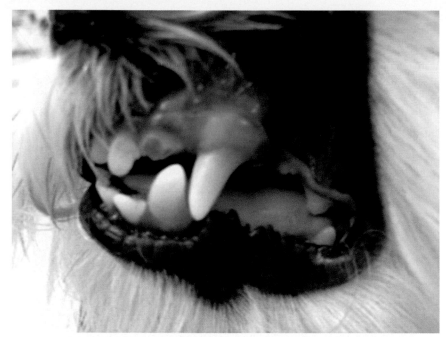

Fig. 2.8 Dentinogenesis imperfecta of left canines and incisors: This patient had dentinogenesis imperfecta, which required extraction of all teeth as the result of continued fractures. (Photo courtesy Dr. Angela Mees.)

the opposing tooth leads to inflammation of the soft tissues, which is called *pericoronitis* or *operculitis*. Treatment is generally exodontics; however, orthodontics can be performed in specialty practices (Fig. 2.9A, B, pericorditis). The mandibular first molar has been trapped by the mandibular fourth premolar. Extraction of the maxillary fourth premolar resulted in complete eruption of the first molar.

Cranial Mandibular Osteodystrophy

Cranial mandibular osteodystrophy is an inherited condition that occurs primarily in West Highland white terriers and occasionally in other breeds. Nonneoplastic bone forms in the region of the temporomandibular joint (TMJ) and occasionally extends into the mandible. Patients with cranial mandibular osteodystrophy are treated symptomatically for pain, which usually lessens as the patient gets older. Fig. 2.10 shows nonneoplastic bone produced in the region of the TMJ.

Mandibular Periostitis Ossificans

Mandibular periostitis ossificans occurs in immature large breed dogs. It causes a unilateral swelling of the ventral portion of the mandible. It is diagnosed radiographically by a two-layered (double) ventral mandibular cortex. This is periosteal new bone formation, which is thought to be an inflammatory condition that spontaneously disappears (Fig. 2.11).

Fractured Deciduous (Primary) Teeth

Fractured deciduous teeth occur fairly frequently. They may be caused by running into objects, catching rocks or other hard substances, or overzealous playing of games such as tug-of-war. If left untreated, fractured primary teeth may result in abscessation, which can cause a defect in enamel production known as *enamel hypoplasia* and may or may not form a fistula. Fig. 2.12 shows a fractured left maxillary canine ([1]c, 604). Note the fistula formation *(arrow)* above the premolar as an extension of the fracture and subsequent abscess. This tooth should be extracted.

Supernumerary Teeth

Supernumerary teeth are primarily incisors, although all types of teeth may be supernumerary. One problem that supernumerary teeth may cause is crowding. The patient

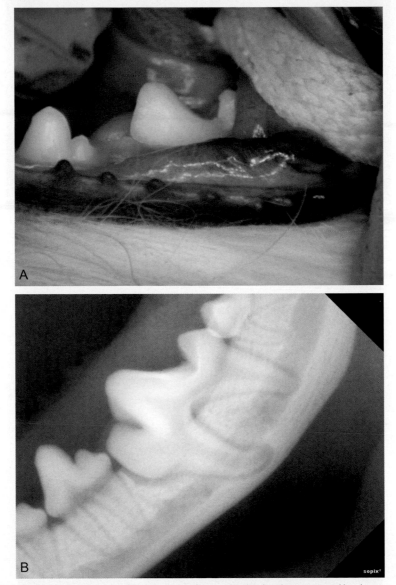

Fig. 2.9 A, Pericorditis. A partially erupted mandibular first molar that has been trapped by the mandibular fourth premolar. B, Pericorditis radiograph: the mesial portion of the mandibular first molar was trapped by the fourth premolar. Extraction of the fourth premolar allowed eruption of the first molar.

in Fig. 2.13 has a supernumerary left mandibular fourth premolar ($_4$P, 308). The patient in Fig. 2.14 has a supernumerary canine tooth.

Supernumary teeth can cause malpositioning and noneruption of other teeth and/or severe plaque accumulation and predispose to periodontal disease owing to the lack of normal cleaning action. Supernumerary teeth that contribute to malocclusion or crowding should be extracted only after intraoral radiographic evaluation to differentiate between deciduous and permanent

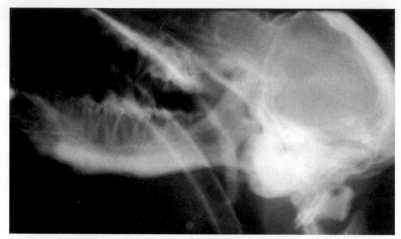

Fig. 2.10 Skull radiograph of a patient with cranial mandibular osteodystrophy.

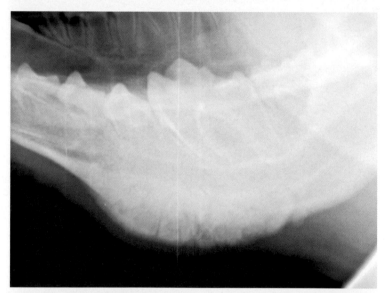

Fig. 2.11 Radiograph of a young dog with periostitis ossificans.

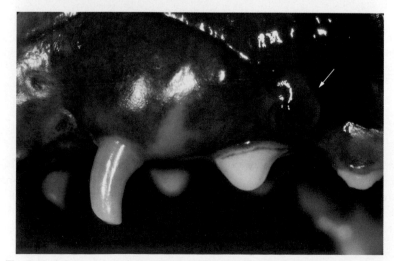

Fig. 2.12 A fractured tooth has caused a fistula *(arrow)* in the mucous membrane.

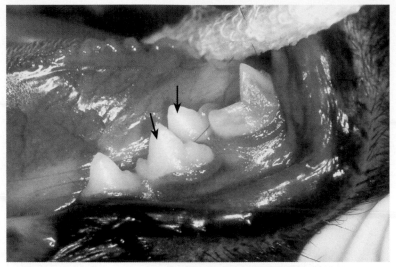

Fig. 2.13 Supernumerary left mandibular fourth premolars in a cat *(arrows)*.

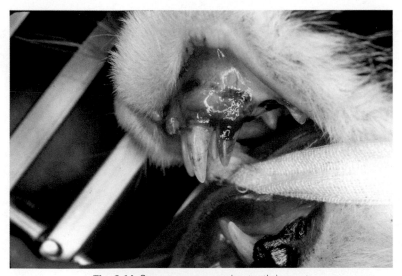

Fig. 2.14 Supernumerary canine tooth in a cat.

teeth. This is important to prevent extracting permanent instead of deciduous teeth. Deciduous teeth are smaller than their permanent counterparts and the roots of deciduous teeth are relatively long in relation to the crown.

Peg teeth. Peg teeth are abnormally formed supernumerary teeth. They generally occur in the canine and incisor regions. The treatment is extraction. The patient in Fig. 2.15 has a peg tooth located lingual to the left maxillary central incisor ([1]I, 201).

Third Set of teeth

Supernumerary teeth may also result from the formation of a third set of teeth. The primary teeth of the patient in Fig. 2.16 fell out at the normal time. The outermost row of teeth are adult teeth. A supernumerary third row of

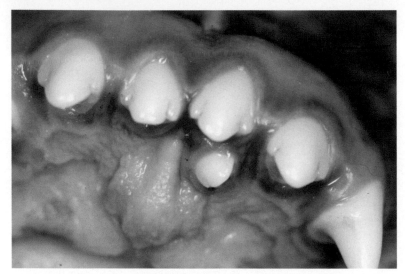

Fig. 2.15 Peg teeth in a dog.

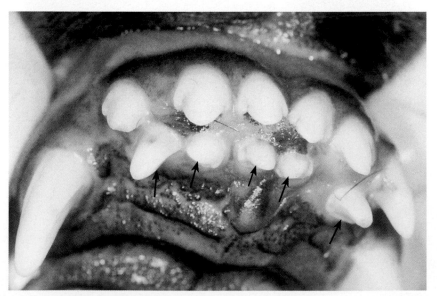

Fig. 2.16 An extreme form of supernumerary teeth in which a complete additional set of teeth has formed *(arrows)*.

teeth is present in this patient. The innermost row of teeth was extracted.

Fused and Gemini Teeth

Fusion is the joining of two developing teeth that have different tooth buds. A gemini tooth is one in which a tooth bud has partially divided in the attempt to form two teeth. The left central incisor ([1]I, 201) in Fig. 2.17 is a gemini tooth. A radiograph is necessary to differentiate between the two. Two roots will be seen with fused teeth, whereas only one root with twin crowns will be seen with gemini teeth.

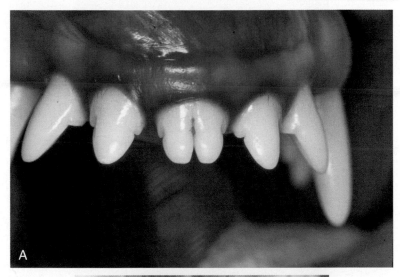

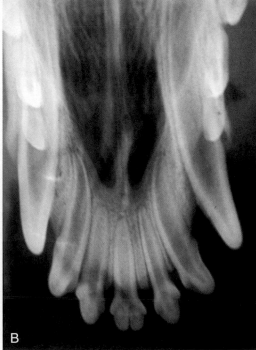

Fig. 2.17 A, This patient has a gemini tooth, as demonstrated by the radiograph (B).

Dilacerated Roots

A dilacerated root is an abnormally formed root, which may be caused by trauma during the tooth's development or by genetic conditions. It may be an unusual finding discovered while taking dental radiographs without pathology or it may be accompanied by severe pathology. The patient in Fig. 2.18, has congenital dilacerations of the mandibular first molars. Treatment was recommended at the time of the discovery, but the client declined. Fig. 2.18B, shows the same patient 4 years later. A severe lytic area around the dilacerated roots has developed. The teeth were extracted.

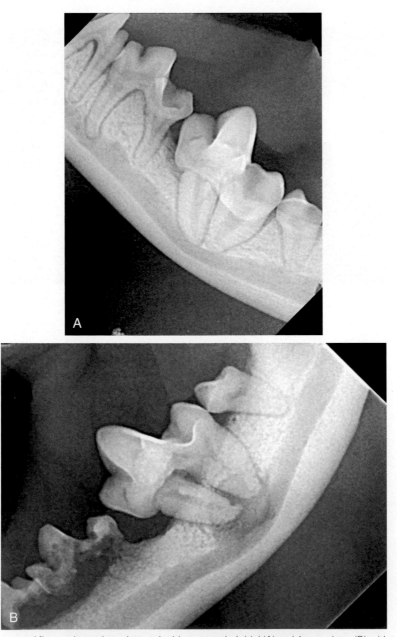

Fig. 2.18 Dilacerated first molar and persistent deciduous teeth. Initial (A) and 4 years later (B) with tooth resorption of the retained deciduous teeth.

Orthodontic Disease

Orthodontic disease is oral disease caused by the malalignment of teeth that is called *malocclusion* (abbreviated MAL). Malocclusion can be caused by dental malocclusion or skeletal malocclusion. There are three classes of malocclusion. Dental malocclusions are class I malocclusions, whereas skeletal malocclusions would cause class II or class III malocclusions. Skeletal malocclusions can be symmetric or identical on each side of the mouth or asymmetric or uneven.

Class I Malocclusions

Patients with class I malocclusions have overall normal occlusions except that one or more teeth are out of alignment. Class I malocclusion occurs in several disease conditions. The abbreviation for a class 1 malocclusion is "MAL1."

Types of class 1 malocclusions include *distoversion* (MAL1/DV), which describes a tooth that is in its anatomically correct position in the dental arch but is abnormally angled in a distal direction, and *mesioversion* (MAL1/MV), which describes a tooth that is in its anatomically correct position in the dental arch but is abnormally angled in a mesial direction.

Spearing (lancing) canines. When the maxillary canines are tipped in a rostral position, they are trapped by the mandibular canines. This class 1 orthodontic condition is known as *spearing canines*. Other terms that are sometimes used are *lancing* and *tusk teeth*.

The condition appears to be genetic and is most prevalent in shelties and Persian cats. Treatment includes orthodontic correction and extraction. Spearing is classified as a buccoversion (MAL1/BV). The cat in Fig. 2.19 has bilateral spearing canines ($^1C^1$, 104, 204).

Spearing (lancing) lateral incisors. Spearing, or lancing, may also occur with the lateral incisors. Occasionally, this condition corrects itself. In Fig. 2.20 the left maxillary lateral incisor (^3I, 203) is spearing and rotated; the left maxillary central incisor (^1I, 201) is also displaced.

Another type of class I malocclusion is *linguoversion* (LV), which describes a tooth that is in its anatomically correct position in the dental arch but is abnormally angled in a lingual direction.

Base-narrowed canines. Base-narrowed canines may be caused by a structural narrowing of the mandible or by the eruption of the canines in an overly upright position. The mandibular canines normally diverge from each other. Base-narrowed canines may cause indentation into and ulceration of the hard palate, or even perforation of the palate. A base-narrowed canine is an LV. The patient in Fig. 2.21A, was not treated for this condition and developed an oronasal fistula that has perforated into the nasal cavity. Fig. 2.21B demonstrates the fistula with a gutta percha point. The patient in Fig. 2.22 is being treated with a metal telescoping incline plane. As the mandibular canines ($_1C_1$, 304, 404) hit the plane, they are deflected buccally.

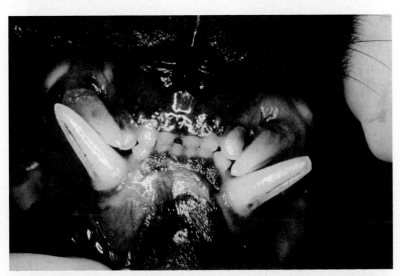

Fig. 2.19 This patient has bilateral mesioversion of the maxillary canine teeth.

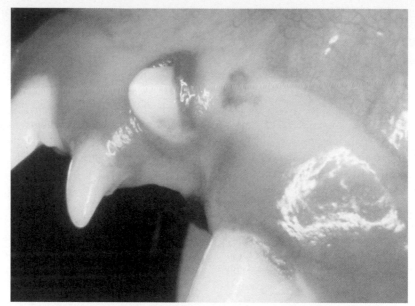

Fig. 2.20 The left maxillary lateral incisor (³I, 203) is spearing and rotated; the adjacent incisor tooth to the left is abnormal and should be evaluated further.

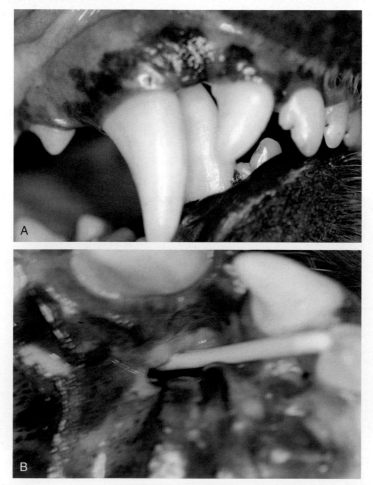

Fig. 2.21 A, This patient has a base-narrowed canine that was not treated. B, Gutta percha has been used to demonstrate the fistula.

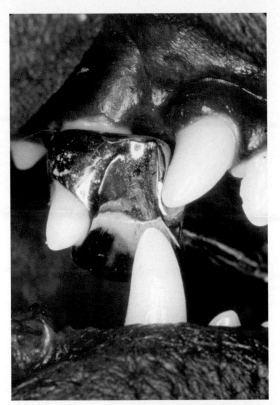

Fig. 2.22 An incline plane has been placed to treat this base-narrowed canine.

Additional class 1 occlusions include *labioversion* (LABV), which describes an incisor or canine tooth that is in its anatomically correct position in the dental arch but abnormally angled in a labial direction. *Buccoversion* (BV) describes a premolar or molar tooth that is in its anatomically correct position in the dental arch but abnormally angled in a buccal direction. *Crossbite* (XB) describes a malocclusion in which a mandibular tooth or teeth have a more buccal or labial position than the antagonist maxillary tooth. It can be classified as rostral or caudal.

Rostral (anterior) crossbite. In *rostral crossbite* (CB/R), which is similar to anterior crossbite in human terminology, one or more of the mandibular incisor teeth is labial to the opposing maxillary incisor teeth when the mouth is closed. A rostral crossbite is a normal occlusion except that one or more of the incisors are malaligned. In the patient in Fig. 2.23, the maxillary central and intermediate incisors are displaced palatally and the mandibular central, intermediate, and lateral incisors are displaced labially. Untreated, these teeth (usually the mandibular incisors) may fall out because of chronic trauma. Several treatment options exist, including extraction of the malaligned teeth and placement of an orthodontic appliance to move the maxillary teeth labially and the mandibular teeth lingually.

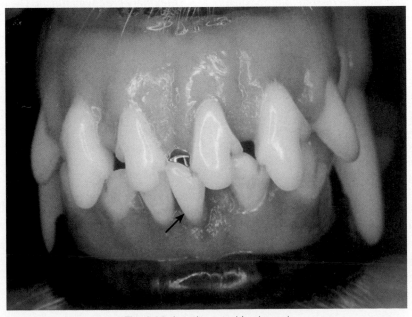

Fig. 2.23 Anterior crossbite *(arrow)*.

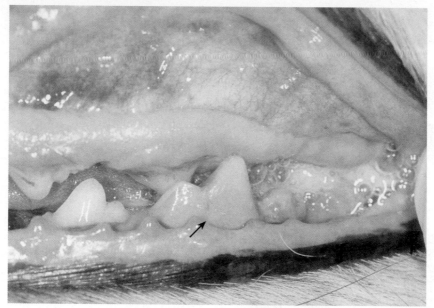

Fig. 2.24 Posterior crossbite causing left mandibular first molar *(arrow)* to occlude buccal to the maxillary fourth premolar.

Caudal (posterior) crossbite. In *caudal crossbite* (CB/ C), which is similar to posterior crossbite in human terminology, one or more of the mandibular cheek teeth are buccal to the opposing maxillary cheek teeth when the mouth is closed. In caudal crossbite, the maxillary premolars are lingual to the mandibular premolars or molars. The left mandibular first molar (₁M, 309) is occluding buccal to the left maxillary fourth premolar (⁴P, 208) in Fig. 2.24.

Class II Occlusion

A class II occlusion (MAL2) occurs when the mandible is shorter than normal. This may cause the adult canines and incisors to penetrate the hard palate, and irritation and ulceration of the hard palate may result. The patient in Fig. 2.25 is in mandibular distoclusion.

Class III Occlusions

Mandibular prognathism. Class III occlusion (MAL3) has several forms. It may be caused by the mandible being too long (mandibular prognathism). As a result, the mandibular incisors occlude labial to the maxillary incisors. With time this may cause excessive wear and injury to both teeth. The shortened maxilla may cause crowding of the teeth. The mandible may be "bowed,"

causing excess space between the premolars, known as *excess freeway space.* In Fig. 2.26, the left mandibular canine (₁C, 304) is occluding against the maxillary lateral incisor (³I, 203).

Maxillary brachygnathism. The other type of class III occlusion is maxillary brachygnathism, which is caused by a shortened maxilla. Typically, the maxillary teeth are rotated as a result of crowding. The lower jaw is normal length, as evidenced by the lack of tooth crowding. The mandible may be bowed, causing excess space between the upper and lower premolars. When charting, the rotated tooth is redrawn over the normal tooth position. In Fig. 2.27, the upper jaw is too short and the mandible appears normal length. In this case, the premolars will be crowded and rotated 90 degrees to their normal position.

Asymmetric Skeletal Malocclusion Class IV Malocclusion (MAL4)

Asymmetric skeletal malocclusion was once called *wry bite;* however, because "wry bite" is nonspecific, the term is no longer used. In this condition, the central incisors of the mandible and maxilla do not align evenly. MAL4 may be caused by uneven mandibular lengths or by the failure of the maxilla to develop evenly. The origin of

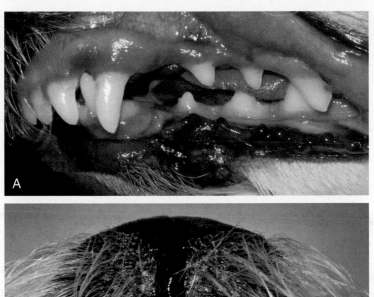

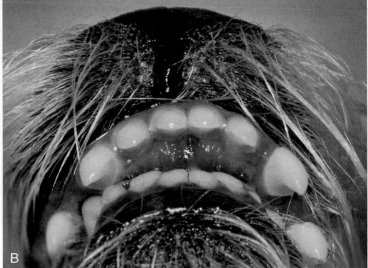

Fig. 2.25 A, The mandible in this patient is much shorter than the maxilla (B). (Copyright AVDC, with permission.)

asymmetric skeletal malocclusion may be genetic (inheritance of uneven jaw lengths) or the condition may be caused by trauma to the bones during development of the facial structure. Treatment ranges from extraction of teeth to placement of orthodontic appliances.

Types of asymmetric skeletal malocclusion include maxillary-mandibular asymmetry, which can occur in a rostrocaudal, side-to side or in a dorsoventral direction.

- Maxillary-mandibular asymmetry in a rostrocaudal direction (MAL4/RC) occurs when mandibular mesioclusion or distoclusion is present on one side of the face while the contralateral side retains normal dental alignment.

- Maxillary-mandibular asymmetry in a side-to-side direction (MAL4STS) occurs when there is loss of the midline alignment of the maxilla and mandible.
- Maxillary-mandibular asymmetry in a dorsoventral direction (MAL4/DV) results in an open bite (OB) that is defined as an abnormal vertical space between opposing dental arches when the mouth is closed.

Iatrogenic Orthodontic Disease

Occasionally, clients (or even veterinarians and office staff) make misguided attempts to correct orthodontic problems. These efforts may cause severe malalignments of teeth.

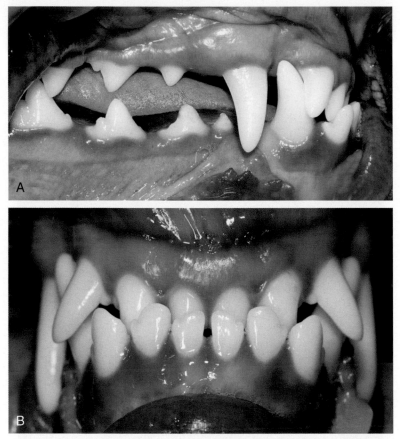

Fig. 2.26 A and B, The mandible of this patient is longer than the maxilla. (Copyright AVDC, with permission.)

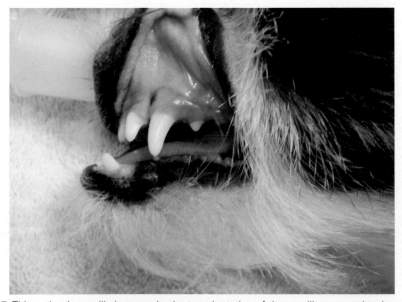

Fig. 2.27 This patient's maxilla is severely short, and rotation of the maxillary premolars is expected.

Oropharyngeal Inflammation

Oropharyngeal inflammation is classified by location, as follows:

Gingivitis: Inflammation of the gingiva that is most often caused by bacterial plaque. A number of conditions should be indicated in the chart of a patient with periodontal disease; these conditions will be discussed in the chapters on prophylaxis and periodontal therapy. Fig. 2.28 shows gingivitis. Gingival inflammation is minimal, however, and the patient is expected to respond positively to professional hygiene and home care.

Periodontitis: Inflammation of nongingival periodontal tissues (i.e., the periodontal ligament and alveolar bone). Periodontitis affects the surrounding tissues of the tooth (Fig. 2.29). This condition is the most common oral disease among dogs and cats. The staging, treatment, and prevention of periodontal disease are discussed in Chapters 7 and 9. The cat may express severe periodontal disease by expansion of buccal bone around the canine teeth, which is caused by alveolar osteitis and is discussed in Chapter 10.

Alveolar mucositis: Inflammation of alveolar mucosa (i.e., mucosa overlying the alveolar process and

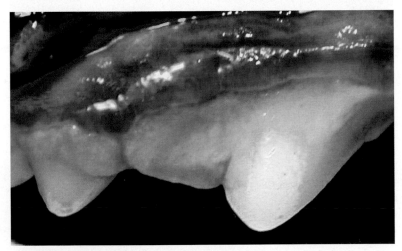

Fig. 2.28 Stage I gingivitis. (Copyright AVDC, with permission.)

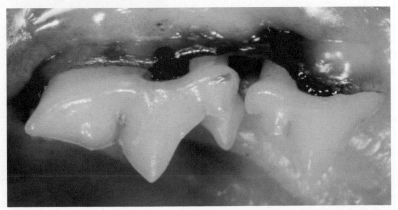

Fig. 2.29 This patient has periodontitis with loss of attached gingiva and pocket formation. (Copyright AVDC, with permission.)

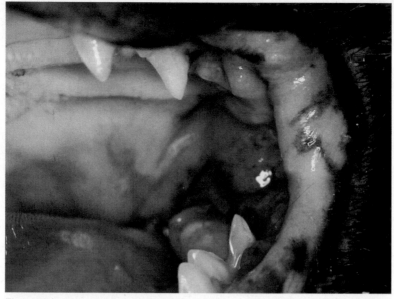

Fig. 2.30 This patient has a caudal mucositis. (Copyright AVDC, with permission.)

extending from the mucogingival junction without obvious demarcation to the vestibular sulcus and to the floor of the mouth).

Sublingual mucositis: Inflammation of mucosa on the floor of the mouth.

Labial/buccal mucositis: Inflammation of lip/cheek mucosa.

Caudal mucositis: Inflammation of mucosa of the caudal oral cavity, bordered medially by the palatoglossal folds and lateral palatine fold, dorsally by the hard and soft palate, and rostrally by alveolar and buccal mucosa (Fig. 2.30).

Contact mucositis and contact mucosal ulceration: Lesions in susceptible individuals that are secondary to mucosal contact with a tooth surface bearing the responsible irritant, allergen, or antigen. They have also been called *contact ulcers* and *kissing ulcers*.

Palatitis: Inflammation of mucosa covering the hard and/or soft palate (Fig. 2.31).

Glossitis: Inflammation of mucosa of the dorsal and/or ventral tongue surface (Fig. 2.32).

Cheilitis: Inflammation of the lip, including the muco-cutaneous junction area and skin of the lip (Fig. 2.33).

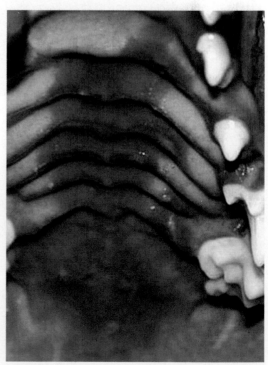

Fig. 2.31 This patient has a palatitis. (Copyright AVDC, with permission.)

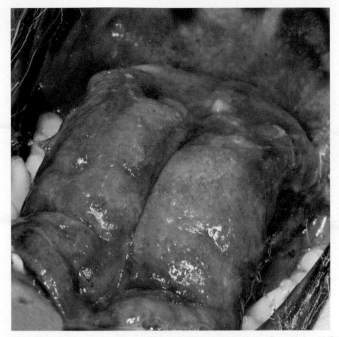

Fig. 2.32 This patient has a severe inflammation of the tongue or glossitis. (Copyright AVDC, with permission.)

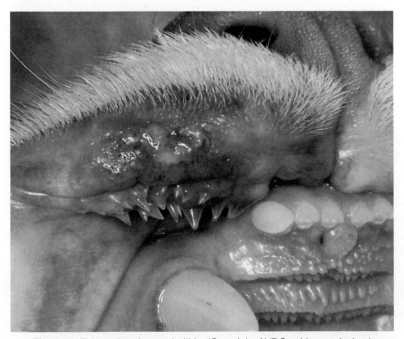

Fig. 2.33 This patient has a cheilitis. (Copyright AVDC, with permission.)

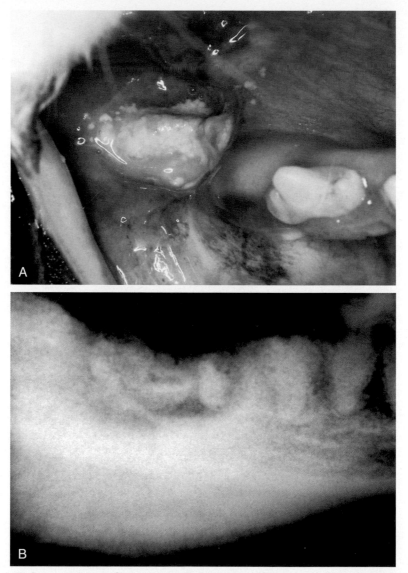

Fig. 2.34 Osteomyelitis. A, Clinical image. B, Radiograph. (Copyright AVDC, with permission.)

Osteomyelitis: Inflammation of the bone and bone marrow (Fig. 2.34). Abnormal looking bone should be biopsied. Bacterial and fungal osteomyelitis have been reported (Fig. 2.35).

Stomatitis (ST): Inflammation of the mucous lining of any of the structures in the mouth; in clinical use, the term should be reserved to describe widespread oral inflammation (beyond gingivitis and periodontitis) that may also extend into submucosal tissues. Marked caudal mucositis extending into submucosal tissues may be termed *caudal stomatitis* (ST/CS).

Tonsillitis: Inflammation of the palatine tonsil (Fig. 2.36).

Pharyngitis: Inflammation of the pharynx.

Examples of the Appearance of Various Regional Oral Inflammatory Diseases

A definitive diagnosis of inflammation often cannot be made based on physical examination findings alone.

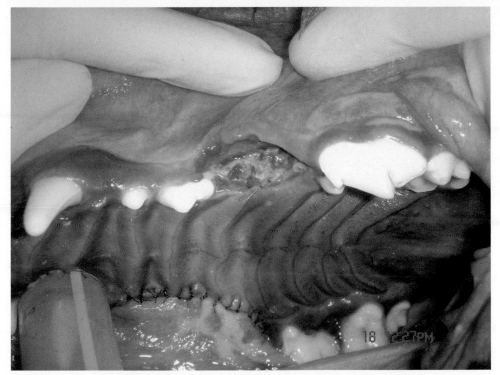

Fig. 2.35 Cryptococcal maxillary osteomyelitis. This patient had a confirmed cryptococcal maxillary osteomyelitis. (Photo courtesy Dr. Katherine Block.)

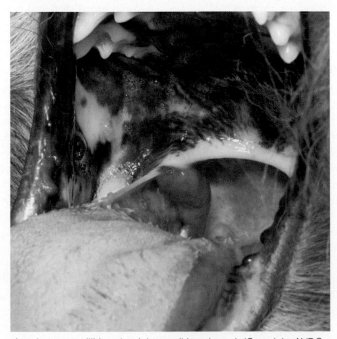

Fig. 2.36 This patient has a tonsillitis—the right tonsil is enlarged. (Copyright AVDC, with permission.)

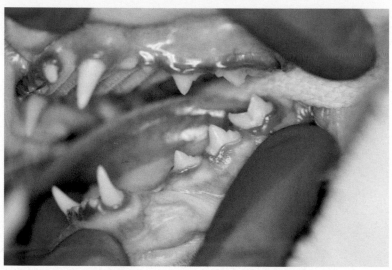

Fig. 2.37 Juvenile periodontitis in a young cat.

Juvenile Periodontitis

Juvenile periodontitis is a condition in young cats, usually less than 3 years of age. It is characterized by minimal plaque and calculus but severe gingival inflammation. Treatment consists of COHAT (see COAPT in Chapter 7) and daily home care (see Chapter 8). These patients should improve; however, if home care cannot be performed, they may progress to chronic ulcerative gingivostomatitis (Fig. 2.37; see Discussion in Chapter 10).

Autoimmune Conditions Affecting the Mouth

Pemphigus vulgaris (PV): An autoimmune disease caused by autoantibodies against components of the protein structures that hold the cells together. As a result, there are oral blisters and/or ulcerative oral and mucocutaneous lesions.

Bullous pemphigoid (BUP): An autoimmune disease caused by autoantibodies against the structures that hold the epithelium to the connective tissue. Clinical findings include erythematous, erosive, blistering, and/or ulcerative oral lesions

Lupus erythematosus (LE): An autoimmune disease caused by autoantibodies against both the nucleus and cytoplasm. In addition to involving the oral cavity, the skin and multiple organs may be involved.

Masticatory muscle myositis (MMM): Masticatory muscle myositis, otherwise known as masticatory myositis, atrophic myositis, or eosinophilic myositis, is an autoimmune disease that affects the temporal, masseter, and medial and lateral pterygoid muscles. The disease mainly affects large breed dogs and Cavalier King Charles spaniels. Acutely, there may be bilateral swelling of the jaw muscles, drooling, and pain on opening the mouth. There may be third eyelid protrusion, red eyes, and exophthalmos. After the acute stage, there is atrophy of the jaw muscles and scarring of the masticatory muscles caused by fibrosis that may result in inability to open the mouth (trismus). The affected muscles include the temporalis, masseter, and pterygoid muscles; as a result, the sagittal crest becomes pronounced.

MMM is caused by the body mistaking 2M fibers in the muscles of the jaw for bacteria; 2M fibers are not found elsewhere in the body. Diagnosis of MMM is by biopsy of the temporalis or masseter muscles or the 2M antibody assay. Treatment is usually with corticosteroids such as prednisone, often with decreasing doses for up to 4 to 6 months; in case the mouth will not open, open the mouth manually under anesthesia. Feeding very soft or liquid food during recovery is usually necessary. Ultimately, the degree of recovery will depend on the extent of damage to the muscle tissue. MMM is often misdiagnosed as a retroorbital abscess, which can lead to inappropriate treatment with antibiotics, which just delays proper treatment.

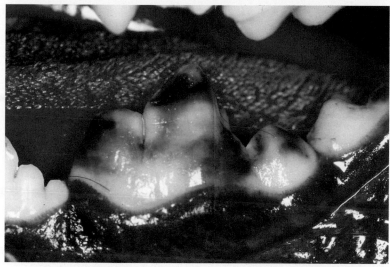

Fig. 2.38 This patient shows staining of dentin.

Adverse Conditions of the Tooth Surface

Stains

Stains result from occlusal wear and exposure of dentine. They are not necessarily pathologic, although many clients ask for a consultation when they think caries are present. Enamel normally resists staining, whereas dentine is porous and stains easily. In Fig. 2.38, the left mandibular first molar (^{1}M, 309) shows wear and a dark dentinal stain.

Abrasions

Abrasions result from the repeated friction of the teeth against an external object such as hair or toys. One common cause of wear is the chewing (and spinning or rolling in the mouth) of tennis balls. Trapped dirt in the fibers covering the tennis ball creates a sandpaper-like surface. The patient in Fig. 2.39 suffers from chronic skin disease and chews its hair as a result. Its mandibular incisors ($_{321}$I$_{123}$, 301, 302, 303, 401, 402, 403) and canines ($_1$C$_1$, 304, 404) show severe wear.

Attrition

Attrition results from the friction of teeth against each other. Attrition can occur in mild class III malocclusion, which results in a level bite. As a result, the incisal edges may have wear, owing to direct contact. In more severe class III malocclusions, grooves may be created in the canine teeth from wear against the opposite canine or incisor. Cases of posterior crossbite may cause wear of the

molars and premolars. Fig. 2.40 shows severe wear of the mandibular canine. The patient in Fig. 2.40 may have had an occlusion similar to that shown in Fig. 2.26 (class III occlusion, mandibular prognathism). The right mandibular canine (C$_1$, 404) shows severe wear resulting from friction against the right maxillary third incisor (I^3, 103).

Abnormalities of Enamel Formation

Amelogenesis imperfecta includes genetic and/or developmental enamel formation and maturation abnormalities, such as enamel hypoplasia and enamel hypomineralization, discussed as follows:

- Enamel hypoplasia refers to inadequate deposition of enamel matrix. This can affect one or several teeth and may be focal or multifocal. The crowns of affected teeth can have areas of normal enamel next to areas of hypoplastic or missing enamel.
- Enamel hypomineralization refers to inadequate mineralization of enamel matrix. This often affects several or all teeth. The crowns of affected teeth are covered by soft enamel that may be worn rapidly.

Enamel Hypoplasia

Cells called *ameloblasts* create enamel. If these cells are debilitated, they stop producing enamel. The area of the crown no longer has a shiny surface; instead, it is dull and susceptible to flaking. This condition is called *enamel hypoplasia*. Conditions that cause a temporary debilitation of the patient, such as high

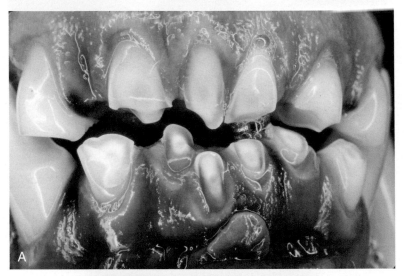

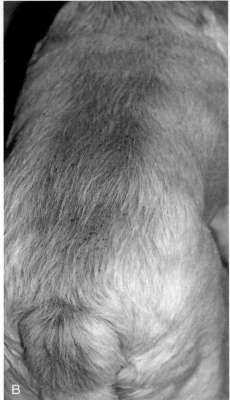

Fig. 2.39 These teeth (A) are worn and the skin (B) is irritated from chronic chewing.

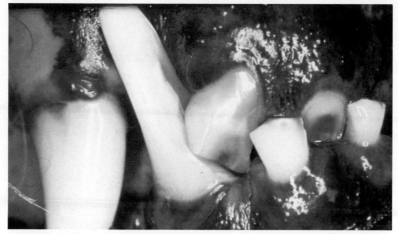

Fig. 2.40 This patient has wear as the result of tooth against tooth.

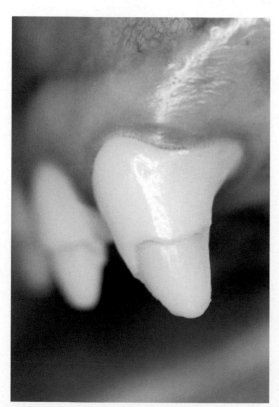

Fig. 2.41 The production of enamel was interrupted at a very young age but then resumed.

fever, may cause enamel hypoplasia. Trauma or traumatic extractions of primary teeth may also be causes. The patient in Fig. 2.41 has enamel hypoplasia of multiple teeth, the result of an infection while the teeth were being formed.

Caries

Caries (also called *cavities*) occur in dogs and cats. The most common types are class I caries, which are pits and fissures on the occlusal surfaces of teeth, and class V caries, which occur on the buccal and labial surfaces. Treatment options depend on the depth of the lesion and include extraction, simple restorations, endodontic therapy, and crown restorations. The patient in Fig. 2.42 has advanced class I caries of the distal cusp of the right mandibular first molar.

Class V caries occur on the gingival third of the crown of the tooth, on the buccal or lingual surface. These are common in cats and are discussed (and classified) in Chapter 13.

Foreign Bodies

Foreign bodies are sometimes caught on the tooth or trapped in the oral cavity. Rubber bands may be wrapped around teeth, and bones may become lodged between teeth. The retention of this foreign material can cause infection and even tooth loss. The patient in Fig. 2.43 had foxtail weed awns lodged behind the right maxillary second molar (M^2, 110). The patient in Fig. 2.44 had a bone wedged between the maxillary fourth premolars.

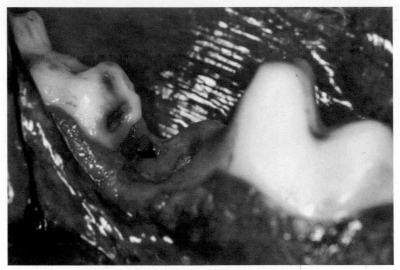

Fig. 2.42 This patient has a class I carious lesion.

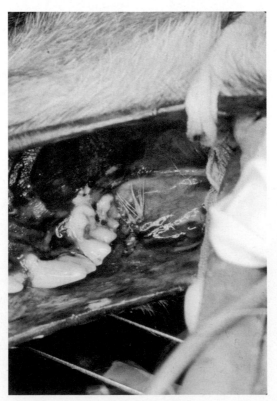

Fig. 2.43 Foxtails, a weed awn, have entered this patient's oral tissues.

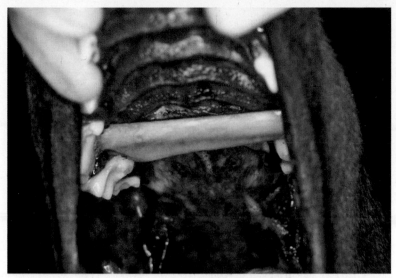

Fig. 2.44 A bone has been wedged between the fourth premolars.

Endodontic Disease

Endodontics is the treatment of diseases inside the tooth. Endodontic disease may be caused by fractures, trauma, and iatrogenic factors (conditions caused by the healthcare provider) such as overheating the tooth during cleaning procedures.

Fracture Classification

Collisions with automobiles and the catching or chewing of hard objects are common causes of fractures. Numerous fracture classification schemes, patterned after those used in human dentistry, exist in veterinary dentistry, as follows:

Enamel fracture (EF): A fracture with loss of crown substance confined to the enamel. Most of these fractures do not require treatment.

Uncomplicated crown fracture (UCF): A fracture of the crown that does not expose the pulp.

Complicated crown fracture (CCF): A fracture of the crown that exposes the pulp (Fig. 2.45).

Uncomplicated crown-root fracture (UCRF): A fracture of the crown and root that does not expose the pulp.

Complicated crown-root fracture (CCRF): A fracture of the crown and root that exposes the pulp.

Root fracture (RF): A fracture involving the root.

Fractures of Specific Tooth Types

Incisors. Incisors can fracture or deteriorate with wear. Fractures of the incisors often result from running into hard objects; catching baseballs, golf balls, and rocks; fighting; and chewing enclosures to escape. Wear occurs most commonly by chewing skin. The friction of teeth against teeth associated with malocclusion also results in wear, as does the chewing of rocks, bones, and other hard objects. Patients who chronically chew certain toys, such as tennis balls and cloth Frisbees, may also wear down their teeth. Practitioners sometimes overlook disease of the mandibular incisors in awake patients because the maxillary incisors cover the labial side when the mouth is closed and the tongue covers the lingual side when the mouth is open. Fractures of the maxillary incisors may be difficult to see because they often occur on the palatal side. Fig. 2.46 shows severe wear of the mandibular canines ($_1C_1$, 304, 404) and incisors ($_{321}I_{123}$, 301, 302, 303, 401, 402, 403).

Canines. The canines are susceptible to trauma because they are the most exposed teeth, located in the front of the oral cavity, and they have long crowns. The canines have several important functions. In addition to their holding and tearing functions, the mandibular canines may act as a guide for the tongue. The maxillary canines serve to hold the lip out and away

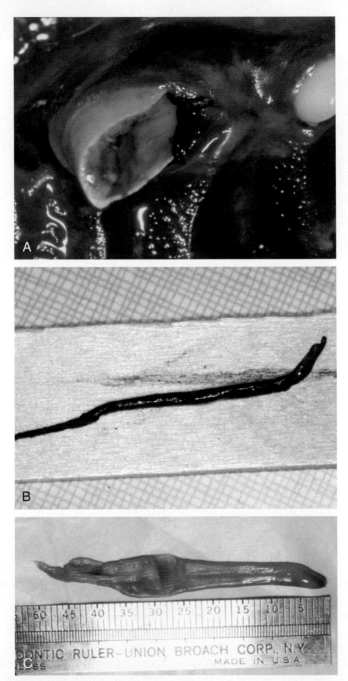

Fig. 2.45 A, Complicated crown fracture. B, Nonvital pulp removed from the root canal in A. Before the microscope was invented, people thought that tooth decay was caused by worms. What they were looking at was the pulp tissue, which consists of blood vascular tissue, nerves, and connective tissue. C, Pulp removed from a more recent fracture.

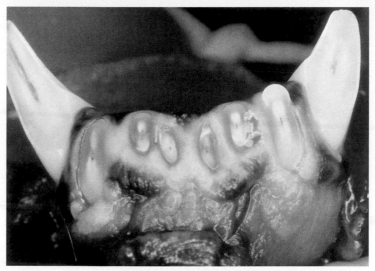

Fig. 2.46 Severe wear of the canines and incisors.

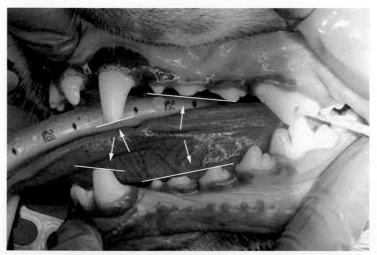

Fig. 2.47 Table wear of the canines and premolars.

from the gums. Without these teeth, many patients pinch or bite their lips between the mandibular canines and gums. Like the incisors, canines are fractured when patients fight and chew, catch, and run into hard objects. Wear occurs by excessive or inappropriate chewing and occlusion abnormalities. The patient in Fig. 2.47, a tennis-ball chewer, exhibits table wear on the crowns of all visible teeth.

Premolars. The most common fracture of the fourth premolar is the "slab" fracture (Fig. 2.48). This fracture results from the force that is placed on a very small area of tooth (cusp) when the patient bites down. The shear force fractures enamel and dentine, exposing the pulp. For this reason the chewing of hard objects, such as hooves, bones, pig's ears, and pressed rawhide products, is discouraged. In Fig. 2.49, the cusp of the right maxillary fourth premolar (P^4, 108) has been compressed into the pulp chamber, moving a slab buccally.

A fractured fourth premolar may also cause fistulous drainage below the eye.

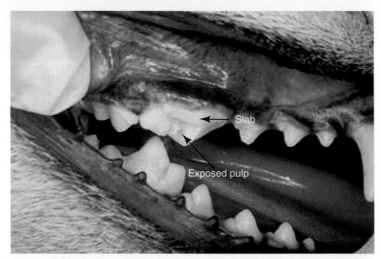

Fig. 2.48 A slab fracture of the right maxillary fourth premolar with the slab attached *(arrow)* and exposed pulp *(arrow)*.

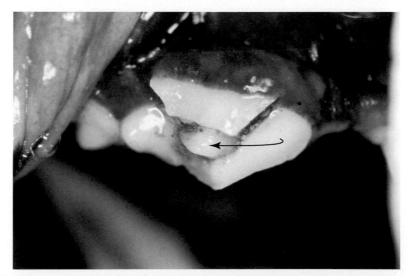

Fig. 2.49 The cusp *(arrow)* of the fourth premolar has been compressed into the pulp chamber.

Fig. 2.50 shows a patient with a chronic draining fistula below the left eye. The patient had been unsuccessfully treated with many courses of antibiotics prior to the current treatment. If the condition goes on long enough, the tooth will start to resorb (Fig. 2.51).

Molars. Fractures of the molars usually occur in combination with fractures of the maxillary fourth premolar.

When patients chew extremely hard objects, the same forces are applied to the mandibular first molar as to the maxillary fourth premolar. Practitioners may miss these fractures during physical examinations because the tongue overlaps the teeth when the mouth is open and the maxillary fourth premolars and molars cover them when the mouth is closed.

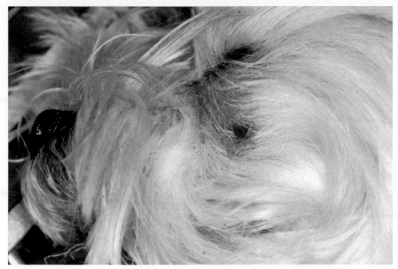

Fig. 2.50 Although this does not always occur, draining fistulas below the eye are often caused by a tooth fracture.

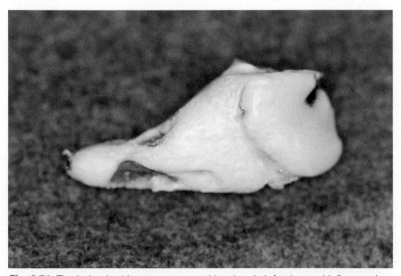

Fig. 2.51 The holes in this root are caused by chronic infection and inflammation.

Tooth Discoloration

The teeth and cusps take on a variety of colors that may indicate a pathologic condition. The normal, healthy tooth is white. If wear has exposed dentine, the exposed portion appears brown. If the pulp has been exposed, it appears black and the tooth loses its translucent appearance. Pink, purple, or tan teeth indicate pulpal hemorrhage.

Purple discoloration indicates pulpal hemorrhage. The most common cause of hemorrhage is trauma to the tooth. This trauma may result from being hit by a car, running into a solid object, or colliding with another dog's tooth. Trauma may lead to pulpitis, which is a pulpal inflammation that may be reversible. If it is irreversible, the pulp hemorrhages and dies as a result of the increased internal pressure in the tooth, which causes

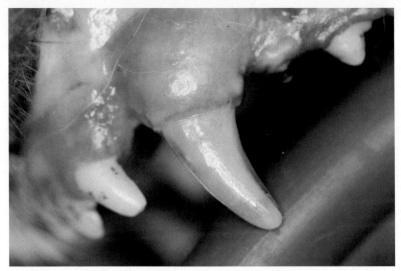

Fig. 2.52 Teeth with pulpal hemorrhage usually start out pink and eventually turn tan.

crushing and death of cells. The odontoblasts that line the pulp chamber and guard the dentinal tubules also die, which allows blood cells to enter the tooth. At first, the result is a pink tooth. As the hemoglobin loses oxygen, the tooth changes to purple and later to tan. The left maxillary canine ([1]C, 204) shown in Fig. 2.52 is purple. The recommended treatment for this tooth is root canal therapy.

Luxations (T/LUX)

Luxation is partial displacement of the tooth from the socket. The tooth may still be vital. Immediate repositioning and splinting is recommended. Root canal therapy may be necessary.

A type of luxation injury that may not be clinically diagnosed is intrusion. Intraoral radiographs are necessary to find the missing tooth that has usually intruded through the alveolar socket into the nasal cavity.

Avulsions (T/A)

Avulsion is complete displacement of the tooth from the socket. If the tooth is to be saved, it must be replaced immediately. Special solutions are available to help preserve the lost tooth, but usually they are not readily available. Clients may place the tooth in milk as a first aid measure. Endodontic therapy is required (see Chapter 12). In Fig. 2.53, the left maxillary canine ([1]C, 204) has been avulsed from the socket. Saving this tooth requires immediate replacement and splinting followed by root canal therapy 6 weeks later.

Electric Cord Shock (TMA/E)

Tooth damage caused by chewing electric cords may not be discovered for days or even months after the injury. If the injury occurs when the patient is very young, severe damage may occur and the affected teeth may require extraction. The maxillary fourth premolar or first molar and the mandibular first molar are usually involved.

Tooth Resorption (TR)

Tooth resorption was formerly called *feline odontoclastic resorptive lesion* (FORL) syndrome. Because this condition occurs in species other than the cat, the name was changed to "tooth resorption." These lesions were first discovered at the neck of the tooth, the area in which the root and crown come together. They were therefore first known as "neck lesions." These lesions have since been given a number of other names: resorptive lesions, cervical line lesions, and feline cavities. The tooth resorbs and is eventually lost. Staging and treatment of this disease are discussed in Chapter 10. The cause in the feline is believed to be excess vitamin D in the diet.

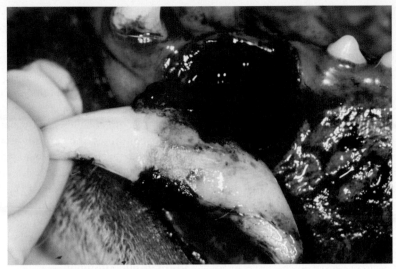

Fig. 2.53 This maxillary canine has been avulsed from the socket.

Oral Medical Disease
Oronasal Fistulas (ONF)

Oronasal fistulas result from advanced periodontal disease on the palatal side of the canines. As the plate of bone between the canine and the nasal cavity breaks down, fistulas develop. They are often present but not diagnosed before the extraction of the canine. Oronasal fistulas are documented by indicating the missing tooth and noting "ONF" in the chart. The patient in Fig. 2.54 has lost its left maxillary canine ([1]C, 204) as a result of chronic periodontal disease. A hole exists that opens to the nasal cavity.

Uremic Ulceration

Patients with advanced renal disease may develop ulcerations on the tip of the tongue. Increased calculus formation and periodontal disease are associated problems—all the more reason that preoperative blood profiles should be run before oral procedures are performed.

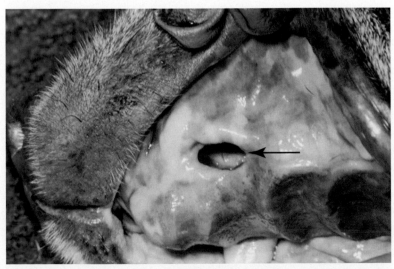

Fig. 2.54 In addition to missing many teeth, this patient has an oronasal fistula *(arrow)* from a previously extracted canine.

Renal Secondary Hyperparathyroidism with Osteodystrophy

Demineralization of maxillofacial bones, loosening of teeth, and pathologic jaw fractures can occur as the result of chronic renal disease. Patients with this condition have very loose teeth and the bone is commonly called "rubber jaw." Blood testing and intraoral radiology are necessary to diagnose.

Oral Neoplasia
Nonclinically Aggressive

Although they may grow locally and, in rare instances, convert to malignant tumors, nonclinically aggressive tumors generally do not spread deep into tissue or metastasize to lymph nodes or lungs. Generally, they respond well to surgical removal. If not completely removed, however, they may return to the same or an adjacent location.

Canine Oral Viral Oral Papillomatosis (OM/PAP)

Canine oral viral oral papillomatosis occurs in young dogs, frequently less than 2 years of age. There are typically warts on the oral mucous membrane, but they also may occur on the lips. This is caused by a virus and generally will go away with time (Fig. 2.55). Occasionally, surgery may be necessary if the warts get large enough to interfere with mastication (chewing) and swallowing.

Granulomas

Benign granulomas are common and usually result from periodontal disease or other irritation. They respond well to local excision and removal of the originating cause (Fig. 2.56).

Cheek chewing granulomas (CL/B). Oral trauma from cheek chewing may result in granulomas. Repeated excision of the masses is often attempted, but as the trauma continues, they do not resolve until the offending teeth are extracted. They may often be bilateral. The patient in Fig. 2.57 is a cat with a granuloma caused by cheek chewing. Extraction of the left maxillary fourth premolars and first molars provided relief. These are also known as *oral pyogenic granulomas* and may be misdiagnosed as squamous cell carcinomas.

Oral Fibromyxolipoma

Fibromyxolipomas are rare, distinct benign soft tissue tumors that have many clinicopathologic features of a spindle cell lipoma and solitary fibrous tumor with myxoid change. They respond to excision (Fig. 2.58).

Gingival Hyperplasia (GH)

Gingival hyperplasia, the proliferation of gingival cells, is common among some breeds, particularly the collie, boxer, and cocker spaniel. Pocket formation and periodontal disease may result from this hyperplastic tissue. Fig. 2.59 shows gingival hyperplasia of the entire left

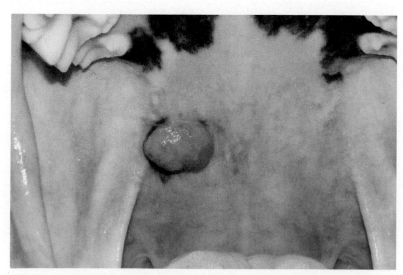

Fig. 2.55 This young patient has an oral viral papilloma, which is in the process of resorbing.

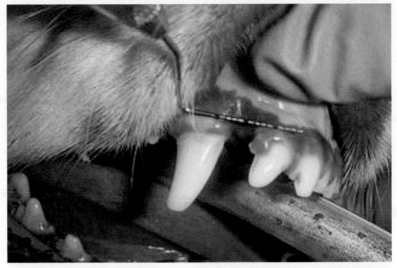

Fig. 2.56 This is a benign gingival granuloma.

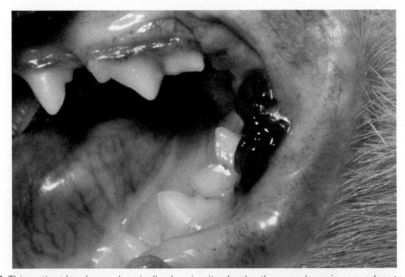

Fig. 2.57 This patient has been chronically chewing its cheek—the granuloma is secondary to chewing.

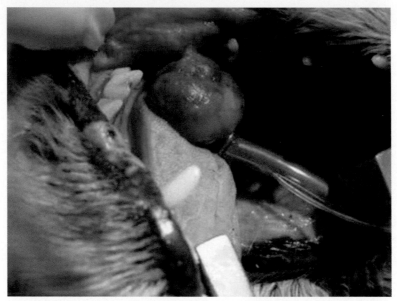

Fig. 2.58 Oral fibromyxolipoma. This was a pedunculated tumor in an asymptomatic 12.5-year-old Cavalier King Charles Spaniel. The tumor was excised without incident. (Photo courtesy Dr. Kristi Adams.)

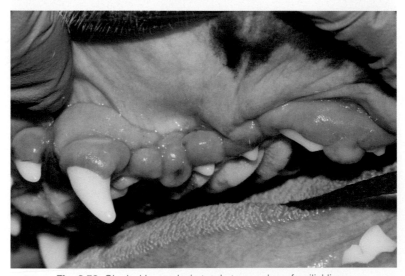

Fig. 2.59 Gingival hyperplasia tends to run along familial lines.

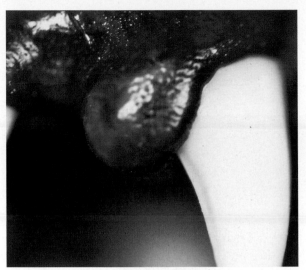

Fig. 2.60 A benign process, the peripheral odontogenic fibroma responds to excision but may recur if not completely removed.

maxilla. The first premolar (^{1}P, 205) and supernumerary first premolar (^{1}Ps, 205S) are completely covered.

Peripheral Odontogenic Fibroma (OM/POF)

Peripheral odontogenic fibroma, also known as *fibromatous epulis,* is characterized by the presence of a tumor in the tissues of the gingiva that contains primarily fibrous tissues. Generally, a peripheral odontogenic fibroma (Fig. 2.60) responds well to excision; however, it may return if the excision is incomplete.

An ossifying epulis resembles a peripheral odontogenic fibroma but also contains large amounts of bone material, which give it a bony quality apparent during excision. Because of the depth of the bone, these tumors sometimes are difficult to remove.

Odontomas

Odontomas are a mass of cells that have enamel, dentin, cementum, and small tooth-like structures. Masses with characteristics resembling normal teeth are considered compound odontomas. Complex odontomas have a more disorganized arrangement. Although these can be fairly extensive and invasive, conservative excision is usually successful. Fig. 2.61A shows a complex odontoma that involves the lower mandible and its radiograph (Fig. 2.61B).

Ulcerative Eosinophilic Stomatitis

Ulcerative eosinophilic stomatitis is a disease of King Charles Spaniels. They tend to be focal raised areas on the palate, but histologically they do not have granuloma formation. The cause of the lesions is unknown (Fig. 2.62).

Sublingual Fibrolipoma

Fibrolipomas are benign encapsulated tumors of fat and connective tissue. Although they can get large, excision is usually curative (Fig. 2.63).

Clinically Aggressive Tumors
Acanthomatous Ameloblastomas (OM/AA)

The acanthomatous epulis is primarily composed of proliferating epithelial cells of dental origin associated with the tissue. Although they are classified as benign, these epulides tend to invade bone, which makes dental radiographic evaluation and aggressive surgery important. Fig. 2.64 is an acanthomatous ameloblastoma that has formed in the region of the left mandibular fourth premolar ($_4$P, 308) and first molar ($_1$M, 309).

Extramedulary Plasmacytoma (EMP)

Extramedulary plasmacytoma is a locally aggressive tumor. A computed tomography scan will help to delineate the tumor; wide excision is indicated (Fig. 2.65).

Fibrosarcomas (OM/FS)

Fibrosarcomas occur in the mandible or maxilla (Fig. 2.66). They may create fleshy, protruding, firm masses that sometimes are friable. As the masses grow, they can become ulcerated and infected. Most of the time, it is the local growth that becomes the problem rather than the spreading of this tumor to the lymph nodes or lungs.

Lingual Mast Cell Tumor (MCT)

Mast cell tumors are the most common cutaneous tumors of dogs; however, they are rarely found in the oral cavity. MCT in the oral cavity can demonstrate an aggressive clinical course. They have a high incidence of lymph node metastasis at the time of diagnosis which results in a poor prognosis. Despite a more aggressive clinical course, treatment can result in remission (Fig. 2.67).

Multicentric Epithelial Lymphoma

Figs. 2.68 and 2.69

In the dog, cutaneous epitheliotropic T-cell lymphosarcoma, also called "mycosis fungoides," occurs in patients over 10 years of age, but it may or not be associated with dermal disease. In the mouth there is

Text continued on page 67.

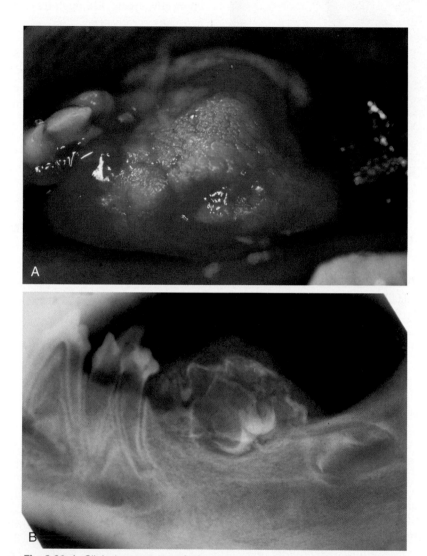

Fig. 2.61 A, Clinical appearance of an odontoma. B, Radiograph of an odontoma.

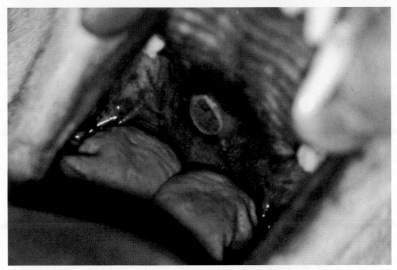

Fig. 2.62 Eosinophilic palatitis in a King Charles spaniel.

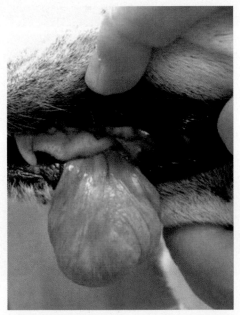

Fig. 2.63 Sublingual fibrolipoma. This slowly growing sublingual fibrolipoma was present for 1.5 years before removal. (Photo courtesy Dr. Alison Powell.)

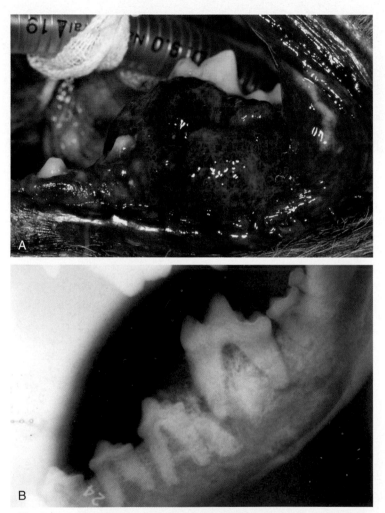

Fig. 2.64 A, Acanthomatous epulis. B, Acanthomatous epulis radiograph.

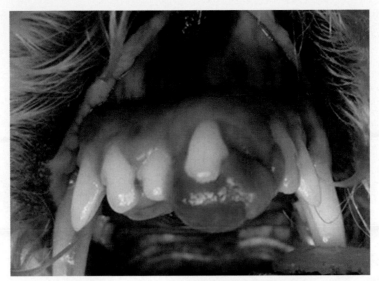

Fig. 2.65 Plasmacytoma. This patient has an extramedulary plasmacytoma, which required surgeries to resolve. (Photo courtesy Dr. Dae Hyun Kwon.)

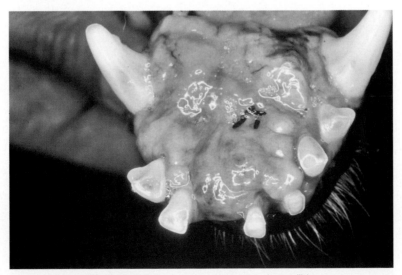

Fig. 2.66 A fibrosarcoma on the rostral mandible.

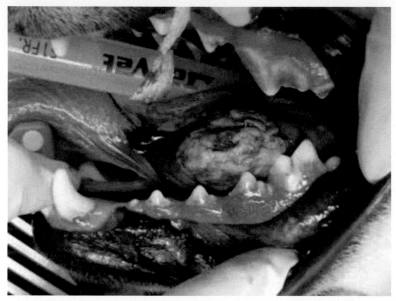

Fig. 2.67 Lingual mast cell tumor. A 4-year-old yellow Labrador presented with bloody saliva. On physical examination, a foul-smelling mass was seen at the left base of the tongue. (Image courtesy Dr. Rebecca Gibilisco.)

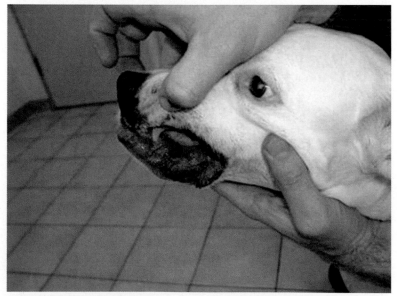

Fig. 2.68 Multicentric epithelial lymphoma. A 13 year old neutered Pitbull, the Tumor had been present for 1.5 years. (Photo courtesy Dr. David Miller.)

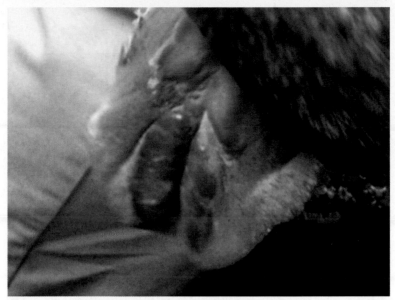

Fig. 2.69 T-cell lymphoma on the tongue. An 8-year-old male neutered boxer with symmetrical and multiple raised tumors on the tongue. (Photo courtesy Dr. Daniel E. Yeulett.)

inflammation, increased blood flow, and an irregular surface. Differential diagnoses include autoimmune diseases, such as pemphigus vulgaris and lupus erythematosus and periodontal disease. Diagnosis is made by histopathology of the affected site, which may be the gingiva, lip, or tongue.

Malignant Melanomas (OM/MM)

Malignant melanomas occur on any site in the oral cavity: gingiva, buccal mucosa, hard and soft palates, and tongue. They are locally invasive and highly metastatic to the lungs, regional lymph nodes, and bone. As with many malignancies, clients may first notice a minor change such as bad breath. Clients also sometimes report oral bleeding. Malignant tumors may appear darkly pigmented or nonpigmented. Loose teeth, caused by bone involvement, are another symptom. The prognosis is poor because recurrence is common. Fig. 2.70 shows a malignant melanoma of the maxilla.

Maxillary Multilobular Osteochondroma

Maxillary multilobular osteochrondromas produce bone and cartilage. Some believe these are a variant of osteosarcoma, and they may be the same tumor. It is a slowly progressive neoplasm that compresses adjacent structures. Metastasis is rare, but can occur. Local recurrence can be expected in about 50% of surgically excised cases (Fig. 2.71).

Odontogenic Fibromyxoma (OM)

Odontogenic fibromyxoma is an uncommon tumor originating from the remnants of connective tissue from which normally lymphatic and circulatory systems are formed within the jaw known as ectomesenchyme. Regrowth is common and may not occur for several years. A biopsy that goes deeper than the superficial gingival inflammation is necessary for diagnosis and additional surgery or radiation therapy may be necessary after obtaining a diagnosis.

Oral Papillary Squamous Cell Carcinoma (PSCC)

Papillary squamous cell carcinoma is an invasive neoplasm affecting the rostral oral cavity in young dogs, usually less than 9 months of age. This is an aggressive tumor and early, aggressive surgery is necessary to treat it (Fig. 2.72).

Salivary Gland Carcinoma (SGC)

Salivary gland carcinomas are rare in cats and dogs; by the time they are diagnosed they have already metastasized

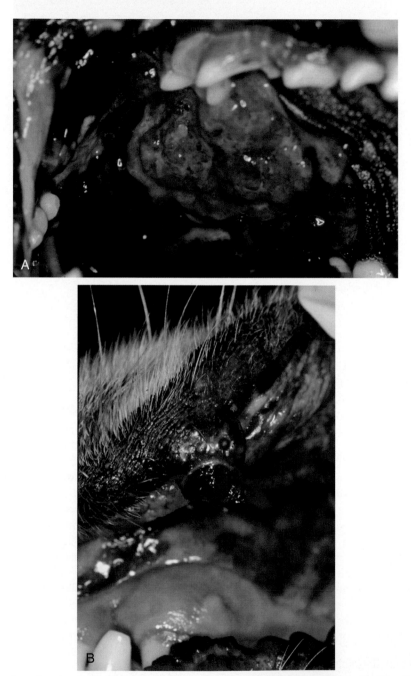

Fig. 2.70 A malignant melanoma can occur anywhere in the oral cavity; here it is on the maxilla (A) and on the lip (B).

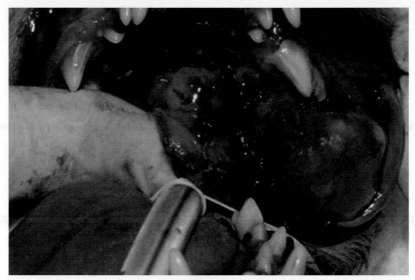

Fig. 2.71 Maxillary multilobular osteochondroma bellows. A 4-year-old dog with a left-sided swollen orbit unable to open its mouth.

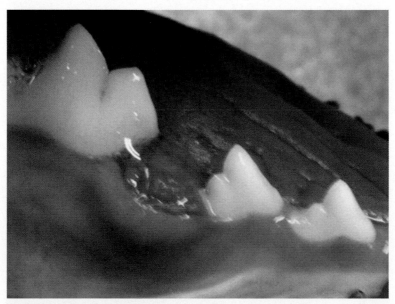

Fig. 2.72 Papillary squamous cell carcinoma. A papillary squamous cell carcinoma on the mandible of a 1-year-old dog. (Image courtesy Dr. Jose Evans.)

to the lymph nodes. Treatment can include surgical excision, radiotherapy, and chemotherapy. Even with these treatments, the prognosis cannot be predicted (Fig. 2.73).

Squamous Cell Carcinomas (OM/SCC)

Squamous cell carcinomas arise in a variety of locations in the mouth. Their cell type is from the epithelium. They can

occur in tonsillar crypts and the gingiva. Their appearance varies, but generally they are nodular, gray to pink, irregular masses that invade the bone and cause tooth mobility. Generally, the farther away from tonsils or the floor of the mouth, the better the prognosis. Fig. 2.74 is a squamous cell carcinoma in the region of a dog's hard palate where the lateral incisor would normally be located. The tooth

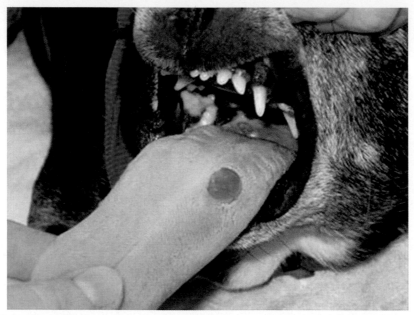

Fig. 2.73 Salivary gland carcinoma. A salivary gland carcinoma on the tongue of an 8-year-old pug. (Photo courtesy Dr. Jenny Elwell-Gerken.)

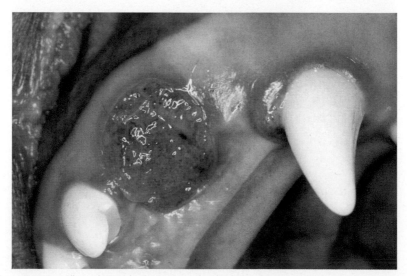

Fig. 2.74 A squamous cell carcinoma in the region of a dog's hard palate where the lateral incisor had been.

had been extracted because it was mobile. The wound did not heal, and a biopsy was taken. While the patient required additional surgery, the prognosis is good. Fig. 2.75 shows squamous cell carcinoma of the right tonsil of a cat. The prognosis is poor. Fig. 2.76 shows advanced squamous cell carcinoma in a radiograph of a cat's mandible.

Other Traumatic Oral Conditions
Mandibular Lip Avulsion

Traumatic lip avulsion injuries occur as a result of caudal force applied to the lip and gingiva. This can be caused by automobiles, falls, bite wounds, trauma from objects, and a number of other causes.

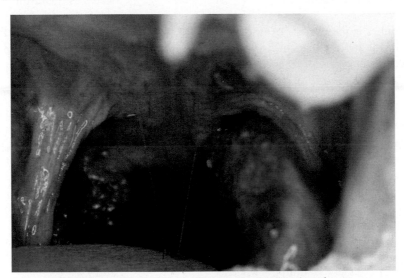

Fig. 2.75 Squamous cell carcinoma in the tonsil region of a cat.

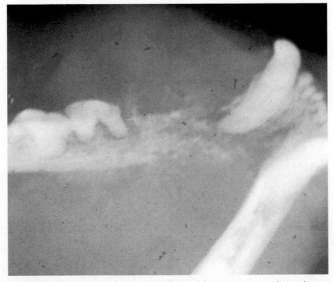

Fig. 2.76 Radiograph of a cat mandible with squamous cell carcinoma.

Temporomandibular Joint Luxation

Temporomandibular joint luxation can present as the inability to close the mouth or malocclusion. Radiology or CT scanning may be necessary to diagnose the condition. Differential diagnosis includes neoplasia and fracture.

CHAPTER 2 WORKSHEET

1. The primary teeth are also known as _____ or _____ teeth.
2. _____ orthodontics is the process of extracting primary teeth when it appears that they will cause orthodontic malocclusions.
3. Cranial mandibular osteodystrophy occurs in primarily _____ _____ _____ _____.
4. A class _____ occlusion is said to occur when the mandible is shorter than normal.
5. The condition known as maxillary brachygnathism is caused by a _____ maxilla.
6. A _____ bite is a condition in which the central incisors of the mandible and the maxilla do not align evenly.
7. _____ is inflammation of the gingiva.
8. _____ disease is disease of the surrounding tissues of the tooth.
9. _____ normally resists staining, whereas _____ is porous and stains easily.
10. _____ result from the friction of teeth against an external object such as hair or a tennis ball.
11. _____ occurs as the result of the friction of teeth against each other.
12. _____ _____ can result from conditions that cause a temporary debilitation of the patient, such as high fever.
13. _____ is the treatment of diseases inside the tooth.
14. A fracture that has penetrated enamel and dentine and involved the pulp chamber should be treated by _____ or _____.
15. The most common fracture of the fourth premolar is the _____ fracture.
16. Purple discoloration indicates _____ in the pulp.
17. An _____ is the displacement of the tooth from its socket.
18. Tooth resorption has been known in the past as _____ _____ _____ _____, _____ _____, and _____ _____ _____.
19. _____ tumors generally do not spread deep into tissue or metastasize to lymph node or lungs.
20. As with many oral malignancies, clients may first notice a minor change such as _____ _____.

Dental Instruments and Equipment

OUTLINE

LEARNING OBJECTIVES

When you have completed this chapter, you will be able to:

- List the hand instruments used in veterinary dentistry and describe the structure and purpose of each.
- Describe the materials used for sharpening hand dental instruments and explain the technique used to sharpen them.
- Explain the principle utilized by the ultrasonic scaler and differentiate between magnetostrictive and piezoelectric devices.
- Differentiate between sonic and rotary scalers.
- Differentiate between electric-powered and air-powered dental polishing units.
- Discuss the types of air-compressor systems used in veterinary dentistry and describe care of the systems.
- Differentiate between the uses and care of low-speed and high-speed handpieces.
- List and describe the types and uses of burs available for low-speed handpieces.

KEY TERMS

Arkansas stone
Bur
Calculus removal forceps
Conical stone
Curette
Explorer
Flat stone
Handle
High-speed handpiece
India stone

Low-speed handpiece
Periodontal probe
Piezoelectric
Pigtail explorer
Power scaler
Rotary scaler
Scaler
Shank
Shepherd's hook
Sonic scaler

Suction
Terminal shank
Three-way syringe
Torque
Turbine
Ultrasonic ferroceramic rod
Ultrasonic instrument
Ultrasonic metal strips/stacks
Working end

Veterinary dentistry is a very instrument- and equipment-intensive profession. An ample assortment of seemingly similar instruments is required for the proper performance of dental procedures. This chapter is devoted to the instruments and equipment required for the prevention and treatment of periodontal disease. The equipment and materials required for dental radiology and other procedures are discussed in subsequent chapters.

ORGANIZATION OF THE DENTAL DEPARTMENT

For the successful treatment of patients, veterinary dentistry requires many instruments and materials. The great number of tools necessitates sufficient shelf space and a practical method for keeping track of each item. A card file or a book with photographs identifying each item's proper place is important for organization.

Organizing the dental equipment into trays that can be pulled from the shelf as needed is a very efficient method of organizing dental equipment (Figs. 3.1 through 3.6).

HAND INSTRUMENTS

Veterinary technicians and practitioners use four main types of hand instruments (Fig. 3.7). Most instruments have four specific parts: handle, shank, terminal shank, and working end. Handles, the parts that are grasped, come in a variety of round, tapered, and hexagonal shapes. The best handle shape for the procedure depends on individual preference. The shank joins the working end with the handle. The length and curvature of the shank determines the teeth that the instrument will be able to access. The terminal shank is the part of the shank that is closest to the working end. The

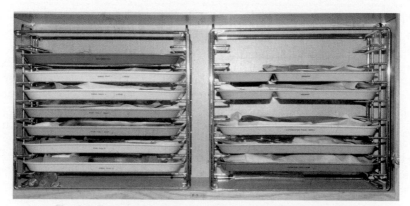

Fig. 3.1 Trays are organized in racks on a shelf in the operatory.

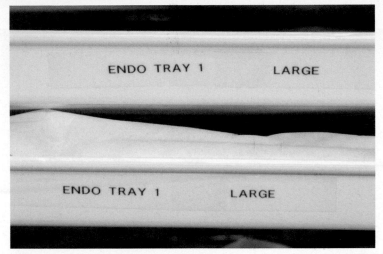

Fig. 3.2 Labels are attached to the edge of each tray for easy selection.

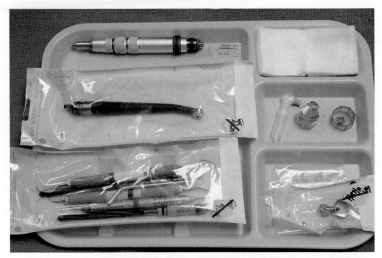

Fig. 3.3 Prophy tray set up for use.

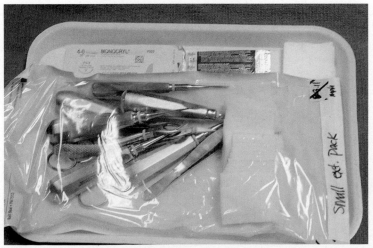

Fig. 3.4 Exodontic tray. An example of one of the trays used for extractions. There may be several trays with different sizes of instruments.

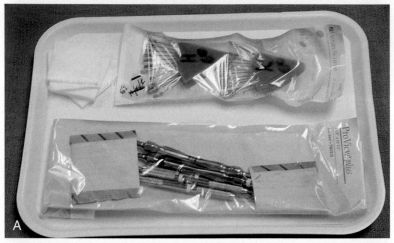

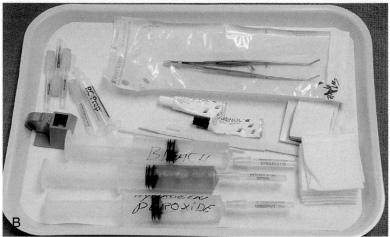

Fig. 3.5 A, Endodontics tray #1. B, Endodontics tray #2. When procedures require more instruments than can be placed on a single tray, multiple trays are used.

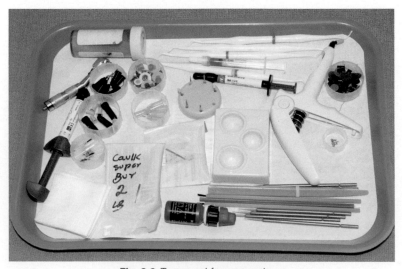

Fig. 3.6 Tray used for restorations.

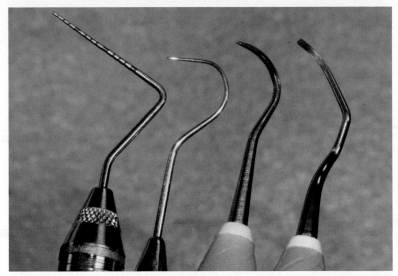

Fig. 3.7 Types of hand instruments: periodontal probe, Shepherd's hook, scaler, and curette.

working end of the instrument is the portion that comes in contact with the tooth.

Explorers

Although explorers and periodontal probes are actually two different types of instruments, they are grouped together because they are usually manufactured as double-ended instruments. One end is the periodontal probe, and the other end is the explorer. Explorers are used to detect plaque and calculus. They are also used to explore for cavities and check for exposed pulp chambers. The design of the explorer increases the operator's tactile sensitivity.

Shepherd's Hook

The shepherd's hook (or crook) is the most commonly found explorer. These instruments are manufactured in combination with the periodontal probe (Fig. 3.8).

Pigtail Explorer

The curved shape of the pigtail explorer allows the operator to use the tip of the instrument and thereby avoid touching with the side of the instruments those parts of the tooth that are not being explored (Fig. 3.9). Pigtail explorers usually come hooked to the right on one end and to the left on the other, allowing for a greater range of exploration. The explorer functions by gliding along the tooth surface in search of irregularities and magnifies the user's tactile sense.

Periodontal Probes

Many styles of periodontal probes are available (Fig. 3.10). The notched periodontal probe has three major notches at 5, 10, and 15 mm. There are intermediate notches at 1, 2, 3 (skip 4), 6, 7, 8 (skip 9), 11, 12, and 13 (skip 14) mm.

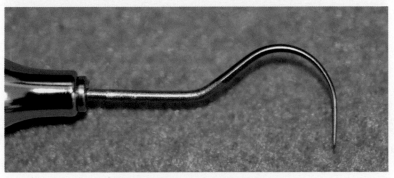

Fig. 3.8 Shepherd's hook explorer.

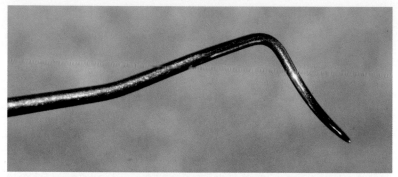

Fig. 3.9 Pigtail explorer.

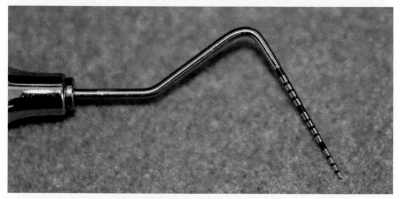

Fig. 3.10 Notched periodontal probe.

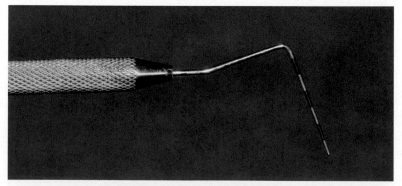

Fig. 3.11 Banded periodontal probe.

Periodontal probes with bands are available in 18-mm lengths. Each band represents 3 mm (Fig. 3.11).

Calculus Removal Forceps

The calculus removal forceps allows for quick removal of large pieces of calculus (Fig. 3.12). The instrument has tips of different lengths and shapes. The longer tip is placed over the crown, and the shorter tip is placed under the calculus. Calculus is sheared off the tooth when the two parts of the handle are brought together. When using this instrument, the technician or practitioner must be careful not to damage the enamel surface or gingiva.

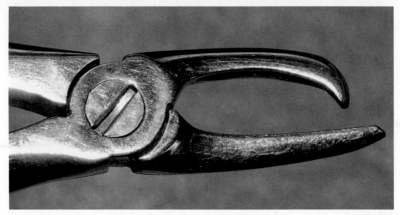

Fig. 3.12 Calculus removal forceps.

Scalers

Scalers have three sharp sides and a sharp tip. These instruments are used for scaling calculus from the crown surface. They are particularly useful in removing calculus from narrow but deep fissures such as those located on the buccal surface of the fourth premolar. Scalers are used for supragingival scaling only. Because they may damage the gingiva and periodontal ligament, scalers should not be used subgingivally. The ends of the instrument are usually mirror images of each other, which allows adaptation to opposite surfaces.

Scalers have a sharp point, or a tip (T). The face (F) is the flat side of the instrument between the two cutting edges. The cutting edge (C), the working portion of the scaler, is the confluence of the face and the sides (Fig. 3.13). To be effective, scalers must be sharpened regularly.

Several types of scalers exist (Fig. 3.14). The scaler in the middle of Fig. 3.14, generally called a *sickle scaler,* is most commonly used. The ends of this scaler are mirror images of each other. Depending on the manufacturer, sickle scalers are denoted H6/7, S6/7, or N6/7. The scaler

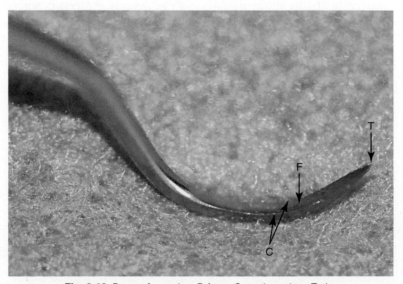

Fig. 3.13 Parts of a scaler: *F,* face; *C,* cutting edge; *T,* tip.

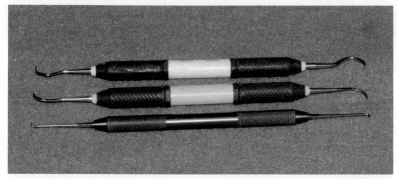

Fig. 3.14 The scaler at the top has a sickle scaler on one end and a 33 on the other. The scaler in the middle is a sickle scaler, with each end being a mirror image of the other. The instrument on the bottom is a fine scaler for extremely small teeth. It is known as a Morris 0-00.

at the top of Fig. 3.14 has a sickle scaler on one end and a #33 on scaler on the other. The instrument on the bottom of Fig. 3.14 is a fine scaler for extremely small teeth. It is known as a Morris 0-00.

Curettes

Curettes have two sharp sides and a round toe. They are used to remove calculus both supragingivally and subgingivally. Curettes are designed so that each end is a mirror image of the opposite end. This allows adaptation to the curved dental surface. If one end does not appear to be adapting to the curvature of the tooth, the instrument can be rotated. There are two types of curettes: the universal curette and the area-specific curette. The universal curette can be adapted to almost all the dental surfaces. The area-specific curette is adaptable to different areas of the mouth. One type of area-specific curette is the Gracey curette. The higher the number of the instrument, the farther back in the mouth it is used.

The point of the curette, called the *toe* (T), is rounded. The *face* (F) of the curette is the concave side. The *cutting edge* (C) is the confluence of the sides and the face. Curettes have a round back (Fig. 3.15).

Curette and Scaler Care

The best practice is to sharpen each instrument after cleaning and disinfecting and before every use. Heavy-duty industrial gloves should be used while cleaning instruments (Fig. 3.16). Alternatively, ultrasonic instrument cleaners may be used. Ideally, the operator should have several instrument packs so that the instruments can be cleaned, sharpened, and sterilized between uses. Sterilization reduces the risks of cross-infection among patients and from patients to staff members (e.g., if staff

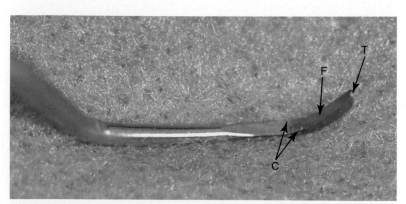

Fig. 3.15 The point of the curette, called the toe *(T)*, is rounded. The face *(F)* of the curette is the concave side. The cutting edge *(C)* is the confluence of the sides and the face. Curettes have a round back.

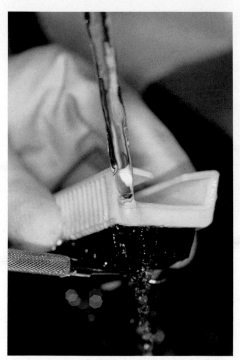

Fig. 3.16 Use of heavy-duty gloves and a brush.

recommended. Visual inspection and sharpening sticks are appropriate methods to check for sharpness.

Testing for Sharpness

Visual inspection. All that is needed to perform a visual inspection is a bright light and sharp eye. The instrument is held and rotated toward the light source (Fig. 3.17). If the instrument is dull, the edge is rounded and reflects light. If the instrument is sharp, the edge does not reflect light.

Sharpening stick. A sharpening stick is an acrylic or plastic rod (Fig. 3.18). A syringe casing may also be used to check for sharpness. To test, the edge of the instrument is drawn across the rod. A dull blade glides over the surface without catching at it. Conversely, a sharp blade easily catches as the instrument is drawn against the surface of the sharpening stick.

Sharpening Equipment

Flat stones. Several types of stones are available for sharpening (Fig. 3.19). The Arkansas stone is used for final sharpening of an instrument that is already close to sharpness. An India stone is used for "coarse" sharpening of an overly dull instrument or for changing the plane of one or more of the sides of the instrument. Sharpening with the India stone is followed by the use of an Arkansas stone. Both the Arkansas and the India stones require oil for effective use. The ceramic stone may also be used for fine sharpening. With ceramic stones, water is generally used as the sharpening medium instead of oil. A conical stone is a round Arkansas stone. It is used to provide a final sharpening to the instrument by working on its face.

members accidentally injure themselves with the instrument). Disinfecting a stainless steel table before placing an animal on it makes little sense if the instrument itself is unclean.

If an instrument is sharp, its two planes come together at a precise angle. In the past, technicians checked for sharpness by performing the "fingernail" test. For reasons of hygiene, this method is no longer

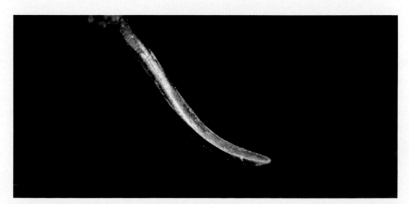

Fig. 3.17 A bright light, such as a surgical light, should be used to perform a visual inspection.

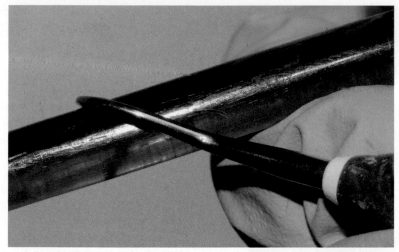

Fig. 3.18 An acrylic rod may be used to check for sharpness. The instrument should "catch" when dragged along the rod.

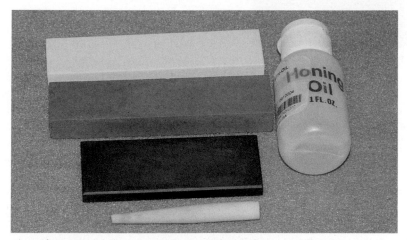

Fig. 3.19 A variety of stones and oil are necessary to sharpen instruments. *Top,* Arkansas stone. *Top middle,* India stone. *Lower middle,* ceramic stone. *Bottom,* conical stone.

Sharpening Technique

Flat stone. Two methods of sharpening with a flat stone are common. One technique is to hold the instrument motionless and move the stone. Because the edge of the instrument is stationary, the blade is highly visible during sharpening. The second method is to move the instrument against a stationary stone (Fig. 3.20). Because the moving instrument technique is less difficult, it is the method demonstrated in this text.

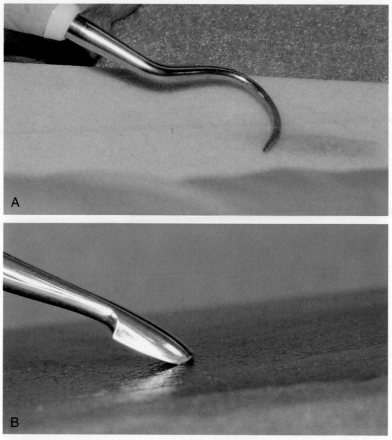

Fig. 3.20 Both curettes and elevator may be sharpened with a flat stone.

A few drops of sharpening (or mineral) oil are placed on the sharpening stone (Fig. 3.21A). The oil is spread out evenly over the stone with tissue paper (Fig. 3.21B). The stone must be lightly coated with oil. The technician must be careful not to wipe off the oil while attempting to spread it. The first step in sharpening the instrument is to hold it firmly against the edge of a table, with the tip facing the operator. The instrument is rotated so that the face is parallel with the ground. This position provides a reference point for the adaptation of the stone (Fig. 3.22).

The stone is held with the thumb and index finger at the top and bottom of the stone (Fig. 3.23).

The operator should exercise caution: the instrument is sharp and can easily cause injury. The stone is first placed at a 90-degree angle to the face of the instrument or straight up and down (Fig. 3.24A).

The upper portion of the stone is rotated approximately 10 to 15 degrees away from the instrument or to the 11 or 1 o'clock positions (Fig. 3.24B). This creates a 75- to 80-degree angle at the edge of the instrument.

The stone is moved up and down approximately 1 inch. As the stone is moved down, a "flashing" should be observed on the face of the instrument. The flashing consists of stone oil, stone particles, and instrument particles (Fig. 3.25).

As the stone moves up, the flashing should recoat the stone. If the stone is tipped too much (e.g., the top of the stone is before 11 o'clock or past 1 o'clock), the stone will miss the convergence of the face of the instrument and the side, and the blade is not sharpened. If the stone is tipped too little (e.g., the top is toward 12 o'clock), the blade may actually become dulled. The sharpening should end on the down stroke,

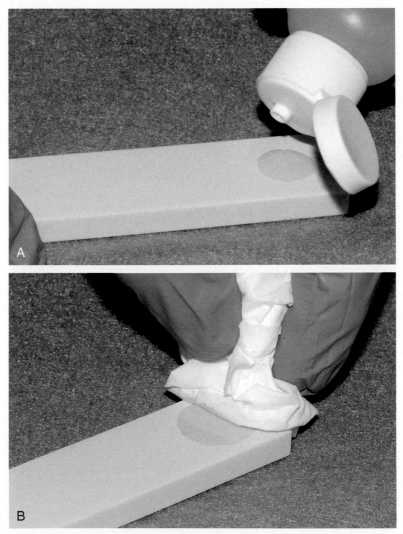

Fig. 3.21 A drop of oil is placed on the stone (A); the oil is then wiped off the stone (B).

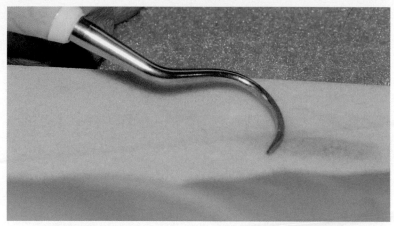

Fig. 3.22 The stone is held firmly against the edge of a table.

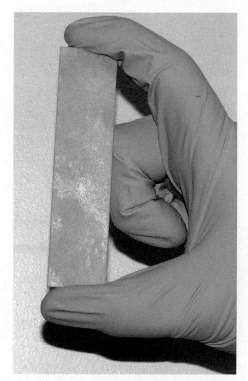

Fig. 3.23 The stone is held with the thumb and index finger at the top and bottom of the stone.

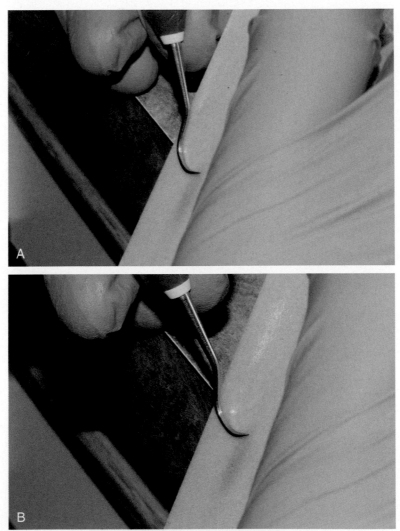

Fig. 3.24 A, The instrument is placed so that the face is 90 degrees to the stone. B, It is then rotated outward 10 to 15 degrees.

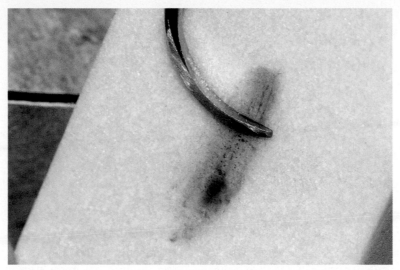

Fig. 3.25 If held at the proper angle, a flashing will be noted on the up stroke.

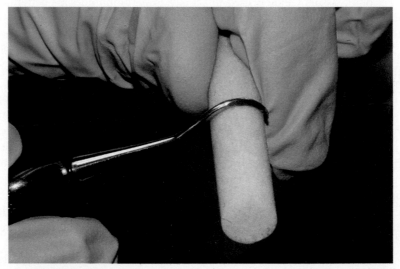

Fig. 3.26 Conical stones may be used for light sharpening of a curette.

which helps prevent the formation of a bur on the sharpened edge.

Conical stone. The conical stone is rolled over the face (Fig. 3.26). Overuse of this technique shortens the life of the instrument, the strength of which lies in the direction from the face to the back. If the face is removed, the instrument becomes weaker. The advantage of sharpening with a flat stone is that the strength of the instrument is maintained even as the sides of the instrument become worn. Thinning of the sides with the flat stone makes it better suited to subgingival work.

Conical stones can be used to sharpen dental elevators when the manufacturer has sharpened the elevator from the concave side (Fig. 3.27).

For further instruction watch: https://www.youtube.com/watch?v=z05sQSYpxJs.

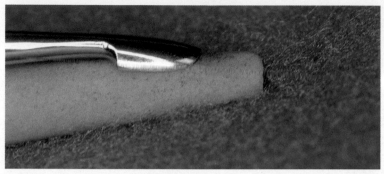

Fig. 3.27 If the elevator was originally sharpened from the inside, a conical stone may be used to sharpen it.

Rx Honing Machine. This unit simplifies sharpening. It consists of the following: a diamond disk to sharpen extremely dull instruments; a carbide disk used to maintain an edge with the removal of a minimal amount of metal; a round hone to sharpen explorers and spoons; a U-shaped hone to round off the edge of curettes and keep them sharp. A Perio & Scissors Guide is used to establish the angle at which the instruments should be sharpened (Fig. 3.28).

POWER SCALERS

Power scalers convert electric or pneumatic energy into a mechanical vibration (Table 3.1). When the power scaler is placed against calculus, the vibration shatters it, freeing it from the tooth surface. Power scalers operate in the range of 8000 to 45,000 cycles per second. There are three types of power instruments. The ultrasonic scalers work by converting sound waves into a mechanical vibration. The sonic and rotary instruments convert air pressure into mechanical vibration.

Ultrasonic Instruments

Ultrasonic instruments work by converting energy from a power source into a sound wave. This sound wave is picked up at the handpiece. Ultrasonic instruments function in a way similar to that of two identically tuned tuning forks: when one is caused to vibrate, the other starts to vibrate in resonance. Two types of devices in the handpiece can pick up the sound wave and turn it into a vibration: *magnetostrictive* and *piezoelectric*. Magnetostrictive devices use either a ferroceramic rod or metal strips (Fig. 3.29).

Magnetostrictive

Ultrasonic metal strips/stacks. Several manufacturers produce flat metal strip units. These vibrate at 18,000, 25,000, and 30,000 cycles per second. The amplitude of tip movement in these units is between 0.01 and 0.05 mm, which is an extremely narrow motion. Generally, lower amplitudes are better because they cause less damage to the tooth. The working tip is all sides, which results in an uneven motion and an elliptic pattern. Two lengths of inserts are available, which is important to remember when ordering and inserting them into the handpiece (Fig. 3.30).

Ultrasonic and combination electric motor handpieces. Several of the manufactured dental units are combinations of ultrasonic scalers and electric motor handpieces. These are used for polishing and simple cutting of teeth. The electric motor handpieces are generally not as effective as the air-powered, high- and low-speed handpieces that use compressed air.

Handpiece inserts need periodic replacement. The handpiece in Fig. 3.31 has fractured welds and will no longer function efficiently.

Ultrasonic ferroceramic rod. Magnetostrictive ferroceramic rods vibrate at 42,000 cycles per second (Fig. 3.32). These instruments have an amplitude of 0.01 to 0.02 mm with a circular-type motion. All sides of the tip are equally active (about 13 mm of the tip).

Inserting ultrasonic inserts. If a metal strip/stack unit is used, the unit must be turned on and the handpiece filled before insertion of the insert (Fig. 3.33). However, with ferroceramic rod units, the handpiece should be drained before insertion of the insert (Fig. 3.34). Forcing the insert into a handpiece that contains water may prevent it from vibrating or cause the tip to fracture.

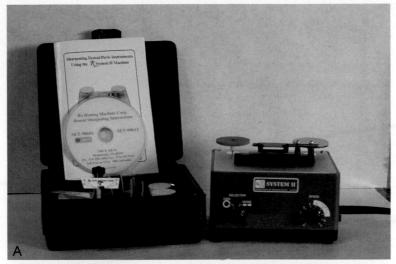

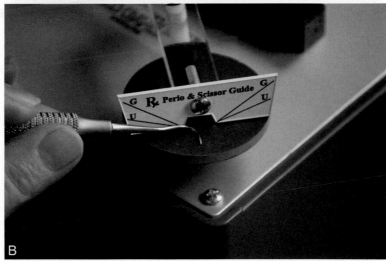

Fig. 3.28 A, The Rx Honing Machine system sharpening unit, with manual and DVD. B, Universal sharpening device. The terminal shank of the Universal curette is lined up with the "U Line" of the Universal scaler. (Photo courtesy Rx Honing. Mishawaka, Indiana.)

TABLE 3.1	**Comparison of Mechanical Scalers**			
Instrument Type	**Cycles per Second**	**Amplitude (mm)**	**Active Tip (mm)**	**Motion**
Magnetostrictive: metal strips	18,000, 25,000, 30,000	0.01–0.05	5–7	Elliptic
Magnetostrictive: ferroceramic rod	42,000	0.01–0.02	13	Circular
Piezoelectric	25,000–45,000	0.2	3	Linear (back and forth)
Sonic	6000	0.5		Elliptic
Rotary			Depends on tip	Circular

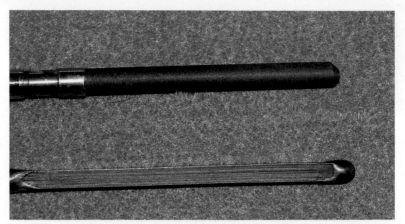

Fig. 3.29 *Top,* Ferroceramic rod as is used in the iM3 42-12 (iM3 Inc., Vancouver, WA, USA) Ultrasonic scaler. *Bottom,* magnetostritive insert as used in a Vetroson Millennium 25/30 Ultrasonic Scaler or a Cavitron type unit (Summit Hill Laboratories New Jersey, NJ, USA).

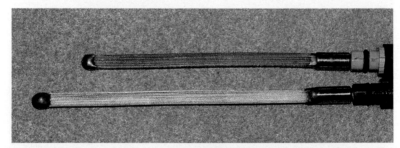

Fig. 3.30 The upper shorter metal strip unit is a 30K (30,000 cycles per second), and the lower longer unit is a 25K (25,000 cycles per second).

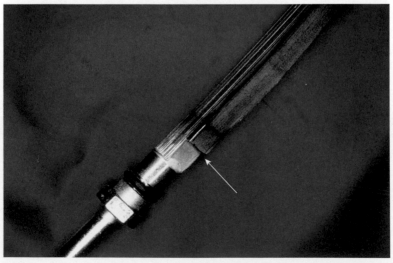

Fig. 3.31 Because of use, this ultrasonic tip has fractured at the weld *(arrow)* and should be replaced.

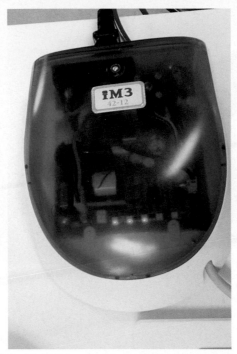

Fig. 3.32 The iM3 unit (iM3 Inc., Vancouver, WA, USA) uses a ferroceramic rod.

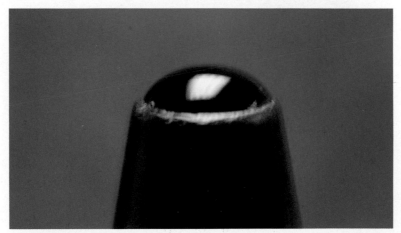

Fig. 3.33 When using the magnetostrictive metal type, the handpiece should be filled with water before inserting.

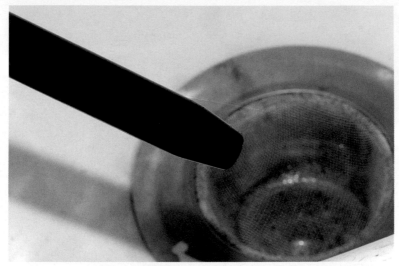

Fig. 3.34 When using the iM3 ferroceramic rod, inserted water should be drained prior to insertion.

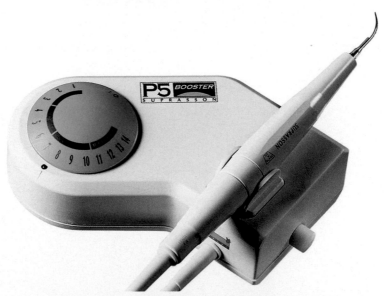

Fig. 3.35 Piezoelectric scaler. (Courtesy Dentalaire, CA, USA.)

Adjust the power prior to use (see Chapter 7). Once the power is adjusted, the scaler is turned on at the ring/switch on the handpiece by pulling it back—there is no foot pedal.

Piezoelectric

Piezoelectric ultrasonic scalers use crystals in the handpiece to pick up the vibration (Fig. 3.35).

The frequency of the piezoelectric units ranges from 25,000 to 45,000 cycles per second. The amplitude of these units is approximately 0.2 mm, which results in a wide, back-and-forth tip motion. Approximately 3 mm of the working tip is active.

Some ultrasonic scalers also come with lights for better visualization (Fig. 3.36).

The vibration energy is not distributed evenly down the tip of piezoelectric ultrasonic scalers (Fig. 3.37).

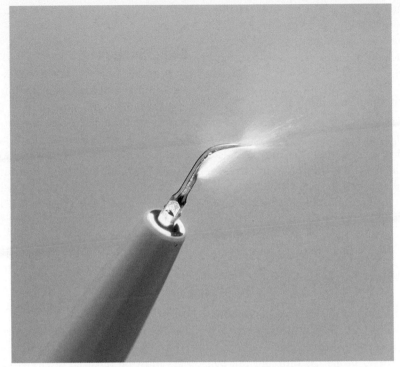

Fig. 3.36 Scaler tip with light. (Courtesy Henry Schein/Kruuse.)

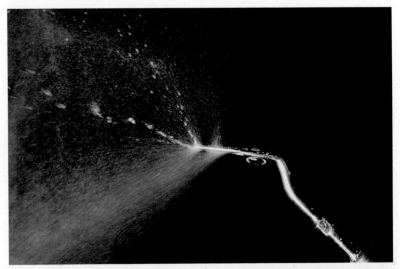

Fig. 3.37 Piezo tip showing the energy nodes.

The motion of the piezo tip is not uniform. The tip moves farther in one direction than in the other, which means that during use the most active side of the tip must be placed on the part of the tooth where the calculus is to be removed.

Medicaments in Irrigating Solutions

Many piezoelectric and magnetostrictive units have reservoirs for an irrigating solution. A variety of solutions may be placed in the containers. The most popular and effective solution is 0.12% chlorhexidine. In-line reservoirs may be spliced onto the water line, allowing irrigation solutions to be used in units that do not have their own containers. Another alternative is to use a garden sprayer, otherwise known as a "bug buster," for the water supply. These units must be pressurized by hand.

Ultrasonic Tips

As shown by the tip on the top in Fig. 3.38, the beaver-tail tip is relatively wide. This tip was the first type of tip developed and it is used for supragingival cleaning. The bottom tip, the "perio probe," is thin and can be used subgingivally. Furcation tips hook to the left or right, which allows them to gain access to furcations around crowns and be used subgingivally. Further information on these units and tips is provided in Chapters 7 and 9.

Sonic Scalers

Sonic scalers operate at 6000 cycles per second and have a 0.5-mm amplitude. Their motion is elliptic—a figure-of-eight motion. All sides of these tips are active during cleaning, although the cleaning action may not be even. One feature of these units is that the compressed air has a cooling effect. They are less likely to cause heat-related damage to teeth than are the ultrasonic scalers.

Air enters the sonic scaler, passes through the shaft, and exits from small holes on the shaft that are covered with a metal ring. The air exits the holes at an angle and causes the ring to start spinning. Because the ring does not fit the shaft tightly, it begins to wobble. This wobbling sets off a vibration that is transmitted down the shaft to the tip (Fig. 3.39).

Rotary Scalers

The use of rotary scalers is discouraged for two reasons. First, rotary scalers can easily damage the tooth. Second, burs must be replaced often because they become dull extremely quickly. For proper functioning, a new bur must be used for each patient, which is prohibitively expensive.

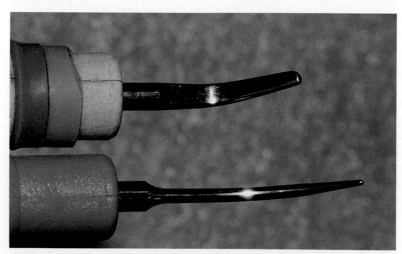

Fig. 3.38 Ultrasonic tips. *Top,* Beaver-tail insert; *bottom,* periodontal insert.

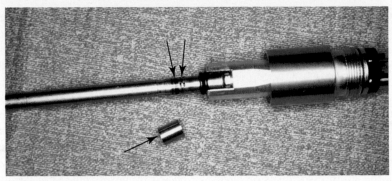

Fig. 3.39 The small metal ring *(arrow)* has been removed from the shaft of the sonic scaler. Air blows out of the small holes *(double arrows)*.

DENTAL UNITS FOR POLISHING AND DRILLING

Two driving mechanisms exist for polishing and cutting teeth: electric power and air power. Electric-powered units generally are the least expensive, although some sophisticated electric systems, used for specialized procedures such as implantation and endodontics, rival the price of the compressed-air systems.

Electric-Powered Systems

Electric-powered systems (Fig. 3.40) operate at lower speeds than air-powered systems and have higher torque, which is the ability to overcome resistance to movement. Water or irrigating systems cannot be used with electric-powered systems, except with fairly expensive models. Generally, air-powered systems are preferable to electric-powered systems.

Air-Powered Systems

Two types of air-powered systems exist. One uses compressed gas from a cylinder, the second uses an air compressor. The air compressor pumps air either directly into the dental unit or into a storage tank for slow release to the dental unit. The compressed gas is either room air or nitrogen. Because of associated hazards, oxygen and carbon dioxide should not be used. Oxygen is explosive, and carbon dioxide may be toxic.

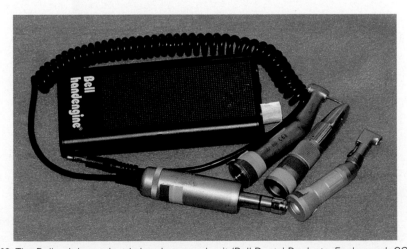

Fig. 3.40 The Bell unit is an electric hand-powered unit (Bell Dental Products, Englewood, CO, USA).

Air-Compressor Systems

Compressors take the room air and compress it to drive the handpieces. Most units work by pumping air into an air-storage tank. The compressor pumps air into the tank until the pressure inside the tank reaches between 80 and 100 pounds per square inch (psi). At this time the compressor turns off. Air is bled from the tank as it is used by the handpiece at a lower pressure, usually 30 to 40 psi. When the pressure drops below the minimum pressure in the tank, approximately 60 psi, the compressor turns on again, filling the tank back up to 100 psi. Newer compressors are quieter than traditional air compressors. To reduce noise, refrigerator compressors were converted so that they pump air rather than refrigerator coolant. The single-unit compressor rate is approximately 5½ hp. If a multistation or sonic-scaler handpiece is to be used, a double-unit, 1 hp compressor should

be considered. These units are available in portable carts, portable cabinets, and countertop units. They can be custom built to the practitioner's needs.

Counter or table top units allow the unit to be stored in cabinets and other areas remote from the place the procedure is performed. They are self-contained and require only a power source to function (Fig. 3.41).

Dental carts with switches, handpiece holders, and suction are available. The compressor may be mounted on the cart or stored in a remote location. The air is connected by hoses (Fig. 3.42). Dental units may also be mounted on walls with the compressor in a remote location, connected by hoses.

The Surgiden system is a complete dental suite, with table, compressor, light, and intravenous (IV) stand built into an ergonomic table with its own water and waste disposal reservoirs (Fig. 3.43). This system can also be wall mounted (Fig. 3.44).

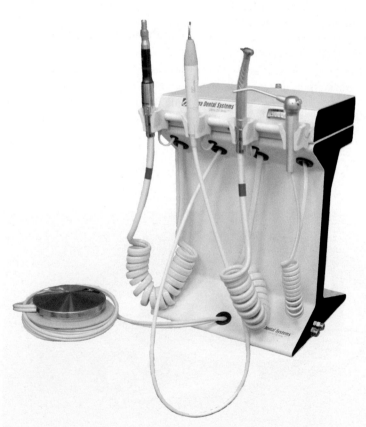

Fig. 3.41 A table or counter top unit can be moved and stored when not in use. (Photo courtesy Shipps Dental & Specialty Products, AZ USA.)

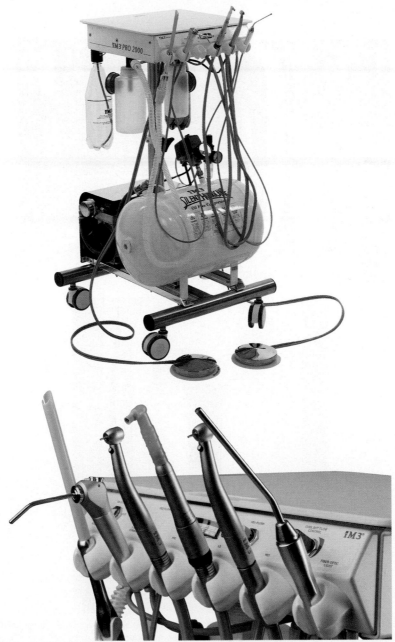

Fig. 3.42 Dental cart. This iM3 unit has low and high speeds, air-water syringe, suction, fiberoptic light, and multiple water bottles. (Photo courtesy iM3 Vancouver, WA, USA.)

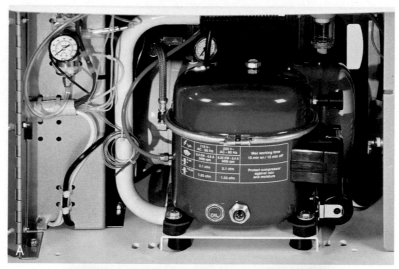

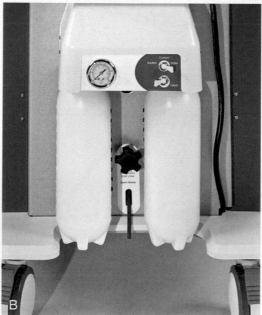

Fig. 3.43 The Surgiden unit includes a dental table, compressor, and water supply. A, Surgiden compressor. B, Surgiden water supply (photo courtesy Surgiden Inc., www.surgiden.com).

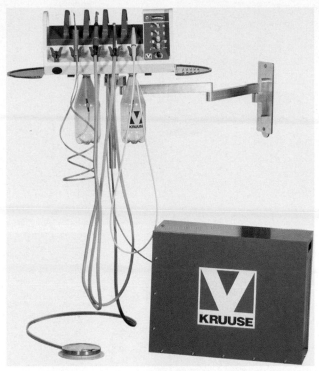

Fig. 3.44 Dental Trio Wallmount. A wall-mounted system with a compressor that can be stored elsewhere (Photo courtesy Kruuse/ Henry Schein Co., NY, USA).

Compressor Care

Most air-compressor systems use oil for lubrication. The oil level must be monitored frequently because insufficient oil could cause the compressor to cease functioning. Some systems use a dipstick, similar to that of an automobile, for checking the oil. Others have a porthole in the side of the oil reservoir. When adding oil, the technician should always use the type of oil recommended by the compressor manufacturer.

The compression of air into the storage tank may cause condensation. Air-storage tanks have a drain cock that can be turned to let the water out of the tank (Fig. 3.45). Failure to do so allows water to fill the tank, decreasing the effectiveness of the system and possibly ruining the compressor.

Handpieces

Different types of handpieces can be attached to compressed-air systems (Fig. 3.46). Low-speed handpieces are used for polishing with prophy angles and for performing other dental procedures with contra angles. High-speed handpieces are used for cutting teeth in extractions and making access holes into teeth in root canal therapy. All handpieces use a rubber gasket to ensure a water- and air-tight seal. Make sure the gasket is connected when connecting the handpiece (Fig. 3.47). (See previous section for discussion of sonic scalers.)

Low-Speed Handpieces

Low-speed handpieces are used for polishing teeth. They have a high torque and a slow speed of 5000 to 20,000 revolutions per minute (rpm) (Fig. 3.48).

low-speed attachments. A prophy angle is an attachment that allows the use of a prophy cup for polishing teeth during cleaning. (Types of prophy angles and prophy cups are discussed in more detail in Chapter 7.) Attachments, such as special files for engine-driven root canals and slow-speed burs for cutting and smooth restoration, are available. A contra angle is an attachment used to change either the direction or speed of rotation (Fig. 3.49).

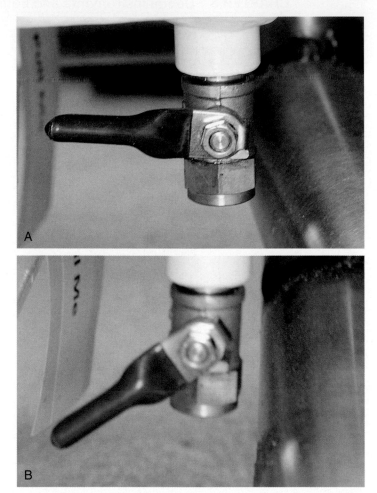

Fig. 3.45 If the compressor has an air-storage tank, it must be periodically drained. A, Valve closed. B, Valve open for drainage.

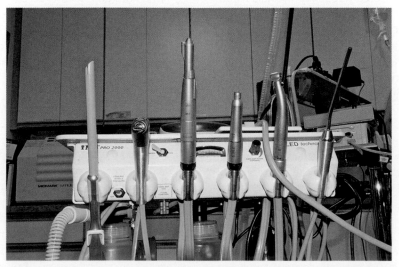

Fig. 3.46 This iM3 unit has a suction, air-water syringe, slow-speed handpiece, second slow-speed handpiece, high-speed handpiece, and fiberoptic light (Photo courtesy iM3 Inc., Vancouver, WA, USA).

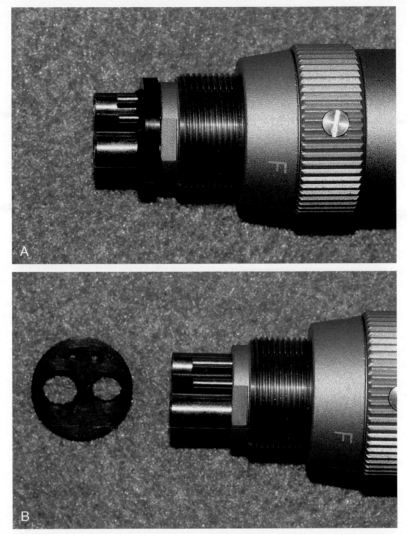

Fig. 3.47 A; Check to make sure the gasket is on. B, Gaskets may come off of the handpiece.

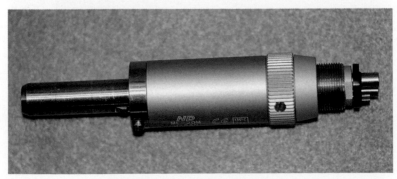

Fig. 3.48 Low-speed handpiece engine.

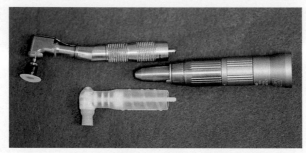

Fig. 3.49 Low-speed attachments. *Upper left,* contra angle; *right,* nose cone; *lower left,* prophy angle.

Care of low-speed handpieces. The low-speed handpiece must be lubricated at the end of each day of use. The technician must first insert lubricant into the smaller of the two large holes, using the oil or spray that comes with the handpiece. WD-40 may be sprayed into the low-speed handpiece once every 2 weeks to remove residues, followed by the recommended lubricant.

Prophy and contra angles. The specific lubrication of prophy and contra angles depends on the instrument. Generally, prophy heads must be lubricated weekly with prophy angle lubricant. For many models the head of the instrument may be twisted off to expose the crown gears that require lubrication. Some prophy angles are self-lubricating. In all cases, the manufacturer's instructions should be consulted for each piece of equipment.

High-Speed Handpieces

High-speed handpieces turn at 300,000 to 400,000 rpm. They are used for cutting teeth for exodontics, making root canal entries, and other procedures. Practitioners who use one of these instruments for splitting a tooth in exodontics will find it difficult to return to (or even imagine) the old methods of extracting. Some high-speed handpieces come with fiberoptic lights that are turned on by the spinning turbine (Fig. 3.50).

Changing high-speed burs. Two styles of high-speed bur heads are available. One uses a push button on the handpiece to open the chuck. The bur may be removed and replaced by simply pressing the button. The second uses a chuck key. The bur may be loosened and removed by twisting the key counterclockwise. The new bur is placed in the handpiece, and the bur key turned clockwise to tighten (Fig. 3.51).

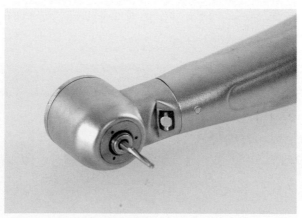

Fig. 3.50 This high-speed handpiece has a fiberoptic light for better visualization of areas being cut. (Photo courtesy Kruuse/Henry Schein Co., NY, USA.)

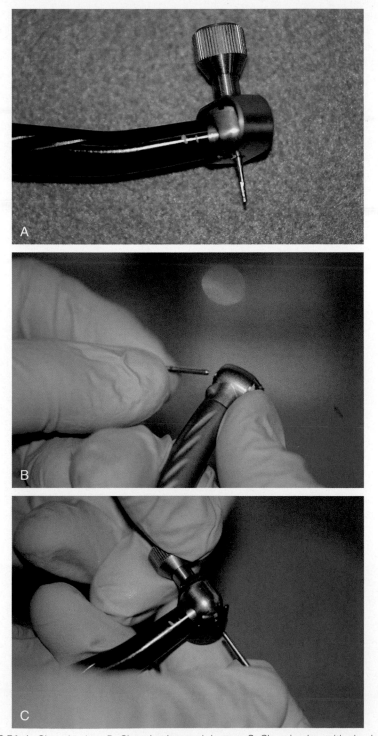

Fig. 3.51 A, Changing bur. B, Changing bur push button. C, Changing bur with chuck key.

Burs should be treated as sharps and disposed of in the sharps container. They should be removed from the handpiece when not in use and when the handpiece is covered. If the bur is removed from the handpiece, a "blank" should be put in its place. If the handpiece is accidentally turned on without a bur in the handpiece chuck, the chuck may be damaged.

Bur selection. Both diamond and carbide operative burs are used with clinical success, and careful clinical technique is more important, than type of bur. When selecting a bur, the practitioner must first know the type of handpiece with which the bur is to be used. At the top of Fig. 3.52 is a straight-shank bur that fits directly into the low-speed handpiece. The bur in the middle is a right-angle (RA) bur that fits into contra angles for low-speed handpieces. The bur on the bottom is a friction-grip (FG) bur that fits into contra angles for low-speed handpieces. Technicians must be extremely careful when selecting a bur. Some slow-speed FG burs resemble high-speed burs. However, when placed in a high-speed handpiece, these slow-speed FG burs disintegrate under the centrifugal forces placed on them.

Types of burs. Fig. 3.53 contains the types of burs.

Pear-shaped burs. Pear-shaped burs, which are numbered in the 320s through 330s. These burs are a cross between the round bur, crosscut bur, and inverted-cone bur. The result is a bur that has a round cutting tip, cutting sides, and a slight taper for undercutting. These are ideal all-purpose burs for cavity preparation. The L after the number indicates a longer-length bur (Fig. 3.54)

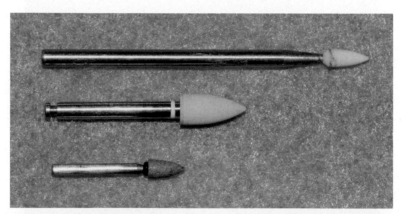

Fig. 3.52 *Top,* Straight-shank bur; *middle,* right-angle (RA) bur; *bottom,* a friction-grip (FG) bur.

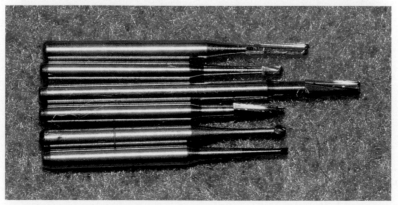

Fig. 3.53 *Top to bottom,* 331 L (long pear), 330 (pear), 701S (surgical length), 701 (crosscut fissure), 2 (round), 33½ (inverted-cone bur).

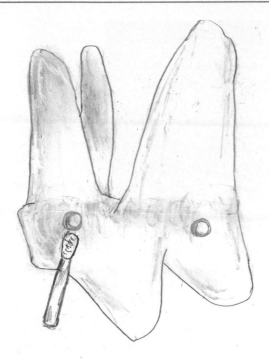

Fig. 3.54 A 330 pear-shaped bur is used to create a slight under-cut for retention. (Sketch by Peter Emily, DDS, HonAVDC.)

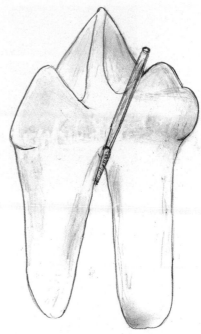

Fig. 3.55 Starting from the furcation and working coronally, a 701 crosscut fissure bur is used to section a canine first molar. (Sketch by Peter Emily, DDS, HonAVDC.)

Crosscut fissure burs. Crosscut fissure burs are numbered in the 500s through 700s. They are used for gaining access to root canals, cutting teeth, and preparing cavities. The crosscut fissure bur is one of the best all-around dental burs. The bur is slightly tapered, with a cutting surface on the side as well as the tip. The letter S after the number indicates a surgical-length bur, which is good for cutting teeth where a long reach is necessary (Fig. 3.55).

Inverted-cone burs. The inverted-cone burs are given numbers in the 30s (e.g., 33½, 34, 35). The larger the number, the larger the bur. Inverted-cone burs are used for undercutting in cavity preparation. They are wider at the tip than at the shank.

Round burs. These are numbered ¼, ½, 1, 2, 4, and 6 and are general, all-purpose burs. They may be used for access into pulp chambers and for cavity preparations, and sectioning small teeth. Fig. 3.56 demonstrates a feline first molar being sectioned with a ½ round bur.

Diamond burs. Diamond burs are used for crown preparation (Fig. 3.57). A wide variety of shapes and degrees of coarseness is available. Selection depends on the preparation to be performed.

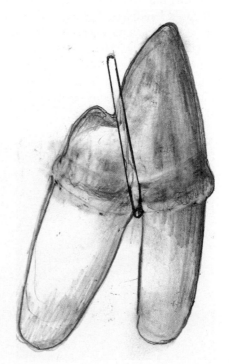

Fig. 3.56 Starting from the furcation and working coronally, using a ½ round bur on a feline first molar. (Sketch by Peter Emily, DDS, HonAVDC.)

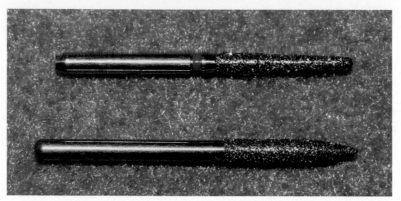

Fig. 3.57 Diamond burs are used for crown preparation.

Finishing burs,. A number of burs are used for finishing restorations. One type is a stone, and another has multiple flutes.

Care of high-speed handpieces

Lubrication. The high-speed and subsonic scalers should be lubricated daily with a spray-type cleaner and lubricant or another product recommended by the manufacturer of the handpiece (Fig. 3.58 and Table 3.2).

Defective turbine. The turbine is the internal portion of the high-speed handpiece that spins at an extremely high speed. It is subject to wear over time and must be replaced periodically. Maintenance may be performed in the office. The signs of a defective turbine cartridge include the following: (1) failure of chuck to tighten around the bur; (2) increased noise or vibration;

(3) roughness felt when spinning bur by hand, with turbine in or out of handpiece; (4) intermittent stopping of handpiece; and (5) failure of handpiece to function. Fig. 3.59 shows a turbine that has fractured.

Changing turbines. To change the turbine, a "blank" bur is placed in the handpiece. If the bur that is in the handpiece cannot be removed, caution should be exercised to keep from cutting the hands on the bur. Next, the small metal ring (wrench) supplied with the handpiece is placed on the cap of the handpiece. The handpiece cap is unscrewed and removed by rotating the wrench counterclockwise. The turbine cartridge is removed from the handpiece head by pressing on the blank or bur (Fig. 3.60). The new turbine cartridge is placed into the handpiece head. Finally, the new turbine cartridge is aligned with the pin side up. If the pin is not

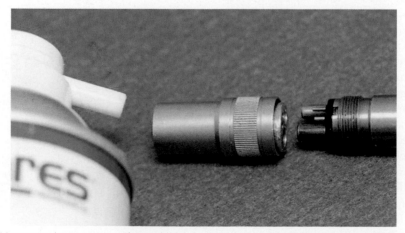

Fig. 3.58 This system has a spray canister with lubricant and a connector that connects with the high-speed handpiece.

TABLE 3.2 **Maintenance Chart**[a]

Procedure	Daily	Weekly	Yearly
Oil in slow speed	√		
Spray in high speed	√		
Check compressor oil level		√	
Drain water out of compressor		√	
Annual compressor maintenance			√

[a]Manufacturers' recommendations supersede this chart.

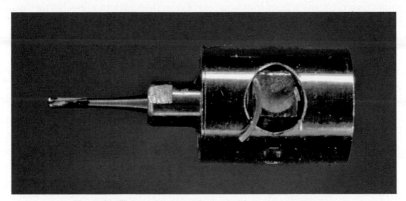

Fig. 3.59 This turbine has fractured from long-term use.

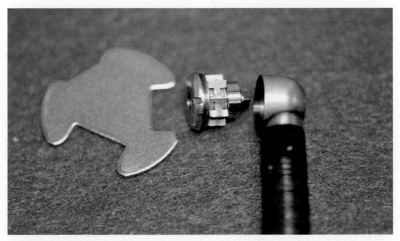

Fig. 3.60 Follow the manufacturer's instructions when changing the turbine.

aligned with the slot, the turbine cartridge will not slide completely into the handpiece head.

Troubleshooting High-Speed Handpieces

Several problems can occur with high-speed handpieces: bur fails to spin, burr falls out, slow cutting.

A bur that fails to spin is likely caused by a defective turbine. Another cause is if the head housing is damaged and not detected. This may have been caused by dropping the handpiece. Even when the heads are pressed back out when damage is noticed, they are never truly 100% right. It is very easy to knock the handpiece out of the holder, or not put it in the holder in the first place.

A bur that falls out can be caused by reusing dull burs, this is not the case here, being heavy handed—pushing too hard on a good bur, bur is not fully seated in turbine. If a longer-length bur is needed, a surgical-length bur should be used; do not pull a bit of the bur out to give the extra length needed. As soon as the bur catches, the turbine will spin (and not the bur) and remove metal off the chuck and the burs will just slip out. Another problem is caused by the use of inexpensive burs that have inconsistent shank diameter, which results from poor engineering of the bur. A bad turbine can wear away the inside of the head, particularly the front where the turbine chuck exits the housing and where the bur is inserted. It may be noticed that the hole is wider than it should be. If that is the case, putting a good turbine in a bad housing will just continue to chew through all future turbines.

Slow cutting is caused by incorrect compressor air pressure setup, a leak in the system or a defective turbine.

Three-Way Syringes

Most dental units come equipped with three-way syringes. These syringes have two buttons. Pressing one button creates a water spray, which can be used to irrigate a tooth surface and clear away prophy paste, tooth shavings, and other debris. Pressing the second button creates an air spray, which can be used to dry the field.

The technician must be careful not to flush air into tissues; air can create subcutaneous emphysema or, even worse, enter a blood vessel and create an embolism. Pressing both buttons together creates a mist. The tip of the three-way syringe can be removed for autoclaving. Other disposable tips are also available (Fig. 3.61).

Suction

Suction units—either combined into a dental cart or separate—are useful in aspirating blood and debris from extraction sites to allow better visualization in the case of retained roots, better visualization of surgical fields, and visualization in performing endodontics.

LIGHTING AND MAGNIFICATION

With a few exceptions, the following statement holds true for veterinary dentistry: "If you can't see it, you can't do it." Lighting and magnification are two very important aids that allow the technician and practitioner to visualize the structures in the oral cavity. Once used, most ask how they were able to work without them.

Lighting

Lighting is available from a variety of sources. A good surgical light produces wide-ranging, even lighting. Spot lighting is obtained by the use of a light mounted to a headlamp. Focal lighting is achieved by the use of fiber-optic lights built into a handpiece.

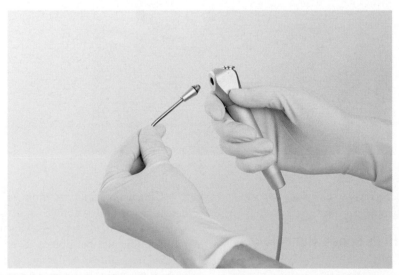

Fig. 3.61 Replaceable three-way syringe tip. Syringe tips can be removed and sterilized. (Photo courtesy Henry Schein/Kruuse.)

There are a number of things to consider when purchasing a light source. Brightness and uniform illumination provide even visualization of the field. Some light sources also have an adjustable spot. The Color Rendering Index (CRI) provides a quantitative measure (up to 100) of a light source that shows colors in comparison to an ideal or natural light sources. The higher the CRI, the better reduction in eye fatigue. There are also cordless and corded LED headlamps. In the cordless versions, the battery is stored on the unit. Whereas it is more convenient not to have a cord attached to a battery pack, three variables to the headlamp include the following: weight, intensity of the light, and battery life. Some will have battery life indicators and some just turn off when out of power. The intensity can also be an important consideration: not intense enough leads to poor visualization; too intense can lead to eye strain.

Magnification

Loupes are available in two types, fixed and flip-up. Fixed has the advantage of being through the lens (TTL) and is the most popular among dentists. They are well balanced and allow a larger field of view, have lower maintenance, can have prescriptions incorporated into the optics, and retain alignment better than the flip-up type. The flip-up type allows for a greater angle for the loupe optics to be inclined downward. By looking down rather than tilting the head down, less eye strain can be obtained. However, looking down causes greater eye strain.

Binocular eyeglasses produce the best type of magnification. Ideally, they should be adjustable so that the operator's head does not tilt forward; rather, the eyes look down and the head is kept squarely above the shoulders. Two and one-half to three-powered magnification, with a focal length of between 15 and 18 inches, enlarges the subject without excess distortion.

There are a variety of systems available. Some are custom made for each user—the distance between your eyes, called the interpupillary distance (IPD), is fixed. Some have adjustable IPD, so multiple users can use the same loupe. Loupes can be custom built for a specific user. Some are attached to lenses that are similar to bifocals or trifocals to allow normal vision or diopter correction. Others have sliding adjustment between the lenses that allow multiple users to use them. Some have locked adjustment that cannot moved inadvertently.

Another consideration is the ability to disinfect the loupe. Some are completely waterproof so they can be scrubbed. If keeping a loupe clean and sterile is important, some loupes have an autoclavable flip handle so you can move the loupe away from your field of vision when the loupe is not needed and then back in play while remaining sterile (Fig. 3.62). Ideally, have an eye examination to determine if any prescriptions should be incorporated into custom loups. Wear loups for short periods each day to let eyes gradually adjust. There are many choices in loops and it is best to try out a few before purchasing. Make sure the frames, nose pads, and other adjustable features are properly adjusted.

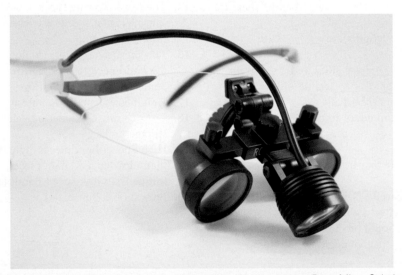

Fig. 3.62 An adjustable Rose Micro Solutions loupe and light. (Photo courtesy Rose Micro Solutions, NY, USA)

When using loupes, occasionally take them off and focus on more distant objects. Consider purchasing additional loupes with greater magnification for more delicate procedures. There are also adjustable magnification lenses.

Suppliers of Telescopic Glasses, Loops and Lights

Clear Optic http://clearoptix.com/
Denlight http://www.denlight.com
Denmat (Perioptic) http://www.denmat.com
Designs for Vision http://www.designsforvision.com
Eclipse Loops and Products http://www.eclipselou pesandproducts.com
Enova Illumination http://www.enovaillumination.com
Orascopic http://www.orascoptic.com
Perioptic http://www.denmat.com
Rose Micro Solutions http://www.rosemicrosolutions.com
Schultz Loop Factory Direct http://www.loupedirect.com
Surgitel http://surgitel.com
Ultralight Optics http://www.ultralightoptics.com
Welch Allyn http://www.welchallyn.com

DISINFECTION AND STERILIZATION

Disinfection and sterilization are both processes to decontaminate instruments, equipment, and surfaces. Disinfection eliminates or reduces harmful microorganisms and sterilization kills all microorganisms and destroys the spores of various organisms. Whenever possible, dental instruments and equipment should be sterilized via steam or gas. However, there are some instances where this is not possible. Disinfection and sterilization are done to protect the patient as well as every member of the veterinary facility. This is part of keeping the workplace safe and free of pathogens.

Saliva, blood, crevicular fluid, biofilm, and hard and soft tissue are spread on everything and everyone. This contamination comes mostly from aerosols, smears, splatters, and spills. Fortunately, microbes are contained within the various fluids and tissues, and are rarely found free on clinical surfaces without whatever has spread them. Unfortunately, when microbes are mixed with complex proteins from the oral cavity, disinfectants do not necessarily kill the bacteria. Therefore, instruments should be cleaned before disinfecting.

CHAPTER 3 WORKSHEET

1. The four types of hand instruments are as follows: _____, _____, _____, and _____.
2. The portions of all instruments are the handle, the shank, the terminal shank, and the _____ _____.
3. Banded veterinary probes have bands that are _____ mm wide.
4. The newer probe lengths are _____ and _____ _____.
5. Scalers have _____ sharp sides and a sharp tip.
6. Scalers are used for _____ scaling only.
7. Curettes and scalers are usually _____ _____; this means that they can adapt to opposite surfaces.
8. The _____ _____ is the working portion of the scaler.
9. The _____ curette may be adapted to almost all the dental surfaces.
10. A _____ blade reflects light, whereas a _____ blade does not reflect light.
11. The instrument should be sharpened so that it has a _____ to _____ degree angle.
12. As the stone is moved down, a "_____" should be observed on the face of the instrument.
13. Powered scalers convert _____ or _____ energy into mechanical vibration.
14. The two following types of devices in the handpiece can pick up a sound wave and turn it into a vibration: _____ and _____.
15. The piezoelectric ultrasonic scalers use _____ in the handpiece to pick up the vibration.
16. Sonic scalers are driven by _____ _____.
17. Handpieces usually operate at _____ to _____ psi.
18. _____ must be periodically drained from air-storage tanks.
19. High-speed handpieces operate at _____ speed than low-speed handpieces, but have _____ torque than low-speed handpieces.
20. Burs should be treated as _____.

Personal Safety and Ergonomics

Steven E. Holmstrom and Laurie A. Holmstrom

OUTLINE

LEARNING OBJECTIVES

When you have completed this chapter, you will be able to:
- List the safety equipment required for use when performing veterinary dental procedures.
- Discuss the rationale for use of eye protection, face masks, and gloves when performing veterinary dental procedures.
- Describe proper handwashing techniques.
- List the information that must be included on the label of a chemical container.
- Describe the symptoms of repetitive motion disorders for which a veterinary dental technician is at risk.
- Define ergonomics and discuss methods to address prevention of workplace injuries in the veterinary dental practice.

KEY TERMS

Anionic detergent
Antiseptic
Composite restoration materials
Dermatitis
Ergonomics

Eye shields
HAZCOM
Material safety data sheet
Neutral position
OSHA

Repetitive motion disorder
Sharps
Substantivity

HAZCOM

The Federal Hazard Communication Standard (HAZCOM, or HCS) is a regulation enforced by the Occupational Safety and Health Administration (OSHA) of the United States Department of Labor. HAZCOM is based on employees' rights and their "need to know" the identities of hazardous substances to which they may be exposed in the work environment. OSHA requires employers to provide workers with preventive safety equipment and ensure that they wear it during dental procedures. To comply with the HAZCOM requirements, employers must also submit a written hazard communication program.

SAFETY REQUIREMENTS FOR VETERINARY DENTISTRY

For the veterinary dentistry practice, OSHA requires that the employer provide safety glasses, masks, and gloves for all employees who perform dental procedures (Fig. 4.1). The employee is responsible for wearing the safety equipment during all procedures. After all, it is the employee's health that is at stake, and flying debris or other substances can easily cause infections if the employee neglects to wear the safety protection provided. Employees must always be careful to take responsibility for their own safety by wearing the necessary safety equipment and should not expect their employers to remind them before each potentially hazardous procedure.

TYPES OF HAZARDS

Veterinary staff risk exposure to several different hazards. Hazards are classified as follows: chemical, physical, biologic, and ergonomic. Chemical hazards are formulations that can act on the skin, eyes, respiratory tract, alimentary system, and other organs and organ systems. Physical hazards are those that can physically harm. Biological hazards in the veterinary dental practice are organic materials that pose a hazard to the health of practitioners and patients. These hazards include pathogenic bacteria, viruses, toxins, spores and fungi. Ergonomic hazards are owing to workplace interactions.

EYE PROTECTION

The importance of eye protection cannot be overstated. Infections from a number of sources can cause

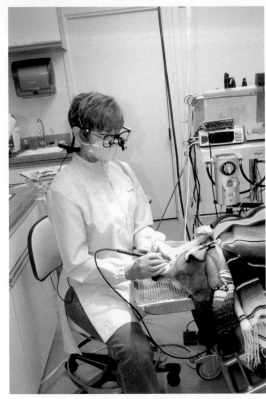

Fig. 4.1 Mask, eye protection, and gloves should be used for every procedure.

permanent visual impairment. Unprotected operators are sometimes struck in the eye by pumice while polishing or by a flying piece of tooth during high-speed drilling. Scaling can also send bacteria-laden calculus into the dental technician's eyes or mouth. The calculus almost always scratches the eye and thereby deposits bacteria directly into the wound. Splatter from rinsing acid etch or sodium hypochlorite is potentially devastating to the eyes and can also cause small lesions on the face.

MOUTH AND LUNG PROTECTION

Use of high-speed equipment, such as ultrasonic scalers and high-speed drills, creates a vapor that contains bacteria, blood, saliva, and tooth dust. This vapor extends up to 3 feet from the source and can irritate and infect the respiratory system of people who are not wearing protective masks. The risk extends to nonemployees, such as clients visiting the dental area while a procedure is in progress.

Masks

Respirator masks offer more protection than surgical masks. All masks must fit tightly to function properly. Some allow for adjustments at the upper (nose) and lower (chin) portions of the mask.

HAND AND SKIN PROTECTION

Gloves protect the patient from cross-contamination and the veterinary staff from the toxic materials used in dentistry. Toxins in resins, such as methyl methacrylate, formaldehyde, chloroform, x-ray chemicals, and cold sterilization chemicals, are all absorbed through the skin. Some are carcinogenic and accumulate in the body with repeated exposure. Most affect the liver and kidneys. Because of the critical importance of these organs, all staff members should wear proper safety protection when handling these materials.

HANDWASHING

Proper handwashing is important for disease control. If employees do not wear gloves and are accidentally stabbed by an instrument or bitten by a patient, they may become infected by the organisms on their own skin. Employees should always wash their hands before putting on gloves in case a glove is torn or otherwise penetrated during the course of a procedure.

Handwashing Agents

A number of handwashing agents are available. Simple anionic detergents (soaps) help by destroying the cell walls of bacteria. Antiseptics, such as alcohol, iodine, iodophors, and hexachlorophene, are also effective. The ability of chlorhexidine, parachlorometaxylenol, and triclosan to stick to surfaces, a property known as *substantivity,* makes these agents superior.

Handwashing Technique

Proper technique in handwashing is important. Rings and other jewelry (e.g., bracelets) should be removed. Hands should be washed for a minimum of 1 minute immediately on arrival to the office and then washed again for 15 seconds between each patient.

Employees should rinse their hands in cold water, making sure to remove all soap. Then, they should dry their hands thoroughly. Many people rinse their hands in hot water, mistakenly believing that if it hurts, it is killing bacteria. In fact, the hot water causes the pores in the hands to open, which draws water from the hands and makes them more susceptible to dermatitis.

GLOVE CONCERNS

Some people develop allergies to latex gloves with time. Three types of hypersensitivity reactions to latex exist. The most common is a contact dermatitis, which is a delayed, type IV allergy. It causes a localized rash and develops 24 to 72 hours after exposure. Next frequent is a contact urticaria, which is an immediate, type I allergic reaction that occurs immediately after exposure. Contact urticaria manifests itself as hives, nasal inflammation, general itching, and wheezing. The worst but rarest type is a systemic reaction, also known as a type I reaction, which results in conjunctivitis, asthma, and systemic anaphylaxis. The fact that latex powder remains in the air for a long time if gloves are snapped on complicates the reaction. Because many conditions mimic these hypersensitivities, employees should consult an allergist if they experience problems.

Proper fit in gloves is also important for preventing hand fatigue that can lead to tendonitis in the wrist. Gloves should be loose through the palm of the hand. If they are too tight, the muscles of the palm will cramp with the effort to maintain a relaxed position.

SHARPS

Needles are another source of potential infection. To keep from accidentally stabbing themselves, employees should never recap needles with both hands. The needle cover should be scooped up with one hand with the needle (Fig. 4.2) or simply discarded in the sharps container. Sharps containers should be disposed of properly when they reach the full line. To prevent punctures when inserting needles, employees should never continue to pack additional needles in the containers after they are full.

EYE SHIELDS

Light-curing guns use an intense white light to cure resins. Because looking at the light can cause permanent retinal damage, employees should use the approved orange shields and refrain from looking at the light, except when necessary.

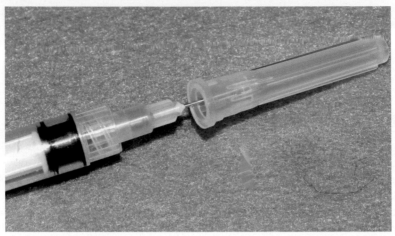

Fig. 4.2 If the cap is placed back on the needle, it should be replaced by scooping the syringe cap.

SAFETY WITH PRODUCTS

Employees should always know the materials in the products used for all procedures. Reading the instructions and following them carefully are crucial steps for safety.

Material Safety Data Sheets

Chemical manufacturers and importers must convey hazard-related information to employers by means of labels on containers and material safety data sheets (MSDSs). In addition, all employers are required to implement a hazard communication program to provide this information to employees. Methods for educating employers include container labeling, MSDSs, and training sessions. Employers must receive sufficient information to design and implement employee protection programs. HAZCOM also provides necessary hazard information to employees so that they can participate in and support the protective measures instituted in their workplaces.

Labels

All hazardous materials in original containers must bear a label from the manufacturer that is legible, in English, and prominently displayed on the container. The following information must be included:

1. Product identity: trade name, product name, or chemical identity.
2. Appropriate hazard warnings: physical and any relevant acute or chronic health hazards.

3. Name and address of the chemical manufacturer, importer, or other responsible party.

Composite Restoration Materials

Most composite restoration materials require an acid etch for maximal adhesion. This solution, which can splatter when rinsed off, is extremely strong and can cause damage if it touches an area other than the enamel. In addition, chemical reactions to the uncured resins are possible. Acid etch should be used with caution. Employees should always wear gloves and glasses and understand the proper way to use this substance.

Toxins

Toxic chemicals, radiographic chemicals, disinfectant surface cleaners, ultrasonic cleaning solutions, and cold-sterilizing chemicals should never be handled without gloves. The toxic substances that cause them to work are absorbed through the skin and can accumulate in the body, causing major health problems in the future. The solutions used in ultrasonic instrument cleaners are not necessarily sterile, and bacteria can enter the hand through small cuts and openings.

REPETITIVE MOTION DISORDERS

Repetitive motion disorders are prevalent in occupations that require repeated small repetitions of a single action. Dental hygienists and computer operators are particularly susceptible to this problem. Veterinary technicians who work exclusively in dentistry are therefore at risk.

Symptoms include stiffness in the neck and shoulders (particularly on the dominant side), soreness in the elbow and/or wrist, hand fatigue, headaches, and tingling or numbness in the fingers of the affected side. Tendonitis may also occur in the elbow and wrist as a result of bad positioning. These symptoms often decrease or disappear completely with increased attention to positioning, stroke and hand placement, ergonomics, and strengthening exercises. Occasionally, the damage to the nerves is so extensive that the technician is no longer able to work in dentistry.

Ergonomics in the Workplace

Prevention of repetitive motion disorders is based on keeping repetitive motions as stress-free as possible. Ergonomics is the science of designing the workplace so that operators remain in the most neutral positions possible. It is a good idea to take photographs or videos of practitioners in the operatory to review and improve ergonomics.

Neutral Position

A neutral position entails sitting with the knees slightly below the hips, the back straight, the elbow at a 90-degree angle, and the thumb relaxed at the top of the hand. The head points straight forward, and the shoulders are relaxed. Feet should be flat on the floor or resting on a full footrest on the chair. The back is as straight as possible, with the head leaning over as little as possible (Fig. 4.3). While working, the employee should be careful to keep the shoulders relaxed (not hunched) and the head level, neither tilted too far forward nor leaning toward either side. (The head weighs 12 pounds and is supported only by the small column of the neck.) Dental personnel should never lean on the table supported by their forearms or bend the wrist from the straight position. A bar rest for the feet provides inadequate support for the lower back; resting the feet on the floor with too great an angle between the hips and knees also puts pressure on the lower back and impairs circulation to the lower leg and feet. The working motion while hand scaling should be a pull stroke that rolls the entire forearm, bending the wrist as little as possible.

Preventive Procedures

Repetitive stress injuries can be prevented in a variety of ways. The types of instruments used can make a significant difference. Use of ultrasonic scalers and hand

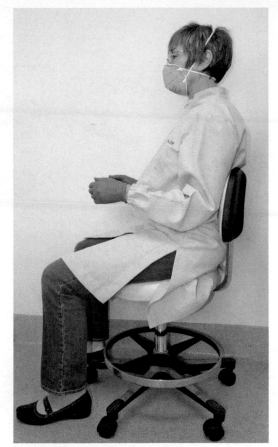

Fig. 4.3 Neutral position.

instruments with the correct types of handles helps. Patient positioning is also relevant. Selecting the correct glove size and regularly performing hand-strengthening exercises are also important preventive measures.

Fitted gloves vs. ambidextrous gloves. The use of ambidextrous gloves can cause fatigue. The thumb may be pulled back to a nonneutral position, which exerts excessive force on the thumb as it moves forward (Fig. 4.4). Left and right gloves keep the thumb in a neutral position (Fig. 4.5).

Mechanical dentistry. Use of mechanical-powered dental instruments in place of manual hand instruments reduces the risk of injury. Therefore, mechanical-powered dental instruments should be used whenever possible. Ultrasonic scalers are an excellent choice for removal of heavy deposits and subgingival root cleaning; these instruments eliminate the need for all but the most cursory scaling.

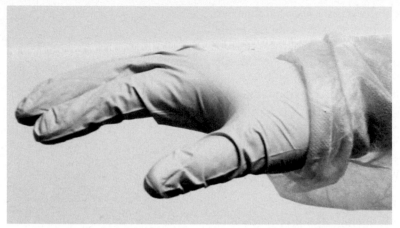

Fig. 4.4 The ambidextrous examination glove pulls the thumb back.

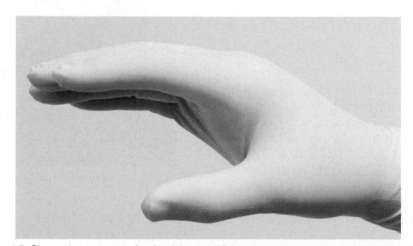

Fig. 4.5 Gloves that are made for the right and left hand are neutral without thumb pull back.

Instrument handles. Because instruments with "fat" handles are easier to hold, they reduce the fatigue caused by pressing the handles with sufficient force to remove deposits (Fig. 4.6).

Patient positioning. Sandbags are used to position the patient for easy access and visibility, which also improves the operator's positioning. Use of a dental operating light, rather than a surgical light, affords greater flexibility in illuminating the deeper parts of the mouth so that the operator does not need to lean excessively to see the back teeth. Technicians should remember that during the course of a procedure they can change their own position or the position of the patient to reduce the risk of injury. Some teeth are more easily reached from over the head, some from the front of the mouth, and some from the patient's mandible side.

Strengthening exercises. Strengthening the muscles opposite the ones used in dental procedures reduces stress on the working muscles by providing more overall support. Employees should remember to stretch during long procedures or whenever they feel fatigued. Alternating hand and mechanical procedures during treatment also helps rest muscle groups. To relax the

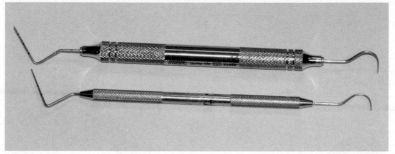

Fig. 4.6 Fat handles are easier to hold on to and less fatiguing than thin handles.

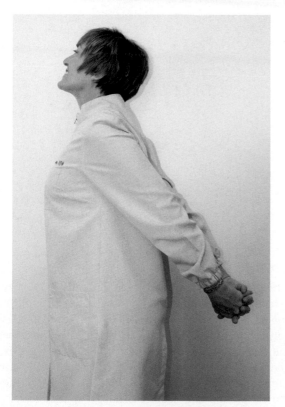

Fig. 4.7 Back shoulder stretch.

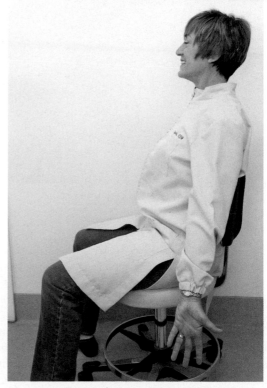

Fig. 4.8 Side shoulder stretch.

shoulders in a standing position, employees can interlace their fingers behind their backs and raise them up as high as possible while leaning forward slightly. This position should be held for 30 seconds (Fig. 4.7).

Another simple way to relax the shoulders while working is to sit up straight, with the hands parallel against the sides. Then, the thumbs should be turned outward as far back as possible while the stomach muscles are tightened. This position should be held for 30 seconds (Fig. 4.8).

To relax the back, the employee should interlace the fingers overhead, with the palms toward the ceiling. With the feet approximately hip width apart and the arms at ear level, the employee should then lean first to the right for 30 seconds and then to the left for another 30 seconds (Fig. 4.9).

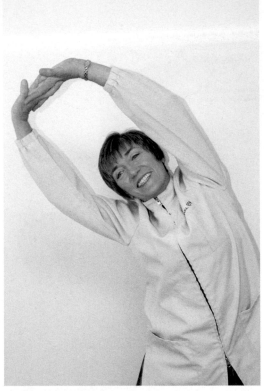

Fig. 4.9 Back stretch.

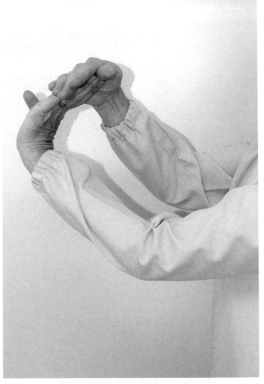

Fig. 4.10 Forearm stretch.

To stretch the forearm muscles, employees should raise one arm almost straight forward and then pull their index, middle, and ring fingers back until they feel resistance, taking care not to lock the elbow. This position should be held for 30 seconds (Fig. 4.10).

To stretch the opposite muscles, employees should bend the hand downward, gently push against the fingers, and hold for 30 seconds (Fig. 4.11). Performing these last two exercises several times a day is recommended, particularly when the technician is especially fatigued (e.g., after scaling the teeth of a patient with an unusual amount of calculus).

Stretching the muscles that go from the outside of your elbow to the wrist is difficult; the best way to accomplish it is to straighten your elbow and rotate your thumb down and out toward the outside while pulling gently on the outside of the palm and pushing on the thumb area toward the rotation at the same time. Spreading your fingers while holding this helps to stretch the entire forearm (Fig. 4.12).

Lifestyle Ergonomics

Attention to muscle groups used in dentistry must also extend into life outside the workplace. Employees should give their bodies a chance to heal and rest between workdays. Regular exercise that does not repeat the same motions frequently performed at work is a good way to maintain health and general well-being. Employees should make an effort to work opposing muscle groups and acquire balanced muscle development as well as working out regularly to relieve the stresses of the day.

Power walking is one of the better ways to maintain overall body toning and relieve stress without overusing injury-prone areas. Using light hand weights (1 pound) while power walking also helps develop upper body strength without stressing the neck or wrist areas. Heavy Hands handles without weights on them allow carrying weight without the need to hold onto them (no "squeeze factor"). Wrist weights also work as long as they are not tight or moving up and down on the wrist. They should

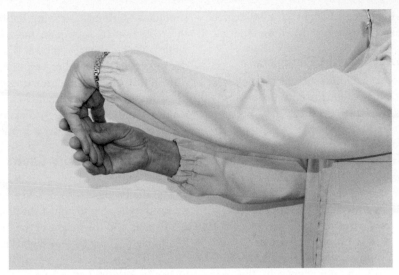

Fig. 4.11 Forearm stretch opposite muscles.

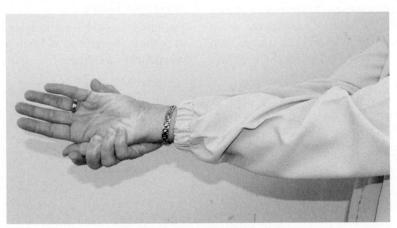

Fig. 4.12 Alternate forearm stretch.

always be carried with the arms bent at a 90-degree angle; straight arms exert pressure on the elbow tendons.

Preventing Injury Away From the Workplace

Performing small-motor activities, such as needlework, prevents the muscles and tendons from relaxing sufficiently after work. Over time, muscles may become sore or irritated. Certain forms of exercise, such as bike riding, put pressure on the wrist, lower back, and neck in much the same way that dental procedures do. Consequently, the body does not have the opportunity to recover from the stresses of the workplace. Carrying heavy items, such as shopping bags, luggage, and large purses, stresses the elbow and wrist tendons excessively and can also cause neck and shoulder pain. Using suitcases with wheels, making frequent trips to deposit shopping bags in the car, and carrying a small purse with only the necessities all help relieve these problems.

Sleeping with the hands curled into the pillow irritates the wrist tendons. People who habitually do this should try tucking their hands flat under the pillow before falling asleep or purchasing braces that hold the wrists in a straight position. These braces should be worn at night until the habit of bending the wrists is broken. Sleeping on the side or back (rather than on the stomach) is also much better for the neck and shoulders. Although sleeping habits are hard to break, the reduction in neck pain makes the attempt worthwhile. Neck-support pillows (the kind that have a depression in the middle) keep the neck in a good position during sleep. Any measures to reduce stress and promote proper alignment in injury-prone areas lengthen the employee's professional life and reduce the pain caused by repetitive motions.

Ergonomic Operatory Chairs and Tables
Dental Chairs

One of the problems faced in veterinary dentistry is that we need to be able to adjust the chair to both the height of the table and the height of the operator choice of cylinder height. If the table is high (and not adjustable) the standard cylinder with a height adjustment of 18¼ inches to 23¼ inches is best. If the table and operator are short, a short cylinder height range is 16¾ inches to 20¼ inches. The ideal dental chair has a lumbar support that adjusts up-down and front-back. The seat tilt should be adjustable (Fig. 4.13). Chairs with arm rests help ease back problems (see Fig 4.13C).

Ergonomic Tables

Ergonomic tables have adjustable heights that allow one to position the table in addition to the chair so that the practitioner can obtain a neutral position (Fig. 4.14).

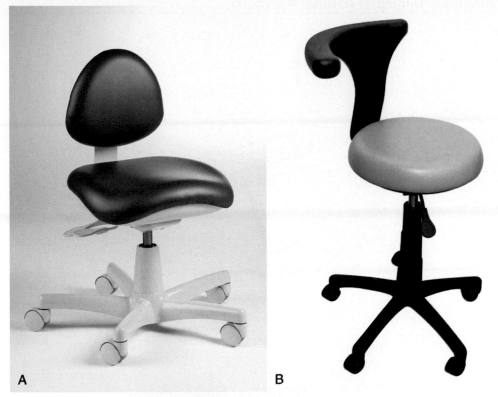

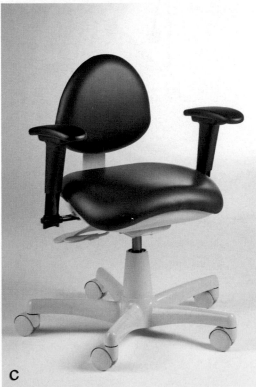

Fig. 4.13 A, Midmark dental chair. B, iM3 dental chair. C, Midmark dental chair with arm rests. (A and C, Courtesy Midmark, Versailles, OH. B, Courtesy iM3, Vancouver, WA.)

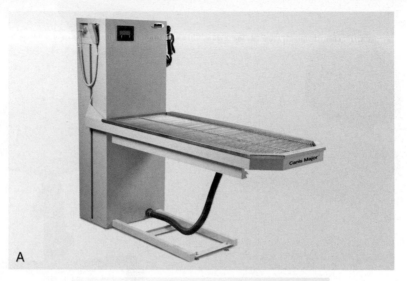

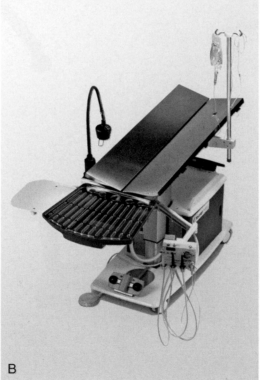

Fig. 4.14 A, Canis Major Wet Dental Treatment Lift Table. B, Surgiden Theramax DX.

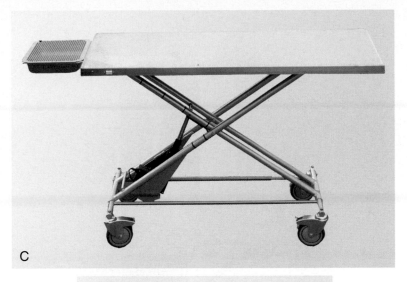

C

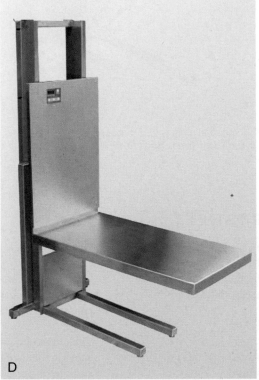

D

Fig. 4.14, cont'd C, Electric Transport Table with dental tray. D, Elsam III Peninsula Table.

Continued

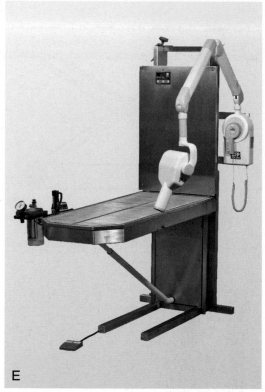

Fig. 4.14, cont'd E, Elsam IV with equipment. (A, Courtesy Midmark, Versailles, OH. B, Courtesy Surgiden, Towson, MD. C and D, Courtesy Technidyne, Toms River, NJ. E, Courtesy Herb Clay.)

CHAPTER 4 WORKSHEET

1. Employers are required by _____ to provide employees with preventive safety equipment and require them to wear it during dental procedures.
2. Employees must always be careful to take responsibility for _____ _____ _____.
3. Hazards are classified as follows: _____, _____, _____, and _____.
4. Scaling can also send _____-laden calculus into the dental technician's eyes or mouth.
5. Proper _____ is important for disease control.
6. Employees should be careful to rinse their hands in _____ water.
7. A type I allergic reaction takes place _____ after exposure.
8. Chemical manufacturers and importers must convey hazard information to employers by means of labels on containers and _____ _____ _____ _____.
9. The ultrasonic solutions are not _____ and contain bacteria that can enter the hands through small cuts and openings.
10. Attention to muscle groups used in dentistry must also extend into _____ outside the workplace.

Local Anesthesia

OUTLINE

LEARNING OBJECTIVES

When you have completed this chapter, you will be able to:

- List possible reactions to local anesthetics used in veterinary dentistry.
- Describe the use of bupivacaine in veterinary dentistry and list time of onset of activity and duration of action for this drug.
- State maximal volumes of local anesthetics that should be administered to dogs and cats.
- Describe the purpose and procedure for performing an infiltration block.
- Describe the purpose and procedure for performing a regional anesthetic block.
- List the four anatomic areas where regional anesthesia is performed before veterinary dental procedures.

KEY TERMS

Bradycardia
Bupivacaine
Caudal mandibular block

Caudal maxillary block
Hypotension
Hypoventilation

Infiltration blocks
Regional anesthesia
Toxicity

This chapter is devoted to local anesthesia, which is used in veterinary dentistry to reduce the depth of general anesthesia that is needed and to control pain after the procedure. This can minimize complications of general anesthesia such as hypoventilation, hypotension, and bradycardia. (For a good understanding of general anesthesia and pain management, the reader is encouraged to read Thomas: *Anesthesia and Analgesia for Veterinary Technicians.*)

State law will vary from state to state as to the legality of the technician performing these procedures. In addition, it is up to the supervising veterinarian to prescribe and determine the appropriateness of the technician performing the procedure.

Nerve cells work by sending small electrical currents through adjacent nerve cells. Simplified, the currents are caused by the exchange of sodium and potassium ions. Local anesthetics work by blocking the channels the sodium ions use to get into the nerve cell. This cuts off any current and therefore any message of pain. This effect wears off as the anesthetic diffuses throughout the body. A number of local anesthetics can do this. In veterinary dentistry, bupivacaine is the drug of choice at a 0.5% solution or 5 mg/mL. Caudal blocks will take care of each arch and as the areas blocked with the rostral blocks are so limited, they are rarely indicated for onset of action and the duration of action is 6 to 10 hours. Bupivacaine may be used with or without epinephrine (adrenaline), which may decrease the chance of toxicity.

Possible, but rare, reactions to local anesthetics include toxicity to skeletal muscle, anaphylactic reactions, and permanent nerve damage. A simple rule of thumb to avoid toxicity is to never exceed 2.0 mg/kg in cats and dogs. Exercise care, especially in smaller patients and cats, so that these maximal doses are not exceeded. The maximal number of sites would be four if the patient requires surgical manipulation in all four quadrants (left and right maxillary and left and right mandibular). Generally, the patient should receive the following at each site: Cats and small dogs = 0.1 mL, medium dogs = 0.2 mL, and large dogs = 0.3 mL. The total volume used depends on the size of the patient and the number of sites that require analgesia. For example, if regional anesthesia is being performed and all four quadrants were blocked in a 10 lb (4.6 kg) cat, the cat would receive 0.4 mL or 2.0 mg, well below the maximal dose of 9.2 mg. Other factors, such as inflammation that causes a reduction of the pH of inflamed tissue, will render local anesthetics less effective.

After administration of the block, the patient should be evaluated for the effectiveness of the block. If respiration rate, heart rate, and blood pressure increase with surgical manipulation, the block either has not had time for onset or was not correctly placed. If the block is not effective and enough time has elapsed, the block may be repeated as long as the maximal total dose is not exceeded. The two types of local anesthesia are infiltration blocks and regional anesthesia.

INFILTRATION BLOCKS

Infiltration blocks, the least effective method of local anesthesia, are used only after the procedure in an attempt to reduce postoperative discomfort. Rather than blocking an entire quadrant, they block only the area where the infiltration has been administered.

Equipment

A 25- or 27-gauge needle and a disposable syringe (Fig. 5.1A) are needed. Alternatively, a dental local anesthesia syringe can be used (Fig. 5.1B).

Technique

A proper dose of the anesthetic is infiltrated around the tissues.

REGIONAL BLOCKS

The advantage of regional anesthesia is the ability to block entire quadrants. The disadvantages of regional nerve blocks include transient loss of sensation and function of the area blocked and the possibility of postoperative self-inflicted injury to soft tissues as a sequel to anesthesia.

Equipment

None of the regional nerve blocks for oral surgery in dogs and cats need any special equipment other than potentially 1¼-inch hypodermic needles. The delivery site is premeasured to determine that the needle length will reach the site.

General Technique

The needle is advanced slowly to the desired location. The syringe plunger is drawn back to perform aspiration. The needle is rotated 90 degrees until a full 360-degree rotation has been accomplished. A small amount of the drug is injected and the aspiration is repeated to ensure that the needle is not in a vessel. If there is no blood drawn back, the agent is slowly injected. If there is blood, digital pressure should be put on the site, and a new syringe and needle should be obtained and the procedure repeated.

The regional nerve blocks are similar for the dog and the cat (Fig. 5.2). The maxilla is blocked either in the rostral or caudal maxilla, but owing to its limitations, the rostral block has few indications. The rostral maxillary

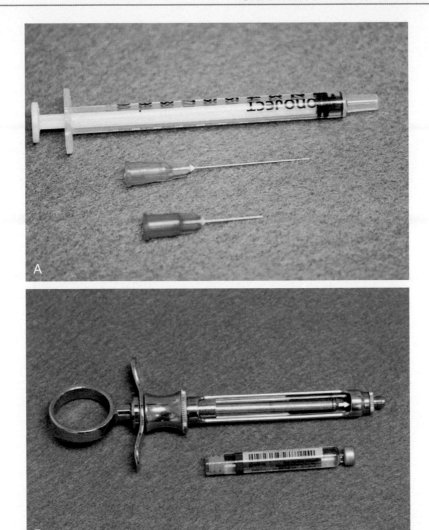

Fig. 5.1 A, A 3-mL syringe with either a tuberculin needle or long needle may be used for local infiltration. B, A dental local anesthesia syringe with carpule.

infiltrates the infraorbital nerve as it exits the infraorbital canal. This block anesthetizes the incisors, canines, and first three premolar teeth as well as the maxillary bone and surrounding soft tissue. The caudal maxillary block anesthetizes both the maxillary nerve (rostrally becomes the infraorbital nerve) and the sphenopalatine nerve/ganglia. It anesthetizes all of the maxillary teeth on the side of infiltration as well as the adjacent bone and soft tissue.

The mandibular blocks are also the rostral and caudal blocks. The rostral mandibular block anesthetizes the inferior alveolar nerve within the mandibular canal via the middle mental foramen. Again, there is limited effectiveness to this block and the caudal block is recommended. The structures anesthetized include the incisors, the canines, and the first two premolars. The caudal mandibular block infiltrates the inferior alveolar nerve on the lingual aspect of the mandible as it enters the mandibular canal. The caudal mandibular block blocks all of the teeth of the mandible on the side of infiltration as well as the adjacent bone and soft tissue.

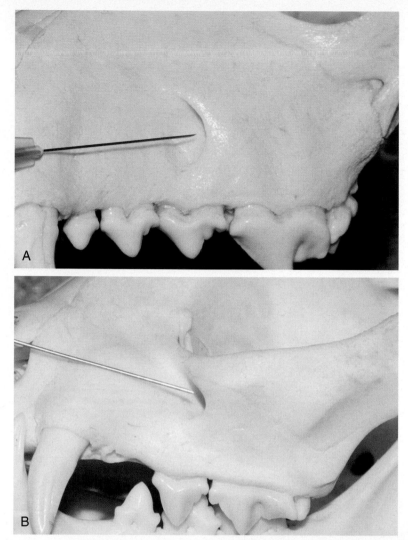

Fig. 5.2 A, Needle placed on the infraorbital foramen in a dog. B, Needle placed on the infraorbital foramen in a cat.

Technique
Rostral Maxillary
To perform the rostral maxillary block, retract the lip dorsally and palpate just dorsal to the distal root of the maxillary third premolar (Fig. 5.3).

The infraorbital neurovascular bundle beneath the vestibular mucosa is palpated as a large cylindric band that exits the infraorbital canal. This bundle is retracted dorsally with a digit of the hand that is not holding the syringe. The needle is advanced close to the maxillary bone ventral to the retracted bundle in a rostral to caudal direction to just inside the canal (Fig. 5.4). The needle should pass without hitting bone around the infraorbital canal. If bone is encountered, the needle is withdrawn slightly and redirected. Proper insertion can be confirmed by gentle movement of the syringe as the needle hits the infraorbital canal wall.

Caudal Maxillary
To perform the caudal maxillary block, retract the lip dorsally and palpate just dorsal to the distal root of the maxillary third premolar. The infraorbital neurovascular

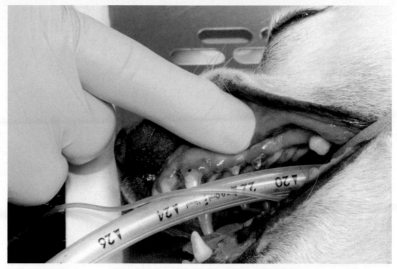

Fig. 5.3 The infraorbital foramen is palpated dorsal to the distal root of the maxillary third premolar.

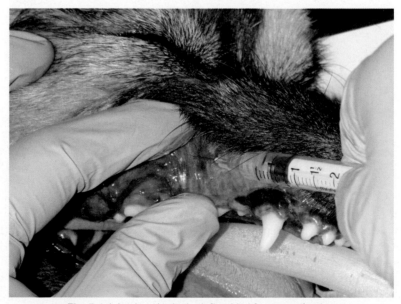

Fig. 5.4 Injection site in the infraorbital foramen of a dog.

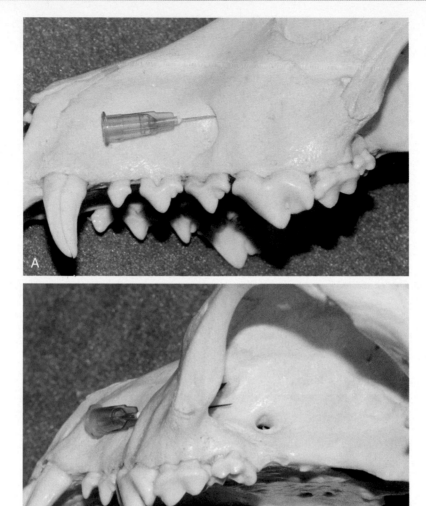

Fig. 5.5 A, Needle advanced for a deep caudal maxillary block in a dog skull. B, Caudal view in a dog.

bundle beneath the vestibular mucosa is palpated as a large cylindric band that exits the infraorbital canal. This bundle is retracted dorsally with a digit of the hand that is not holding the syringe. The needle is advanced close to the maxillary bone ventral to the retracted bundle in a rostral to caudal direction to just inside the canal. The needle should pass without hitting bone around the infraorbital canal. If bone is encountered, the needle is withdrawn slightly and redirected. Proper insertion can be confirmed by gentle movement of the syringe as the needle hits the infraorbital canal wall. The needle is advanced more caudally via the infraorbital canal (Fig. 5.5). The proper size needle must be used; in cats and brachiocephalic dogs the infraorbital canal is very short and therefore it is important to keep the syringe and needle parallel to the dental arch line of the maxilla (Fig. 5.6).

Rostral Mandibular

The rostral mandibular block infiltrates the rostral extent of the inferior alveolar nerve just before it exits the middle mental foramen (Fig. 5.7). The landmark

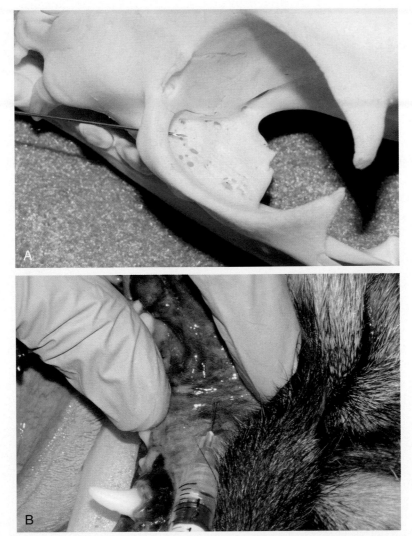

Fig. 5.6 A, Caution should be used because there is very little space between the entrance of the infraorbital foramen and the orbit in the cat. B, Caudal maxillary nerve dog injection.

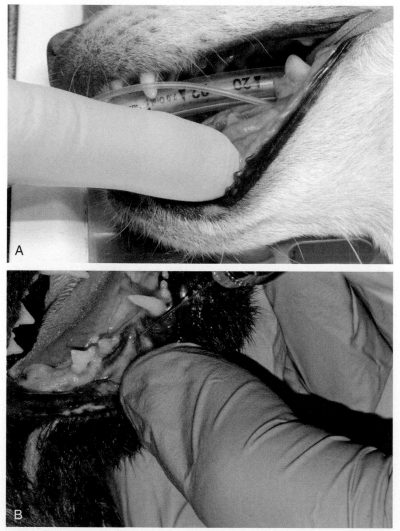

Fig. 5.7 A, Palpation for the rostral mandibular injection just distal to the frenulum in the dog. B, Palpation for the rostral mandibular injection just distal to the frenulum in the cat.

for infiltration is the mandibular labial frenulum. The frenulum is retracted ventrally.

The needle is inserted at the rostral aspect of the frenulum and advanced along the mandibular bone (at about a 30-degree angle to the body of the mandible) to just enter the canal, which is located ventral to the mesial root of the second premolar at one-third of the distance between the ventral and dorsal mandibular borders (Figs. 5.8 and 5.9). If bone is encountered, the needle should be backed out and redirected until the needle passes freely into the foramen. The syringe is then moved laterally to encounter the lateral aspect of the canal to confirm proper placement. The patient's jaw, rather than the alveolar mucosa, will move slightly if the needle is within the canal. Unlike the infraorbital block, the needle is unlikely to thread the canal.

Caudal Mandibular

The caudal mandibular block is performed by palpating extraorally the notch just dorsal to the angle of the mandible and ventral to the condylar process (Fig. 5.10).

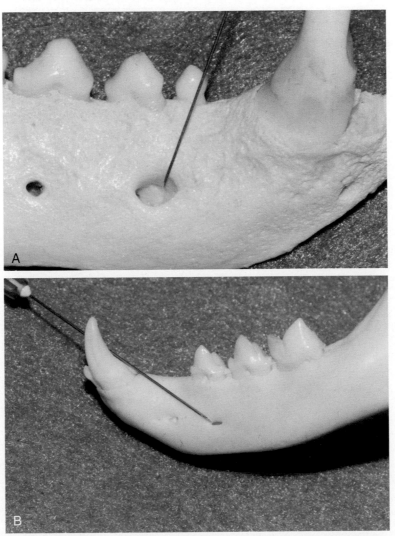

Fig. 5.8 A, Injection site for rostral mandible in the dog skull. B, Injection site for rostral mandible in the cat skull.

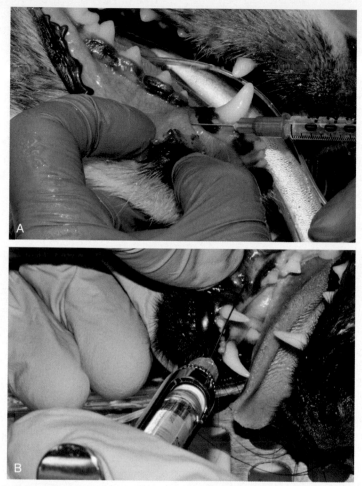

Fig. 5.9 A, Injection of rostral mandible of a dog. B, Injection of rostral mandible in a cat.

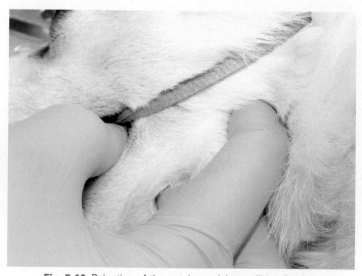

Fig. 5.10 Palpation of the notch caudal mandible of a dog.

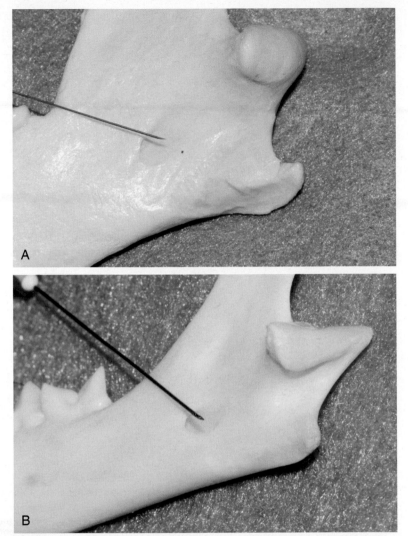

Fig. 5.11 A, Intraoral mandibular needle placement in the dog skull for caudal mandibular block. B, Intraoral mandibular needle placement in the cat skull for caudal mandibular block.

The needle is advanced intraorally along the mandible from just caudal to the third molar in the dog (Fig. 5.11A) or first molar in the cat (Fig. 5.11B). Because the inferior mandibular nerve is located outside of the mandibular canal in this region, it is important that the needle tip is located caudal to the foramen and rostral to the angular process of the mandible (Fig. 5.12). Because the mandibular first molar is missing in the cat in Fig. 5.12B, the mandibular notch is palpated, the position of the first molar is approximated, and the needle is directed to the injection site, midway between where the tooth was and the notch.

An alternative method is to use the lateral canthus of the eye as the landmark. An imaginary line is drawn from the lateral canthus of the eye directly to the ventral mandible. The index finger is used to palpate the foramen notch on the inside of the ramus. Depending on the size of the patient, a 25-g ⅝- or 1½-inch needle is advanced up from the ventral mandible, aiming the point of the needle toward the index finger, which is in position over the foramen. The needle is advanced along the lingual surface of the ramus. When the needle is felt by the index finger, without actually puncturing the skin, the plunger is pulled back to make

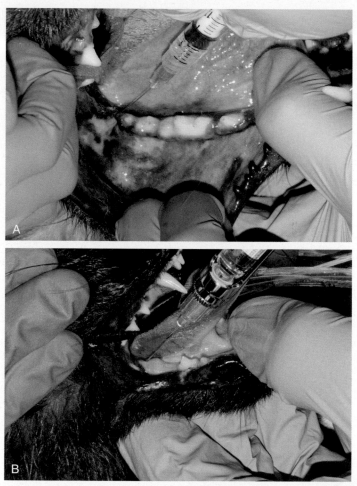

Fig. 5.12 A, Intraoral mandibular needle placement in a dog. B, Intraoral mandibular needle placement in a cat.

sure a blood vessel is not hit and that the local anesthetic is injected. The bleb of local anesthetic should be felt developing under the index finger as the local anesthetic is injected to confirm proper needle placement. This should be about one to one-third of the distance from the ventral to the dorsal mandible. This is in the vicinity of the mandibular foramen where the inferior alveolar nerve enters the mandibular canal. Be careful that the needle does not venture out into the tissues of the tongue. Anesthetizing the tongue could have disastrous results when the patent awakens and cannot sense its tongue (Fig. 5.13). Treatment ranges from distraction of the patient to sedation and general anesthesia until the regional anesthesia wears off or the dysphoria stops. The best treatment is prevention, keeping the bevel of the needle pointed toward the

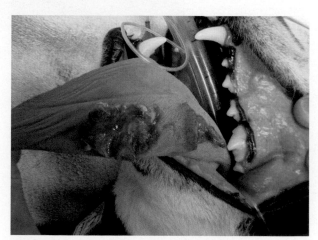

Fig. 5.13 Injured tongue by local anesthesia. This patient awoke and could not feel its tongue and, as a result, chewed its tongue.

mandible and staying right on the mandible as the needle is advanced.

Increasing the Duration of Local Anesthesia

Opioids inhibit the pain signal at multiple steps along the pain pathway. There are opioid receptors in the peripheral nervous system. Because of these receptors, buprenorphine has been shown to effectively double the analgesic duration when combined with bupivacaine. To mix, 0.05 mL of 300 µg/mL buprenorphine is added to 1 mL bupivacaine with the following doses administered as previously described in this chapter.

CHAPTER 5 WORKSHEET

1. It is up to the _____ _____ to prescribe and determine the appropriateness of the technician performing the procedure.
2. Bupivacaine is the drug of choice at a _____% solution or _____ mg/mL.
3. Epinephrine is added to bupivacaine to _____ _____ _____ _____ _____.
4. Possible, but rare, reactions to local anesthetics include _____ _____ _____ _____, _____ _____, _____ _____ _____ _____.
5. The dose for each site should be: cats and small dogs = _____ mL; medium dogs = _____ mL; and large dogs = _____ mL.
6. The total dose should never exceed _____ mg/kg in dogs and cats.
7. If respiration rate, heart rate, and blood pressure _____ with surgical manipulation, the block either has not had time for onset or was not correctly placed.
8. Regional anesthesia blocks the _____ quadrant.
9. The four main areas where regional anesthesia is performed are the _____ _____, _____ _____, _____ _____, and _____ _____.
10. The site for the rostral maxillary block is just dorsal to the _____ root of the maxillary _____ premolar into the _____ foramen.
11. To perform the caudal maxillary block, the needle is advanced more _____ via the _____ canal.
12. The landmark for infiltration is the mandibular labial _____.
13. The caudal mandibular block is performed by palpating extraorally the _____ just dorsal to the angle of the mandible and ventral to the _____ _____.
14. To perform caudal mandibular block, the needle is advanced intraorally along the mandible from just caudal to the _____ molar in the dog or _____ molar in the cat.
15. Always _____ prior to injecting.

Pathogenesis of Periodontal Disease

OUTLINE

LEARNING OBJECTIVES

When you have completed this chapter, you will be able to:

- List the factors that contribute to the development of periodontal disease in dogs and cats.
- Define periodontal disease and describe the appearance of the gingival and other supporting tissues when periodontal disease is present.
- Discuss the etiology of periodontal disease and define the terms plaque and calculus.
- Characterize the bacterial colonization present with periodontal disease and explain how the patient's immune response contributes to damage to periodontal tissues.
- Differentiate between class 1, class 2, and class 3 furcation exposure.
- Describe the staging of periodontal disease using the American Veterinary Dental College (AVDC) classification system.

KEY TERMS

Anaerobic bacteria
Biofilm
Calculus
Endotoxins
Epithelial attachment

Furcation
Gram-positive aerobic bacteria
Halitosis
Pathogenesis
Periodontal disease

Plaque
Pocket
Sulcus
Tartar

Clients often ask, "Why does my pet have periodontal disease when all the pets I have had in the past had no dental problems?" Many factors determine the reason one patient develops periodontal disease and another does not (Box 6.1). These factors are as follows: age, species, breed, genetics, chewing behavior, diet, grooming habits (which can cause impaction of hair around the tooth and in the gingival sulcus), orthodontic occlusion, health status, home care, frequency of professional dental care, and bacterial flora of the oral cavity.

PERIODONTAL DISEASE

Periodontal disease is an inflammation and infection of the tissues surrounding the tooth, collectively called the *periodontium* (Fig. 6.1). Periodontal disease is characterized by movement of the gingival margin toward the apex (exposing more crown and root) and migration of the attached gingiva with associated loss of the periodontal ligament and bone surrounding the tooth. An older term, *pyorrhea,* which indicates discharge of pus from the periodontium, is no longer used.

Systemic Effects of Periodontal Disease

The systemic effects of periodontal disease are fairly well documented in humans. Research in veterinary medicine is still ongoing. Theoretically, bacteria from infected tissues enter the bloodstream. Organs such as the lungs, kidneys, and liver are most susceptible to infection.

Etiology

A glycoprotein component of saliva, known as the *acquired pellicle,* attaches to the tooth surface. The pellicle, which takes only 20 minutes to form, helps bacteria attach to the tooth surface. Approximately 6 to 8 hours after pellicle formation, bacteria start to colonize the tooth surface. This bacterial layer is known as *plaque.* The bacteria that have colonized the tooth surface die. The bacteria that are attached to the tooth absorb calcium from saliva and become calcified. This new substance is known as *tartar* or *calculus.*

Types of Bacteria

The healthy gingival flora is made up of mostly Gram-positive aerobic bacteria. These bacteria require oxygen to survive. As periodontal disease progresses, Gram-negative bacteria begin to colonize the tooth surface. The aerobic bacteria metabolize oxygen, creating an environment in which the anaerobic (those that live without oxygen) bacteria start to develop. As the condition progresses, spirochetes begin to colonize. The bacteria are arranged in what is called a *biofilm,* which is an aggregate of bacterial colonies protected by a polysaccharide complex. It is the disruption of this biofilm, more than anything else, that is important in the control of periodontal disease.

Location of Plaque

Plaque is found in a number of areas around the tooth. Plaque can be supragingival, and it can be subgingival in four different areas. It can be free-floating in the pocket or sulcus, and it can be attached to the tooth or gingiva. Perhaps the worst plaque is the type that infiltrates the gingiva itself (Fig. 6.2).

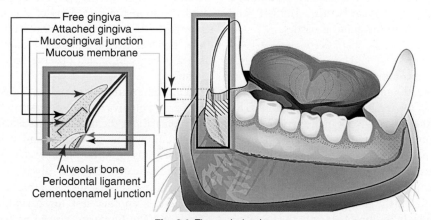

Free gingiva
Attached gingiva
Mucogingival junction
Mucous membrane

Alveolar bone
Periodontal ligament
Cementoenamel junction

Fig. 6.1 The periodontium.

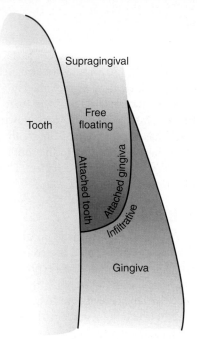

Fig. 6.2 Types of plaque: supragingival, free-floating subgingival, attached to tooth or gingiva, and invasive into gingiva.

Patient Response

As the bacteria infiltrate and colonize the sulcus and invade the gingival tissues, the patient attempts to fight the infection. (In veterinary dentistry, sulcus, which means groove, usually refers to the gingival sulcus present in healthy patients with healthy gingiva between the free gingiva and the surface of the tooth and extending around the tooth's circumference.) White blood cells produce antibodies and send chemical signals into the system to stimulate other cells to come in and attack the bacteria. The bacteria often contain endotoxins (sometimes called *lipopolysaccharides* [LPSs]) and enzymes that are toxic to the gingival tissues.

Pathogenesis

As the inflammation continues, the gingiva loosens from the tooth. As a result, the gingiva separates from the tooth and a space between the tooth and gingiva develops. This space is known as the *pocket*. Deeper in the periodontium, loss of tissue and bone support indicates the beginning of the disease. If the patient is not treated and the disease is allowed to progress, deeper pockets form.

Without the gingival epithelial attachment, which is the epithelium attaching the gingiva to the tooth, the gingiva begins to recede. In multirooted teeth, the furcation

(the area at which the roots join the crown) begins to be exposed. Furcation exposure is classified by depth (Box 6.2). Class 1 furcation exposure is less than 1 mm; class 2 exposure is greater than 1 mm but not fully through; and class 3 is complete furcation exposure. As bone loss proceeds, the tooth may become mobile. Finally, if the loss of attachment is sufficient, the tooth may fall out.

Systemic Inflammatory Response

Periodontal disease is a local inflammatory disease that can also have systemic effects. The relationship between periodontal disease and systemic health is well recognized through studying the relationship of periodontal disease and other systemic diseases such as bacterial endocarditis and liver, kidney and respiratory disease through the response to a protein known as C-reactive protein.

Initial Signs

Most commonly, clients report halitosis (bad breath) as the patient's periodontal disease progresses. This is often mistakenly called "doggy breath." This condition, however, is not normal. It is caused by periodontal disease and is one of the first signs of this condition. Clients may report that their pets are not eating well. Occasionally, patients drool, and blood may be noted in the saliva. Clients may also observe the patient pawing at its mouth.

On oral examination, red, inflamed gingiva may be noted. The gingiva may bleed easily when probed. Fragile capillaries in the inflamed tissue cause this bleeding. An accumulation of plaque and calculus is evident. However, it is important to note that the amount of plaque and calculus does not always correspond to the degree of periodontal disease present.

There is another test for periodontal disease—the OraStrip. The OraStrip is used to test for thiols. The presence of thiols indicates the presence of periodontal disease, but does not stage it.

The OraStrip is first removed from its protective pouch, taking care not to touch the small pad on the top of the strip. Next, the patient's upper lip is lifted while supporting the pad end of the test strip with the index finger on the nonpad side. The pad is gently glided against the upper gum line. Salivary fluid is drawn into the pad and should take no longer than 5 to 10 seconds. Care should be taken not to cause bleeding because this may interfere with the results (Fig. 6.3). Once the sample has been collected, remove the strip from the patient's mouth and wait 10 seconds before reading the result. The strip is held near the colors shown on the comparator card color chart, and the number of the color closest to the color on the pad is noted. The color should be based on the most intense color seen on the pad. A numerical result of 1 or above is associated with active periodontal disease. A score of 0 is not associated with active periodontal infection. For dogs with a history of periodontal disease, a score of 0 reflects favorable ongoing management of existing disease (Fig. 6.4).

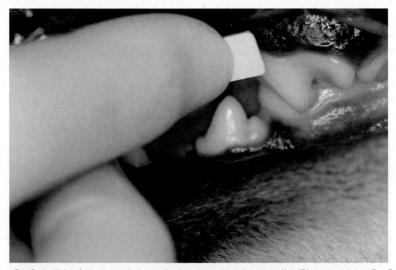

Fig. 6.3 Using OraStrip (Manfra): the strip is applied to the patient's upper lip. (Photo courtesy Dr. Sandra Manfra Marretta.)

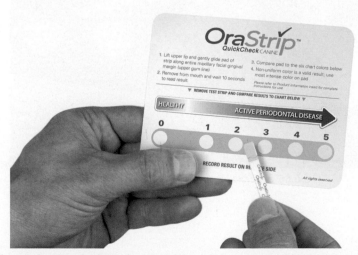

Fig. 6.4 Reading OraStrip: the color of the strip is compared with the color on the chart.

PERIODONTAL DISEASE CLASSIFICATION

The American Veterinary Dental College (AVDC) has created a classification system for periodontal disease. It differs from the system presented in the previous edition of this text. This system is a radiographic system and not a clinical grading system. To use this system, you must have radiographs to evaluate the state of periodontal health with the AVDC's system. Staging is performed only after the radiographs have been taken. The degree of severity of periodontal disease relates to a single tooth; a patient may have teeth that have different stages of periodontal disease (PD), as follows:

Normal (PD 0): Clinically normal: No gingival inflammation or periodontitis clinically evident (Figs. 6.5 and 6.6).

Stage 1 (PD 1): Gingivitis only without attachment loss. The height and architecture of the alveolar margin are normal (Figs. 6.7 and 6.8).

Stage 2 (PD 2): Early periodontitis: Less than 25% of attachment loss or, at most, there is a stage 1 furcation involvement in multirooted teeth. There are early radiologic signs of periodontitis. The loss of periodontal attachment is less than 25%, as measured either by probing of the clinical attachment level or by radiographic determination of the distance of the alveolar margin from the cementoenamel junction relative to the length of the root (Fig. 6.9).

Stage 3 (PD 3): Moderate periodontitis: 25% to 50% of attachment loss, as measured either by probing of the clinical attachment level or by radiographic determination of the distance of the alveolar margin from the cementoenamel junction relative to the length of the root, or there is a stage 2 furcation involvement in multirooted teeth (Fig. 6.10).

Stage 4 (PD 4): Advanced periodontitis: More than 50% of attachment loss as measured either by probing of the clinical attachment level or by radiographic determination of the distance of the alveolar margin from the cementoenamel junction relative to the length of the root, or there is a stage 3 furcation involvement in multirooted teeth (Fig. 6.11).

Patients may have teeth with mixed stages of periodontal disease (Fig. 6.12). In Fig. 6.12A, the premolars are stage 4 and the canine is stage 2. Taking the worst tooth's grade, this would be considered stage 4 (PD 4).

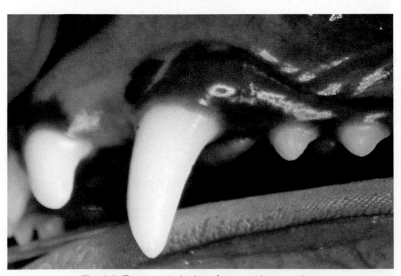

Fig. 6.5 Teeth and gingiva of a normal young dog.

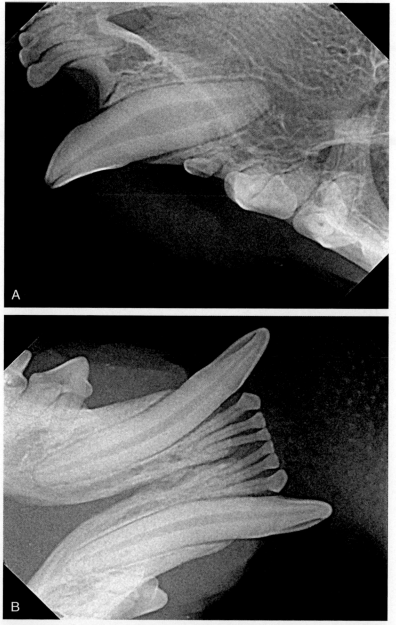

Fig. 6.6 A, Radiograph of a normal young cat: left maxillary incisors and canine teeth; premolars are foreshortened so they cannot be evaluated on this view. B, Normal young cat: incisors and canine teeth.

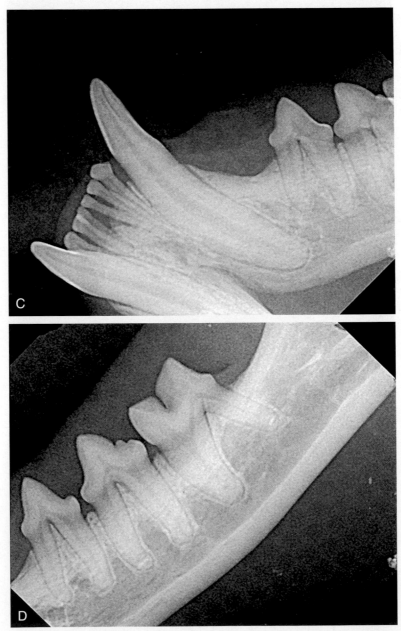

Fig. 6.6, cont'd C, Normal young cat: left mandibular incisors and canine third, fourth premolar. D, Normal young cat: left mandibular third, fourth premolar, first molar.

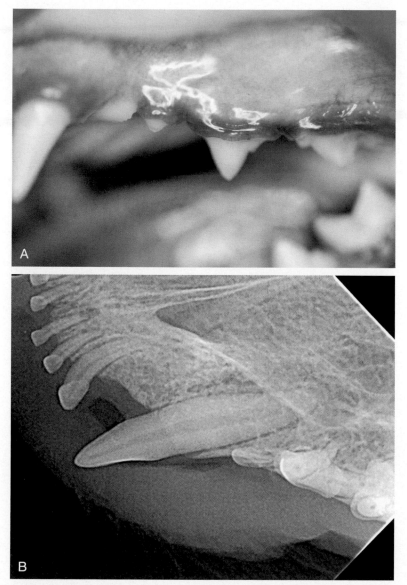

Fig. 6.7 A, Periodontal disease stage 1 (PD 1) in a cat. B, PD 1 radiograph of a cat.

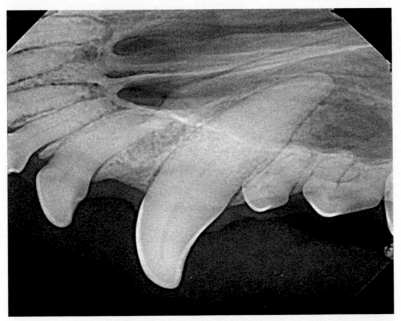

Fig. 6.8 PD 1 radiograph of a dog.

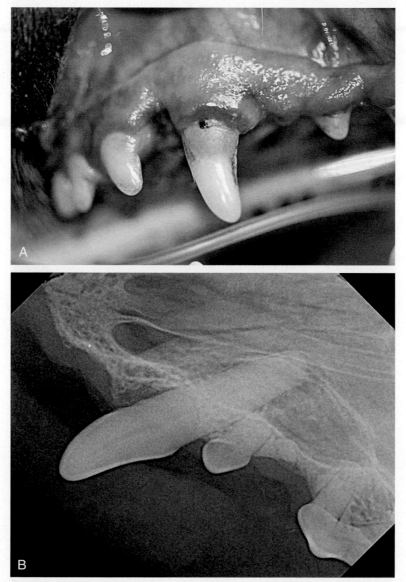

Fig. 6.9 A, Periodontal disease stage 2 (PD 2) in a dog. B, PD 2 radiograph of a dog with a missing left maxillary second premolar.

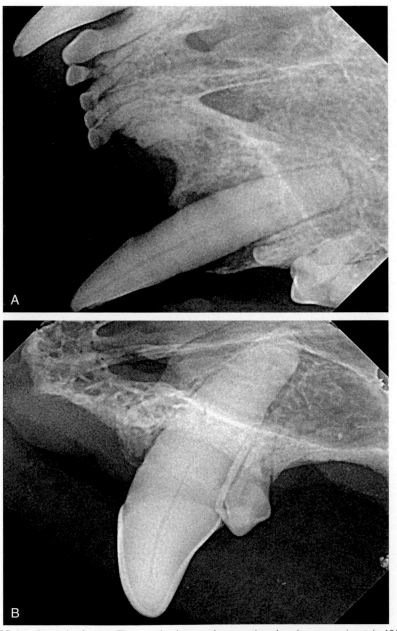

Fig. 6.10 A, PD 2 radiograph of a cat. (The cat also has tooth resorption showing approximately 40% bone loss around the canine tooth.) B, Radiograph of periodontal disease stage 3 (PD 3): left maxillary canine tooth and first premolar.

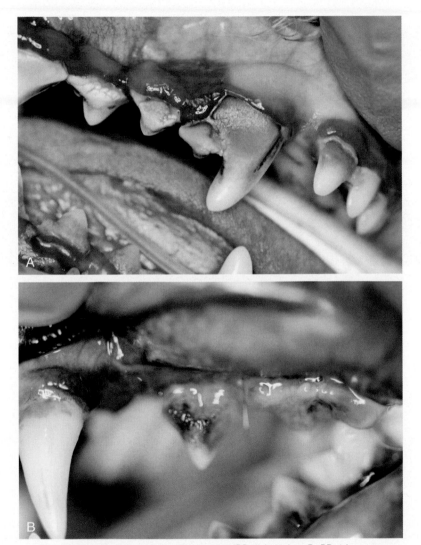

Fig. 6.11 A, Periodontal disease stage 4 (PD 4) in a dog. B, PD 4 in a cat.

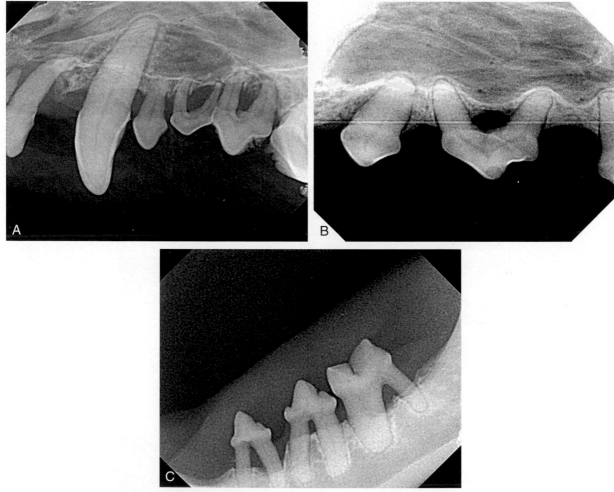

Fig. 6.12 A, Periodontal disease stage 4 (PD 4) radiograph. B, PD 4 radiograph of a dog: left maxillary first premolar and second premolar with stage 4 and class 3 furcation exposure. C, PD 4 radiograph of a cat: left mandibular third premolar (stage 4), fourth premolar (stage 3), and first molar (stage 4).

FURCATION INDEX

Stage 1 (F1): Furcation 1 involvement exists when a periodontal probe extends less than halfway under the crown in any direction of a multirooted tooth with attachment loss.

Stage 2 (F2): Furcation 2 involvement exists when a periodontal probe extends greater than halfway under the crown of a multirooted tooth with attachment loss but not through and through.

Stage 3 (F3): Furcation exposure exists when a periodontal probe extends under the crown of a multirooted tooth, through and through from one side of the furcation out the other.

Tooth Mobility Index (from https://www.avdc.org/Nomenclature/Nomen-Perio.html#periostages)

Stage 0 (M0): Physiologic mobility up to 0.2 mm.

Stage 1 (M1): The mobility is increased in any direction other than axial over a distance of more than 0.2 mm and up to 0.5 mm.

Stage 2 (M2): The mobility is increased in any direction other than axial over a distance of more than 0.5 mm and up to 1.0 mm.

Stage 3 (M3): The mobility is increased in any direction other than axial over a distance exceeding 1.0 mm or any axial movement.

The problem with the AVDC system is that many practices do not have intraoral radiology. Intraoral radiology is the keystone of the AVDC system. Although practicing without intraoral radiology is not ideal, it is the reality for many areas. In this case, there is another system for staging which is based on clinical staging. There are difference in the two systems. The first two types are gingivitis and the second two types are periodontitis. It suggests how periodontal disease looks when discussing it with the client.

HEALTHY GINGIVA

Healthy gingiva has a knife-like margin and is coral pink or a pigmented color. It is important to note the smooth gingival topography. Topography is the surface features of the gingiva as it flows from tooth to tooth. Generally, as periodontal disease progresses, the surface features become irregular and the even flow from tooth to tooth is lost. Healthy gingival tissue is firm. Close observation will reveal that blood vessels can be seen out to the margins. When probing with a periodontal probe, there is a normal minimal sulcular depth of 2 to 3 mm in dogs and 0.5 to 1 mm in cats. There may or may not be evidence of previous disease.

Type 1 Early Gingivitis

A redness of the gingiva at the crest of the gingiva and a mild amount of plaque are noted. There is loss of visualization of the fine blood vessels at the gingival margins. Radiographically, there is no change from healthy periodontium. The condition is reversible with treatment. Type 1 can appear 2 to 4 days after plaque accumulation in previously healthy gingiva and is localized to the gingival sulcus, including the junctional epithelium and the most coronal part of the connective tissue.

Type 2 Advanced Gingivitis

Type 2 is similar to the early type in that it is still reversible. There is an increase in inflammation, including edema and subgingival plaque development. Amounts of supragingival plaque and calculus are increased. The gingival topography has started to become irregular, but is still good. Root exposure has not yet occurred. Radiographically, there is little noticeable change. Plaque-induced gingivitis can be reversed with the initiation of plaque control measures (e.g., dental scaling and prophy, home care).

Type 3 Early Periodontitis

In type 3, there is a moderate loss of attachment or moderate pocket formation with 10% to 30% loss of bone support. Furcation exposure may be present as well as inadequate gingival topography, recession, and/or hypertrophy and there may or may not be mobility. The gingiva will bleed with gentle probing. Radiographically, subgingival calculus may be visualized and a rounding of the alveolar crestal bone at the cervical portion of the tooth can be seen upon careful examination.

Type 4 Established Periodontitis

In type 4, the teeth have advanced breakdown of the support tissues, with severe pocket depth or severe recession of the gingiva. Some of the signs that may be associated with type 4, or advanced periodontal disease, are the presence of severe inflammation, deep pocket formation, gingival recession, bone loss, pus, and mobility. The gingiva usually bleeds easily upon probing and there is loss of gingival topography; radiographically, subgingival calculus and bone loss are noted.

CHAPTER 6 WORKSHEET

1. Periodontal disease is an _____ and _____ of the tissues surrounding the tooth. It is characterized by movement of the gingiva toward the apex and migration of the junctional epithelium, with associated loss of the periodontal ligament and bone surrounding the tooth.

2. A glycoprotein component of saliva, known as the _____ _____, attaches to the tooth surface.

3. As periodontal disease progresses, _____ _____ bacteria begin to colonize.

4. Plaque may be found in which four areas?_____, _____, _____, and _____.

5. _____ _____ is not normal.

6. The amount of _____ and _____ may not always correspond to the degree of periodontal disease that is present.

7. A healthy periodontium has no _____ _____ and is coral pink or a pigmented color.

8. Stage 1 periodontal disease is gingivitis only without _____ _____.

9. Stage 2 is known as _____ _____.

10. The stage with advanced breakdown, severe pocket depth, bleeding easily on probing, pus, bone loss, and mobility is stage _____.

The Complete Prophy

LEARNING OBJECTIVES

When you have completed this chapter, you will be able to:

- List the instruments and equipment needed to perform a complete dental prophy.
- List the steps in performing a complete dental prophy.
- Explain the rationale for performing endotracheal intubation prior to anesthetizing a patient for a dental prophy.
- Describe circumstances under which the veterinarian may prescribe antibiotics for dental patients.
- Describe the proper use of a mouth gag during the dental prophy.

- Explain the purpose of the water flow through the ultrasonic dental scaler.
- Describe the general technique used for scaling teeth with an ultrasonic scaler.
- Describe the instrument used and general technique for evaluating depth of the sulcus.
- Describe the modified pen grasp for holding dental instruments.
- Describe the general technique used for polishing teeth.

KEY TERMS

Cementoenamel junction
Closed position
Disclosing solution
Furcation
Iatrogenic slab fracture
iM3 42-12 unit
Junctional epithelium
Lateral recumbency
Modified pen grasp

Open position
Periodontal probe
Prophy
Prophy angles
Prophy cup
Prophy paste
Prophylaxis
Pseudopocket
Pull stroke

Sealer
Sonic scaler
Subgingival scaling
Sulcus
Supragingival gross calculus
Supragingival scaling
Ultrasonic scaler

Veterinarians and technicians often speak of performing a "prophy" or "dental." This usage is incorrect and may often mislead the client with regard to the patient's true condition. Because the word *prophylaxis,* which means prevention of or protective treatment for disease, is sometimes confused with "prophylactic" or "condom," the dental profession shortened the word to prophy. The difference between performing a prophy and periodontal therapy is extremely important. The term *prophy* is often used incorrectly to indicate the treatment of periodontal disease rather than its prevention. This important distinction must be kept in mind when discussing treatment plans with the client. One analogy is to compare a prophy with a vaccination for a disease rather than the treatment for that disease. Once the patient has periodontal disease, far more extensive treatment is required. In this case the clinician should discuss with the client the necessary steps and options (which may include extractions) to treat the condition. Rather than "prophy" or "dental," a more appropriate term may be COAPT: Complete Oral Health Assessment and Prevention or Treatment. A complete prophy requires several important instruments and pieces of equipment (Box 7.1).

The reader should review and implement the American Animal Hospital Association (AAHA) Dental Care Guidelines for Dogs and Cats, using this text as a reference (see Appendix: AAHA Guidelines).

PREPARATION FOR THE PROCEDURE

Before performing the prophy, the veterinarian should discuss the procedure with the client and provide a written estimate of its cost. After obtaining the client's

---

BOX 7.1   Instruments and Equipment Needed for the Complete Prophy

Sickle scaler: H6/7, S6/7, N6/7, SH6/7, or Cislak P-12
Curette: Barnhardt 5/6, Columbia 13/14, or Cislak P-10
Calculus-removing forceps
Periodontal probe/explorer: double-ended, Williams type with 1-mm markers (sizes go up to 15 mm [Hu-Friedy] or 18 mm [Cislak])
#2 Pigtail explorer
Ultrasonic or sonic scaler
Low-speed handpiece
Prophy angle
Prophy cup
Prophy paste
Sharpening stones
Disclosing solution
Chlorhexidine rinse

---

consent, the veterinarian should develop a contingency plan in case additional problems are discovered under anesthesia and the client must be contacted. The client should provide instructions so that the veterinary staff knows how to proceed in case the client is unavailable during the procedure. Options include the following:
1. Proceed with recommended procedures.
2. Attempt to call first; if the client cannot be reached, proceed with recommended procedures.
3. Do nothing if the client cannot be contacted.

Consideration should also be given to preoperative blood profiles, intravenous fluids, preoperative antibiotics (if indicated), and anesthetic protocol (including preoperative agents, induction, anesthesia, and patient monitoring). Inhalation anesthesia with an endotracheal tube is necessary to prevent the aspiration of fluids, dental calculus, and other debris.

ANESTHESIA INDUCTION

After anesthesia is induced, the patient is intubated with a cuffed endotracheal tube and stabilized. An overview of the oral cavity should take place to establish that the initial diagnosis (stage 1 periodontal disease [PD 1]) was correct and revision of the treatment plan is not necessary.

STEPS TO THE COMPLETE PROPHY

The complete prophy entails several steps (Box 7.2). According to the general sequence, the oral cavity is evaluated, large pieces of calculus are removed, and the periodontal area is probed for pocket depth and the presence of subgingival calculus. Next, the subgingival calculus is removed, and the teeth are evaluated to ensure that they and the entire periodontal area are completely clean. Then, the degree of disease is evaluated, and further diagnostic tests are performed. Any pathologic condition of the oral cavity should be noted and charted. Home-care instruction should be given to the client either before (to assess compliance) or after the procedure.

When to Use Antibiotics

Ultimately, the decision to administer antibiotics is the veterinarian's. The veterinarian evaluates the patient and prescribes antibiotics, if indicated. Generally, antibiotics are not necessary for healthy patients with periodontal disease. Antibiotics are indicated for patients who are compromised by health conditions (e.g., disease of the liver, kidney, or heart) or viral infections (e.g., feline leukemia virus or feline immunodeficiency virus).

Patient Care

Once anesthetized, the patient should be positioned in lateral recumbency on a grate over a table sink or on a specially designed dental table that allows the fluids used in the dental procedure to drain. Mouth gags should not be used for more than a few minutes; when they are used, care should be taken not to overextend the mandible. Overextension of the mandible may lead to stretching and tearing of the ligaments and muscles of the jaw. Instead, the mouth should be propped open with the nonworking hand (Fig. 7.1).

Step 1: Preliminary Examination and Evaluation

Ideally, the patient has allowed the practitioner to perform a preliminary examination of the oral cavity before induction of anesthesia. However, some patients may not allow this examination at all or, at best, only for a brief time. Therefore, the first step in a prophy is a more complete evaluation of the necessary diagnostic and treatment measures.

Step 2: Supragingival Gross Calculus Removal

The next step of the procedure is to remove supragingival gross calculus. Many types of instruments may be used to perform this step.

Hand Scalers

Hand scalers are used for supragingival removal of calculus. They should not be inserted below the gumline. Scalers are particularly effective in removing calculus from the developmental groove of the fourth premolar. A pull stroke (a stroke pulling the calculus toward the coronal aspect) is used to remove calculus.

Calculus Removal Forceps

Use of calculus removal forceps is a fairly quick method for removing supragingival calculus. The longer tip is placed over the crown, the shorter under the calculus. The calculus is cleaved off when the tips are brought together (Fig. 7.2). When using calculus removal forceps, the operator should be extremely careful not to damage the gingiva or create an iatrogenic slab fracture.

BOX 7.2 Steps to the Complete Prophy

1. Preliminary examination and evaluation
2. Supragingival gross calculus removal
3. Periodontal probing (and periodontal charting)
4. Subgingival calculus removal
5. Detection of missed plaque and calculus
6. Polishing
7. Sulcus irrigation and fluoride treatment
8. Application of a sealer
9. Periodontal diagnostics
10. Final charting
11. Home care

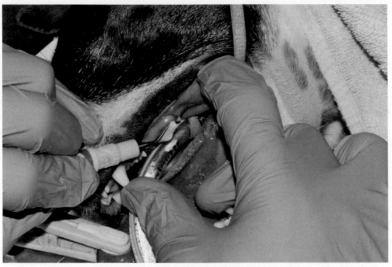

Fig. 7.1 Holding mouth open.

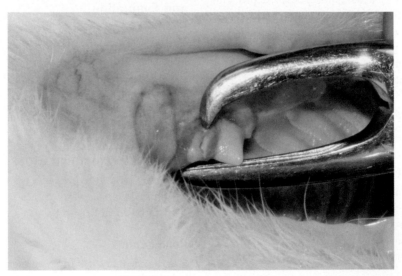

Fig. 7.2 Calculus removal forceps.

Ultrasonic or Sonic Scalers

Ultrasonic or sonic scalers are used to quickly remove the smaller deposits of supragingival calculus. Ultrasonic scalers vibrate in the range of 18,000 to 45,000 cycles per second. When properly applied, this vibration breaks up or pulverizes calculus on the surface of teeth. Because ultrasonic instruments can damage teeth by mechanical etching or thermal heating, they should be used with caution (Fig. 7.3). For supragingival scaling, use of the side of a beavertail tip is preferable rather than the end of the tip. This section of the chapter discusses supragingival scaling, but the same principles apply to the use of ultrasonic or sonic scalers in subgingival scaling. Often, supragingival and subgingival scaling are performed at the same time.

Power instrument grasp. The ultrasonic instrument should be grasped lightly, not tightly. It should feel balanced in the hand, with minimal pull from the handpiece cord. The handpiece, not the hands, must be allowed to do the work (Fig. 7.4A). The handpiece is balanced on the index or middle finger. A modified pen grasp is not as important in holding the ultrasonic or

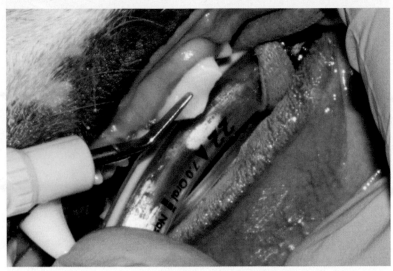

Fig. 7.3 Supragingival scaling.

sonic scaler as it is with hand instruments (Fig. 7.4B). To decrease stress on the hand from the pull on the handpiece cord, the cord may be looped over the little finger (Fig. 7.4C). As opposed to hand instruments, in which a fulcrum is used to provide leverage for the pulling stroke, ultrasonic scalers do not require a fulcrum. The hand is used as a guide for the ultrasonic handpiece.

Water flow. Water flow is required to prevent overheating of the teeth and damage to the pulp. With the broad-based, beaver-type inserts, an ample supply of water is necessary for irrigation (Fig. 7.5A). Less water is required to cool the smaller tips. The water flow can be adjusted to a smaller halo, almost a drip, just enough to cool the tip (Fig. 7.5B).

Insertion. Turning on the handpiece before insertion provides a water supply and thereby eases the insertion of the tip in the sulcus should subgingival scaling be performed at the same time as supragingival scaling.

Pressure. The operator should use a light touch, keeping the tip moving while traveling around the circumference of the tooth and not stopping in any area.

Adaptation. Unlike hand instruments, ultrasonic and sonic instruments do not need cutting edges. However, the tip motion of the instrument must be understood to take advantage of the maximal cleaning stroke. The side of the tip should be held parallel to the tooth surface. The tip of the ultrasonic instrument should not be pointed at the tooth surface or held at a 90-degree angle to the tooth. Doing so could damage the tooth surface by

heating up the pulp; it also provides less cleaning surface and therefore is less effective (Fig. 7.6). The instrument tip is kept parallel with the long axis of the tooth. A straight shank can be used when working straight down the tooth (Fig. 7.7). A curved shank will allow working around a crown or in a furcation.

Ultrasonic technique. The ultrasonic technique includes the following steps:
- Start out with sweeping cross strokes.
- Next, work in various directions (i.e., coronal to apical, oblique, circumferential).
- To reach furcations, use oblique or corkscrew tips. Different tips have been created to reach different difficult areas.
- Avoid pressing the scaler tip on the tooth surface too hard; excessive force can result in thermal damage and render the equipment tip ineffective because it dampens the vibrations.

Power settings—dial type units. Higher power settings should be used for the broad-based, beavertail-type tips. The power should be decreased to lower settings when thin subgingival tips are used. Failure to decrease the power may cause fracturing of the tip or render it ineffective because tips are manufactured to operate in optimal frequency ranges (Fig. 7.8 and Box 7.3).

Adjusting power with the iM3 42-12 unit. The power is turned on at the back of the unit. On the top of the blue cover just behind the iM3 42-12 logo is a silver button. *Text continued on page 162.*

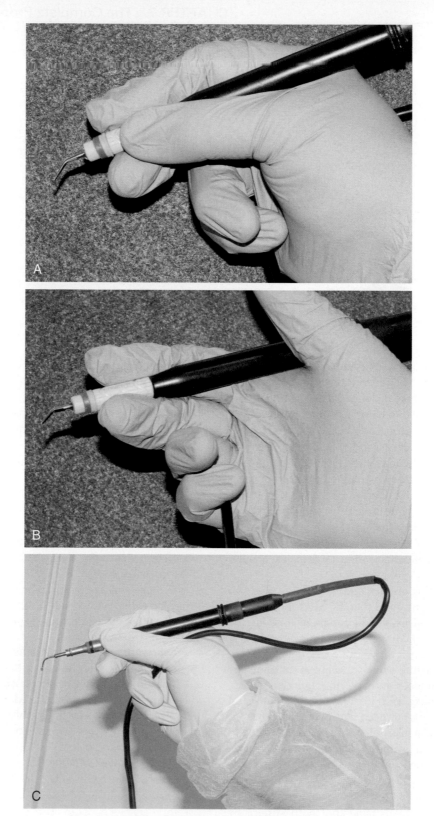

Fig. 7.4 A, Holding ultrasonic. B, Balanced ultrasonic. C, Loop.

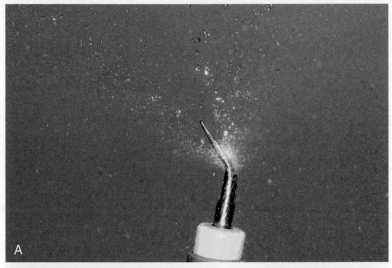

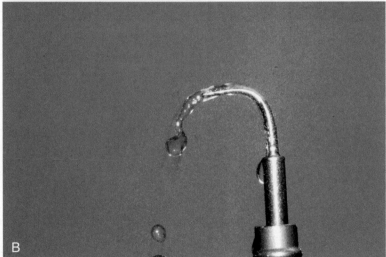

Fig. 7.5 A, Large flow. B, Drip.

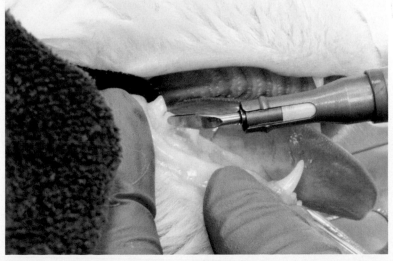

Fig. 7.6 Pointing directly at a tooth is not as effective as using the side of the instrument.

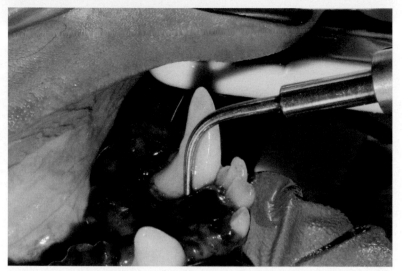

Fig. 7.7 Straight-shank subgingival.

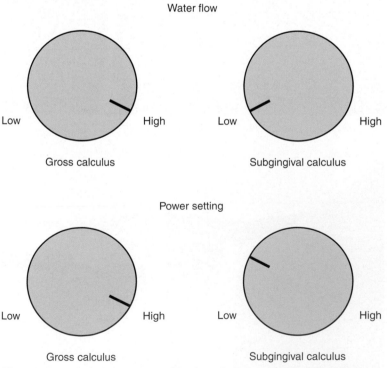

Fig. 7.8 Water flow and power settings must be adjusted according to the use.

BOX 7.3 Ultrasonic Technique (Remember DENTAL)

Digits
- An extraoral finger rest is useful for maxillary posterior teeth.
- Fingers should rest on the teeth for maxillary anterior and mandibular areas.
- A stable fulcrum is not always necessary.

Engage
- Activate the tip of the instrument and direct the tip subgingivally.
- Water lavage will facilitate a comfortable entry into the sulcus.

Neutral
- Use a balanced instrument grasp; the instrument should feel balanced in the hand with no pull from the cord.
- Use a light pen or modified pen grasp.

Technique
- Brush away the calculus, using sweeping cross strokes.

Adaptation
- Unlike curettes, which have a specific cutting edge, ultrasonic and sonic instruments are active on at least two sides when in contact with the tooth surface.
- The side of the tip is held parallel to the tooth surface.
- The end of the tip should not be adapted to the tooth surface at a 90-degree angle.

Light touch
- Apply extremely light pressure, equivalent to that used when blanching the tissue on the back of the hand.

Touching the silver button increases the power by 1 light/level. The power lights can be seen through the front of the unit. The power adjustment is 1 to 5 lights. Use a power setting of 4 to 5 when using the beavertail tip or universal tip (Fig. 7.9A) and reduce the power to 1 to 2 when subgingival scaling using the perio tip (Fig. 7.9B).

Rotary Scalers

Since its introduction to veterinary medicine, the rotary scaler has been very controversial. Its acceptance in human dentistry has been limited because the rotary

scaler can easily damage teeth and requires a great deal of training and practice for safe use. Rather than scaling the teeth, this bur frequently ends up burnishing the calculus. Ineffective removal or burnishing of calculus can lead to a periodontal abscess. Veterinarians who insist on using rotary scalers should discuss them with their own dentists and hygienists. Before using the rotary scaler on their patients' teeth, veterinarians should undergo the experience first (assuming their dentists are willing, which hopefully they are not!). Some of the damage caused by a rotary scaler is shown in Fig. 7.10.

Step 3: Periodontal Probing (and Periodontal Charting)
Probing Technique

A periodontal probe should be used to measure the depth of the sulcus or pocket. Caution is necessary when applying the periodontal probe. A healthy sulcus will bleed if more than 20 gm of pressure is applied to the probe. If too much pressure is applied, the probe can puncture the junctional epithelium. The probe should be held parallel to the long axis of the tooth for an accurate reading (Fig. 7.11A). Holding the probe at an angle results in an inaccurate measurement (Fig. 7.11B). The measured depth must be carefully evaluated when using a periodontal probe. The measurement of sulcular or pocket depth is not necessarily the same as that of attachment loss. If the marginal gingiva is at the normal cementoenamel junction, the probed depth will correspond to attachment loss. Recording sulcular/pocket depth is discussed in Chapter 1.

If previous recession of gingiva has occurred and the marginal gingiva has moved apically, the pocket depth will be less than the actual loss of attached gingiva. If gingival hyperplasia and a pseudopocket are present as a result, the probed depth will be greater than the actual attachment loss.

Charting

Record keeping is an important part of the dental procedure. Dental charts or stick-on labels are used for dental charting and record keeping. Because periodontal disease is progressive, charting is an important aid for follow-up visits. Accurate records establish a baseline: Subsequent measurements of the pockets, furcation exposure, and mobility are compared at each

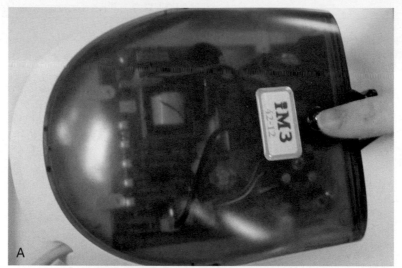

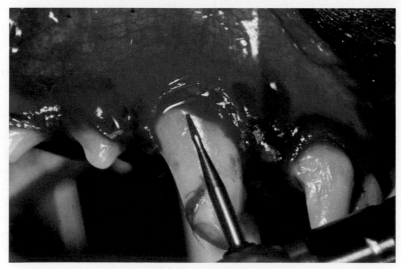

Fig. 7.9 A, High setting. B, Low setting.

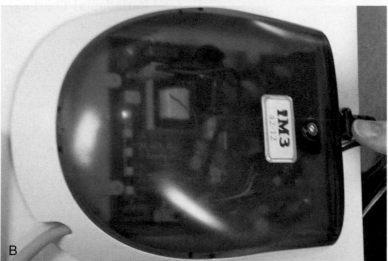

Fig. 7.10 Rotary scaler.

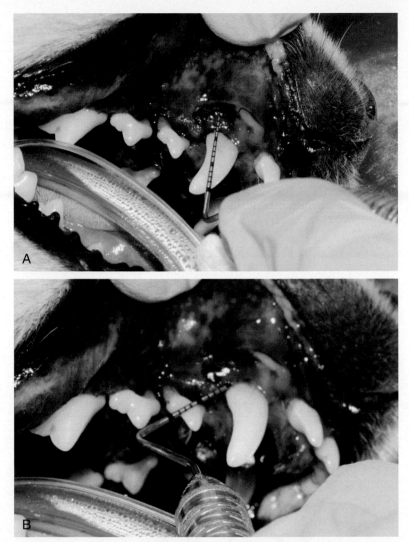

Fig. 7.11 A, Probe correct. B, Probe incorrect.

appointment, which is useful in evaluating treatment and client compliance.

The method used to chart teeth should be consistent (Fig. 7.12). The following starting order is recommended: buccal of right posterior maxilla, lingual of left posterior maxilla, lingual of left posterior mandible, and buccal of right posterior mandible. From the starting point the probing is conducted to the opposite side. Dental abnormalities, such as missing or fractured teeth, are noted. Points on each side should be measured while charting the sulcular/pocket depth. The distal, midsection, and mesial portions of the tooth are measured. One easy, quick method to chart teeth is to record the measurements with a tape recorder. This technique allows continuous measurement, and the tape can be played back later when documenting the information in the chart.

Fig. 7.13 is an example of a dental chart with the following probing depths: 110, 109: 2 mm; 108: 4 mm with 2 mm attachment loss; 107: 1 mm; 106, 105: missing; 104: 3 mm pocket with 2 mm attachment loss; 103, 102, 101: 1 mm. This would be dictated as follows: two slash two, two slash two, three slash five, one slash one, missing, missing, four slash six, one slash one, one slash one, one slash one. Extracted 108 is indicated with an X and the missing teeth are circled.

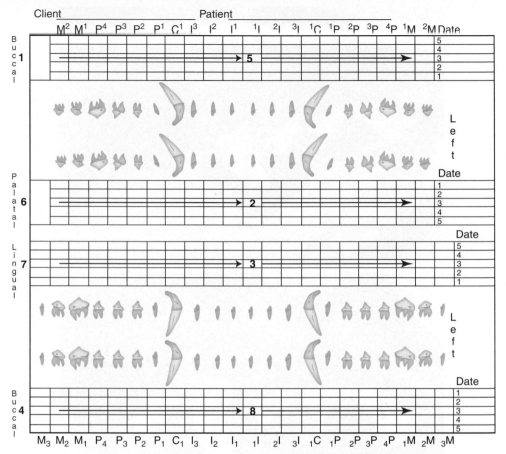

Fig. 7.12 A consistent technique should be used to probe and chart teeth.

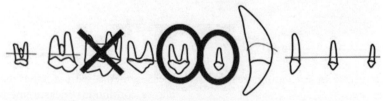

Fig. 7.13 Charting example.

Step 4: Subgingival Calculus Removal

A curette or select ultrasonic scaler should be used to remove the calculus below the gumline. Ultrasonic scalers with subgingival tips can be used to scale and remove calculus below the gumline. Several companies make specialized inserts that can be used subgingivally. Removal of subgingival calculus is an extremely important part of the procedure. If subgingival calculus remains, the patient will not receive long-term benefits from treatment and bacterial plaque will continue destroying the periodontium, leading first to bone deterioration and eventually to tooth loss.

Hand Instrument Technique

The modified pen grasp is the preferred method for holding hand instruments. To obtain the modified pen grasp, first hold the instrument with the thumb and index finger. The instrument should be resting on

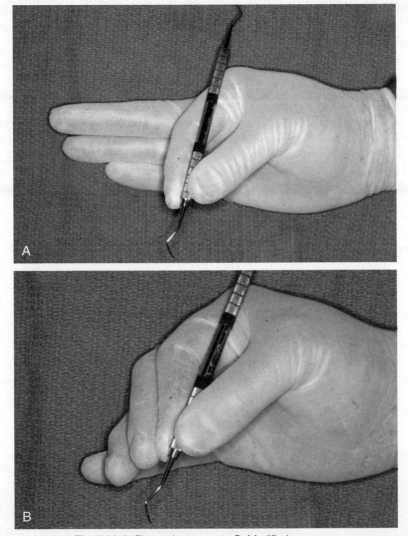

Fig. 7.14 A, First grab pen grasp. B, Modified pen grasp.

the index finger and the middle, ring, and little fingers are extended (Fig. 7.14A). The middle ring and little fingers are then placed alongside the index finger (Fig. 7.14B). In contrast to the pen grasp, in which the working end of the instrument ends up on the back side of the hand, with the modified pen grasp, the working end is on the palm side. The use of a fulcrum and pull stroke results in removal of calculus.

Modified pen grasp. The thumb and forefinger are placed at the junction of the handle and the shank of the instrument. The index finger is placed on the shank. The ring finger is held straight and placed on the surface closest to the tooth being worked on. The position of the fingers creates a "triangle of forces" that provides stability and control when the wrist-rocking motion is initiated. The middle finger, ring finger, or index finger is placed on the tooth to be scaled or an adjacent tooth. The closer the fulcrum is to the tooth being scaled, the more effective the working stroke, as a result of its greater power. This grip can be practiced by holding a pencil and drawing a small circle by rotating only on the fulcrum (ring finger) and moving the wrist. The fingers should not flex at all during this motion.

Adapting to the Tooth

The curette is adapted to the tooth root surface (Fig. 7.15A). If the instrument does not fit the curvature of the tooth, the opposite end of the instrument is adapted (Fig. 7.15B).

As the curette is inserted into the pocket, the face of the instrument should face the root surface. This is called the *closed position*. The instrument is moved over the calculus and then repositioned so that the cutting surface is under the calculus ledge. This is called the *open position*. With a rocking pull or oblique stroke, calculus is cleaved from the root surface.

Step 5: Detection of Missed Plaque and Calculus

An explorer is used to evaluate the tooth surface while checking for subgingival calculus. The tooth is inspected for missed plaque and calculus by the application of disclosing solution or by air-drying, which makes the deposits appear chalky white.

Application of Disclosing Solution

Do you remember the dental hygienist who came to your class in elementary school to demonstrate proper tooth brushing? In such demonstrations, the hygienist gives the students disclosing tablets to chew after brushing their teeth. After rinsing their mouths, the students can see plaque they missed while brushing, which shows up brightly pigmented. Similarly, disclosing solution can be used to maintain quality control of the teeth-cleaning procedure. Painting a small amount of disclosing solution on the teeth with a cotton-tipped applicator allows detection of plaque and calculus that were missed while scaling (Fig. 7.16A). After being rinsed with water, areas where plaque remains assume a red or blue pigment, depending on the brand of the disclosing solution (Fig. 7.16B). Clean teeth do not retain the stain. Care should be exercised when using disclosing solution because it can stain hair and clothing.

Air-drying

Another technique to detect plaque and calculus is to dry the tooth with compressed air. Plaque and calculus appear chalky white when dry (Fig. 7.17). This technique should not be used if the integrity of the periodontium is in question because air could be blown into tissues, resulting in air being trapped in the subcutaneous tissues or possibly entering the bloodstream.

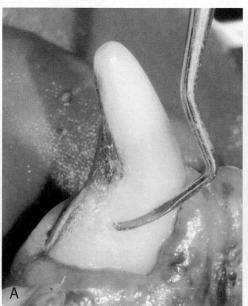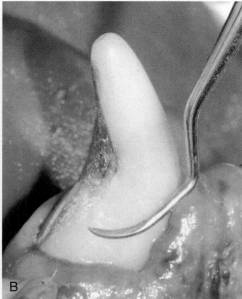

Fig. 7.15 A, Nonadapting. B, Adapting.

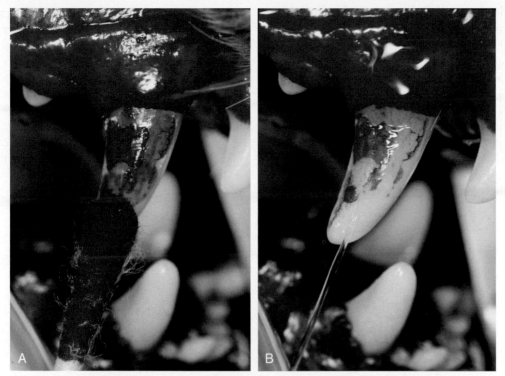

Fig. 7.16 A, Apply disclosing solution. B, Rinse disclosing solution.

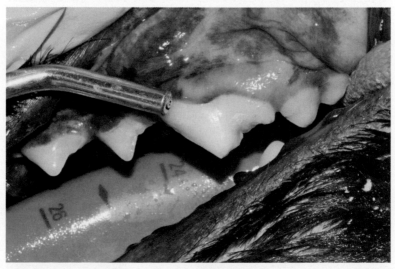

Fig. 7.17 Air-drying.

Step 6: Mechanical Polishing or Air Polishing
Mechanical Polishing

Mechanical polishing is the use of a prophy angle and abrasive paste. Polishing with an electric- or air-powered polisher removes any plaque that may have been missed and smooths the tooth surface. Because polishing generates considerable heat, a liberal amount of prophy paste should be used and only a brief period of time should be spent on each tooth (Fig. 7.18). Some researchers have expressed concern that excessive polishing could cause enamel loss. Risk of enamel loss may be a factor with humans, whose teeth may be polished 3 or 4 times a year for many years; however, most veterinary patients are lucky to have their teeth cleaned 10 times over the course of their lives.

Prophy angles are attachments on slow-speed or electric-motor handpieces that are used to polish teeth. Either screw-on types or pop-on rubber cups can be used with the prophy angle. Prophy angles used in human dentistry come in nonreusable plastic models, inexpensive nonrepairable versions, and expensive non-lubricating sealed units. The disadvantage of these circular units is that hair can get wrapped in the prophy angle (Fig. 7.19).

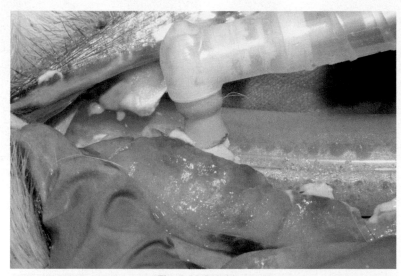

Fig. 7.18 Polishing.

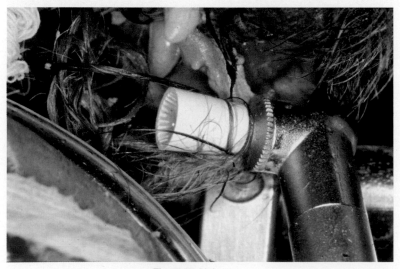

Fig. 7.19 Hair wrap.

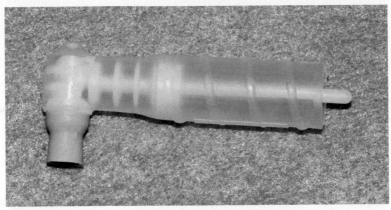

Fig. 7.20 Oscillating prophy angle.

One advantage with disposable plastic prophy angles is that they are relatively inexpensive and do not need to be cleaned after use; they are simply discarded. They should not be cleaned and used on multiple patients. The rubber in the prophy cup cannot withstand multiple uses. The phrase "prophy cup" has multiple meanings. In this text a prophy cup is the rubber cup used on the prophy angle for polishing teeth, and a prophy paste holder is the cup used to hold prophy paste.

Sealed nonrotary prophy angles are also available. They oscillate back and forth at 90 degrees. Because they do not rotate 360 degrees, they will not wrap hair around the prophy cup, which is an advantage (Fig. 7.20).

The most economic (but messiest) means of making prophy paste is to mix flour pumice with a slight amount of water. Many different brands of fine commercial prophy paste are available, in many different flavors. Most contain fluoride, which should not be substituted for the final irrigation. Prophy paste helps reduce the heat that is generated while polishing. Fine paste is used to smooth down the tooth surface. Coarse paste is used to remove stains and should be followed up with fine prophy paste.

Before the teeth are polished, prophy paste is transferred from the prophy paste holder to the teeth with the prophy cup. A small amount of paste is placed on each tooth in a quadrant before turning on the unit. The teeth are polished with a low-speed handpiece at approximately 3000 to 8000 rpm. The prophy cup must be kept moving and should never linger over one area. A slight flare of the prophy cup is used to polish teeth subgingivally.

Air Polishing

Air polishing uses an air, water, and powder projection method on the dental surface with a specialized handpiece (Fig. 7.21). This should not be confused with air abrasion that is used for cavity preparation. Its advantages are that it is faster and less demanding, reducing the operator's hand fatigue; it is less abrasive than abrasive pastes; there is no production of heat; and it gives better access to the teeth and no direct contact with the dental surface treated. It can be used supra- or subgingivally with the perio nozzle (Fig. 7.22). The disadvantage is that it is more expensive than a mechanical polisher and without the judicious use of suction it can be messier (Figs. 7.23 and 7.24).

Step 7: Sulcus Irrigation and Fluoride Treatment

Gentle irrigation of the sulcus flushes out trapped debris and oxygenates the intrasulcular fluids. A saline, stannous fluoride, or diluted chlorhexidine solution may be. A blunted 23-gauge irrigation needle with syringe is effective for this. The full-strength disinfectant chlorhexidine that is commonly found in veterinary hospitals should never be used as a disinfectant without proper dilution. Alternatively, a fluoride gel may be applied to slow the reattachment of plaque after the prophy; it is then wiped (not washed) from the tooth surface.

Step 8: Application of a Sealer

There are two types of sealers available, Sanos and Ora-Vet. At the time of publication, Sanos has Veterinary Oral Health Council (VOHC) approval.

Sanos is a locally active antimicrobial that is applied in a thick coat into the gingival sulcus for antimicrobial activity for up to 6 months (Figs. 7.25 and 7.26). Sanos is designed to work on the gingiva; it is a self-hardening liquid bandage. It should be applied as thick as possible

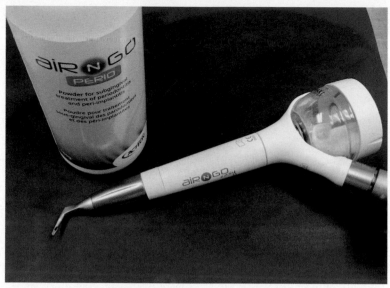

Fig. 7.21 The Air N Go air polisher.

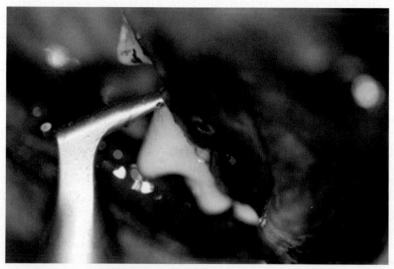

Fig. 7.22 The air polisher can be used subgingivally with a perio nozzle. (Photo courtesy Dr. Thoulton W. Surgeon.)

into the gingival sulcus to inhibit plaque contact with the gingiva. The brush is dipped into the single-use vial after every one or two tooth circumferences. Sanos should not be used in combination with fluoride, Doxirobe, or other products. If there is sulcular bleeding, the area should be gently wiped, pressure lightly applied, and a waiting period for sulcular bleeding to subside. Sanos should be the last product applied.

OraVet is a waxlike product that is applied to the clean tooth surface with a sponge applicator or gloved fingers (Fig. 7.27). It reduces plaque and tartar formation by repelling water and preventing bacteria from

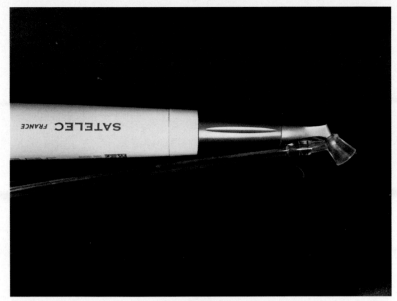

Fig. 7.23 Air n Go with Cavijet vacuum attachment. A Cavijet vacuum attachment is placed over the Air N Go nozzle to clean up the spray as it comes out. (Photo courtesy Dr. Thoulton W. Surgeon.)

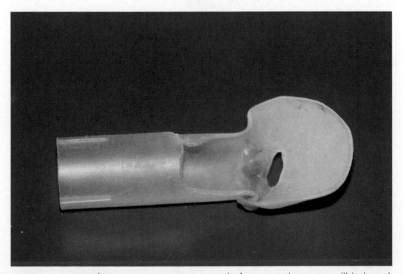

Fig. 7.24 Overspray protector. An overspray protector made from a syringe cap will help reduce the mess (Photo courtesy Dr. Thoulton W. Surgeon.)

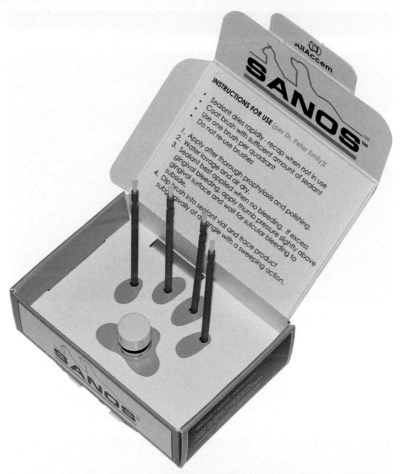

Fig. 7.25 SANOS Box 2012 (Photo courtesy Allaccem Inc., CA, USA).

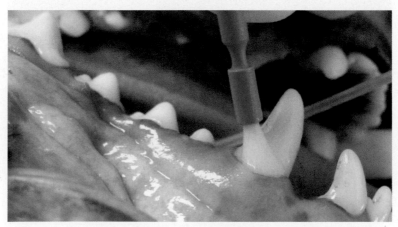

Fig. 7.26 Sanos application.

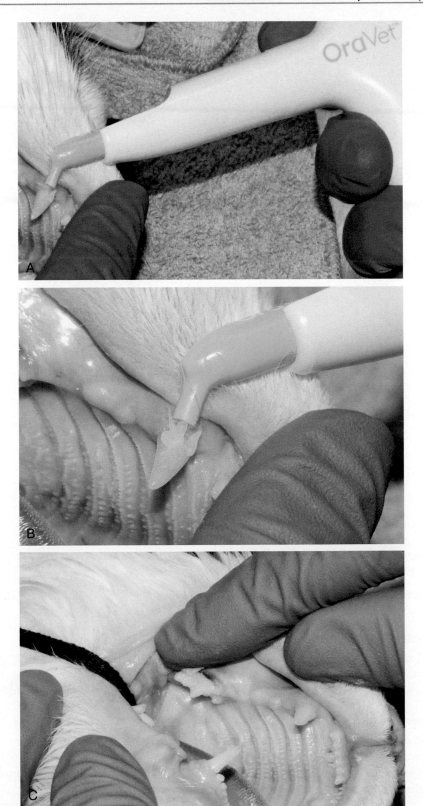

Fig. 7.27 A, OraVet applicator. B, OraVet close. C, OraVet (Merial Inc., GA, USA) being applied with fingers.

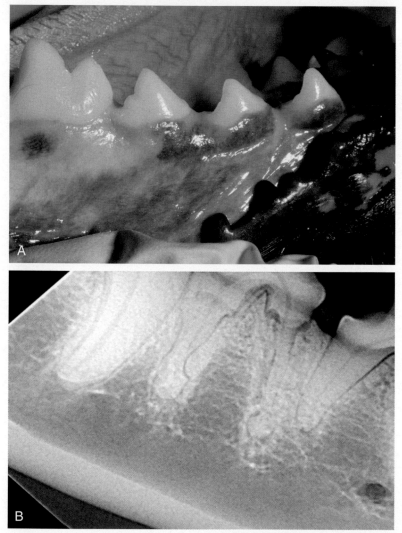

Fig. 7.28 A, Healthy-appearing gingiva and teeth. B, Radiograph of severe subgingival tooth resorption.

attaching to the teeth. This is followed with a weekly application at home.

Step 9: Periodontal Diagnostics

Diagnostics should always include periodontal probing (if not already performed) and intraoral radiology as indicated.

Periodontal Radiographs

Radiographs should be taken to evaluate the dental and bony structures for periodontal bone loss, root canal disease, and other conditions The patient in Fig. 7.28A, has healthy-appearing gingiva and teeth; however, the dental radiographs in Fig. 7.28B show severe subgingival tooth resorption.

Step 10: Final Charting

Final charting involves a review of the previously performed diagnostic and periodontal charting. This final review should include any additional treatment performed.

Step 11: Home Care

The last step to complete prophy is home-care instruction. This subject is discussed in detail in Chapter 8.

NONPROFESSIONAL DENTAL SCALING (NPDS)

Unfortunately, many clients have been misled into thinking they can have their pet's teeth cleaned without anesthesia. It is impossible to do a thorough job in this situation, and dental disease is missed. This procedure is sometimes carried out in grooming clinics and pet stores. In this case, the practice is illegal in most states because it constitutes the practice of veterinary medicine without a license.

Unfortunately, several companies have been formed to also come into veterinary offices and persuade the veterinarian to allow this service. In this case the practice is legal; however, without intraoral radiographs, dental probing, and charting, it is below the standard of practice and the veterinarian may be held guilty of neglect.

The AVDC has a position statement on nonprofessional dental scaling, available at www.AVDC.org. It is provided in its entirety in Box 7.4. Dr. Peter Bates has created the handout shown in Fig. 7.29.

BOX 7.4   American Veterinary Dental College (AVDC) Position Statement on Nonprofessional Dental Scaling: Dental Scaling Without Anesthesia

In the United States and Canada, only licensed veterinarians can practice veterinary medicine. Veterinary medicine includes veterinary surgery, medicine, and dentistry. Anyone providing dental services other than a licensed veterinarian, or a supervised and trained veterinary technician, is practicing veterinary medicine without a license and shall be subject to criminal charges.

This position statement addresses dental scaling procedures performed on pets without anesthesia, often by individuals untrained in veterinary dental techniques. Although the term *anesthesia-free dentistry* has been used in this context, AVDC prefers to use the more accurate term *nonprofessional dental scaling* (NPDS) to describe this combination.

Owners of pets naturally are concerned when anesthesia is required for their pet. However, performing NPDS on an unanesthetized pet is inappropriate for the following reasons:

1. Dental tartar firmly adheres to the surface of the teeth. Scaling to remove tartar is accomplished using ultrasonic and sonic power scalers, plus hand instruments that must have a sharp working edge to be used effectively. Even slight head movement by the patient could result in injury to the oral tissues of the patient, and the operator may be bitten when the patient reacts.

2. Professional dental scaling includes scaling the surfaces of the teeth both above and below the gingival margin (gumline), followed by dental polishing. The most critical part of a dental scaling procedure is scaling the tooth surfaces that are within the gingival pocket (the subgingival space between the gum and the root), where periodontal disease is active. Because the patient cooperates, dental scaling of human teeth performed by a professional trained in the procedures can be completed successfully without anesthesia. However, access to the subgingival area of every tooth is impossible in an unanesthetized canine or feline patient. Removal of dental tartar on the visible surfaces of the teeth has little effect on a pet's health, and provides a false sense of accomplishment. The effect is purely cosmetic.

3. Inhalation anesthesia using a cuffed endotracheal tube provides three important advantages—the cooperation of the patient with a procedure it does not understand, elimination of pain resulting from examination and treatment of affected dental tissues during the procedure, and protection of the airway and lungs from accidental aspiration.

4. A complete oral examination, which is an important part of a professional dental scaling procedure, is not possible in an unanesthetized patient. The surfaces of the teeth facing the tongue cannot be examined, and areas of disease and discomfort are likely to be missed.

Safe use of an anesthetic or sedative in a dog or cat requires evaluation of the general health and size of the patient to determine the appropriate drug and dose, and continual monitoring of the patient.

Veterinarians are trained in all of these procedures. Prescribing or administering anesthetic or sedative drugs by a non-veterinarian can be very dangerous, and is illegal. Although anesthesia will never be 100% risk-free, modern anesthetic and patient evaluation techniques used in veterinary hospitals minimize the risks, and millions of dental scaling procedures are safely performed each year in veterinary hospitals.

To minimize the need for professional dental scaling procedures and to maintain optimal oral health, the AVDC recommends daily dental home care from an early age in dogs and cats. This should include brushing or use of other effective techniques to retard accumulation of dental plaque such as dental diets and chew materials. This, combined with periodic examination of the patient by a veterinarian and with dental scaling under anesthesia when indicated, will optimize life-long oral health for dogs and cats. For information on effective oral hygiene products for dogs and cats, visit the Veterinary Oral Health Council web site (www.VOHC.org).

For general information on performance of dental procedures on veterinary patients, please read the AVDC Position Statement on Veterinary Dental Healthcare Providers.

Courtesy American Veterinary Dental College (AVDC) at www.AVDC.org.

Λnimal Dental News

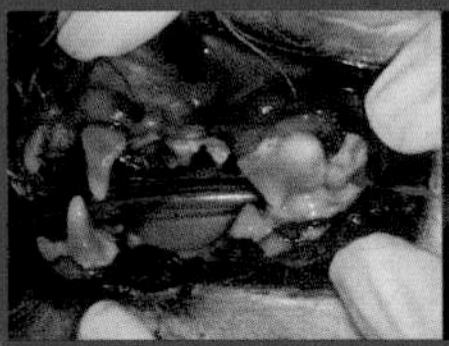

End-stage periodontal disease associated with heavy calculus.

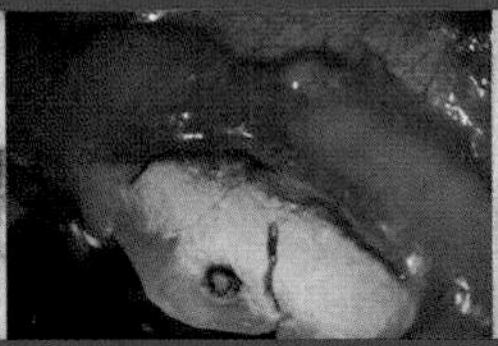

Heavy calculus associated with a fractured and abscessed tooth.

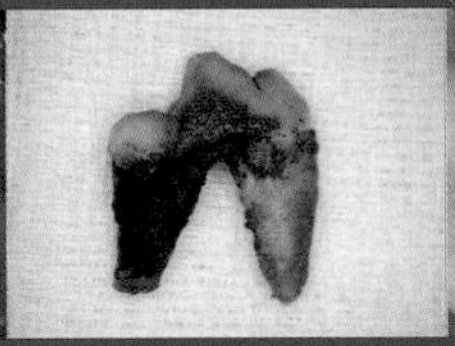

Heavy calculus located below the gingival margin. Abscessed tooth.

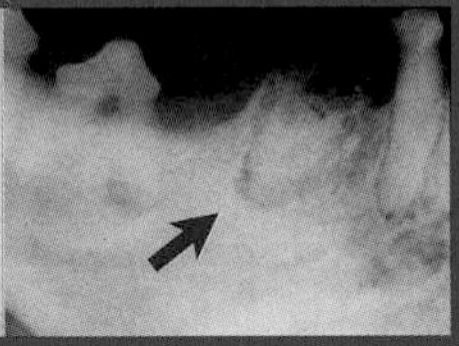

X-Rays are needed to find hidden problems like this buried tooth root.

Anesthesia-Free Dental Cleaning: What You Need to Know

Periodontal disease is the most common ailment of dogs and cats. Regular home care and professional treatment are the first and best means of preventing and combatting this problem. Anesthesia-free methods DO NOT provide the opportunity for thorough cleaning or for proper examination of the oral cavity. Pet owners who rely on anesthesia-free dentistry are leaving a smoldering problem that may well cause chronic pain and become manageable only by extraction.

Questions to Ask:

Whether or not anesthesia is used, when you consider having your pet's teeth cleaned, ask these questions of the provider:

Will you clean all sides of every tooth?

Will you clean below the gingival margin (gum line) as well as above it?

Will you probe around each tooth to find any areas of attachment loss?

Will you take dental x-rays of any areas that have pocketing, loose, missing, discolored or fractured teeth?

If the answer to any of these questions isn't "Yes," look elsewhere for your pet's dental care.

In addition, ask who will be doing your pet's dental cleaning. What are their qualifications? How will the doctor be involved? Who will do the oral examination? If someone other than the doctor is involved, is this person an employee? Who is responsible if there is a problem? If extractions are needed, who will do this?

What About Anesthesia Risks?

No one should pretend that anesthesia doesn't entail some risk. Fortunately, today these risks are very low for healthy animals, even those of advanced age. Underlying medical conditions may increase the risks associated with anesthesia. You should discuss these issues with your veterinarian, along with his or her plans to minimize risk.

Things to Remember:

Periodontal disease is the most common disease of dogs and cats. it is caused by infection below the gingival margin (gum line). It has little to do with the calculus (tartar) that is seen on the crowns of the teeth. Simply removing calculus does nothing to address periodontal disease and it creates a false sense of security.

Signs of Periodontal Disease:

Calculus: While not the primary problem, calculus may accumulate at an abnormally high rate when an animal is not chewing its food. This often indicates underlying pathology.

Halitosis: Probably the most common sign of periodontal disease, halitosis is caused by the bacteria that cause periodontal disease and the associated tissue decomposition.

Gingivitis: Inflammation, or redness of the gingiva indicates the presence of periodontal disease. It is important to intervene early if this symptom is seen.

Loose Teeth: When teeth loosen, it often indicates end-stage periodontal disease.

For More Information, Call:

Fig. 7.29 This handout may be reproduced and used in your practice. (Reproduced with permission of Dr. Peter Bates.)

CHAPTER 7 WORKSHEET

1. _____ is performed for patients with healthy, stage 1, or stage 2 periodontal disease. _____ _____ is performed for patients with stage 3 or stage 4 periodontal disease.

2. The second step of the procedure is to remove supragingival _____ calculus.

3. Use of _____ _____ _____ is a fairly quick method of removing supragingival calculus.

4. Ultrasonic instruments can damage teeth by _____ _____ or _____ _____.

5. The ultrasonic instrument should be grasped _____, not _____.

6. _____ _____ is required to prevent overheating of the teeth and damage to the pulp.

7. The operator should use a _____ touch, keeping the tip moving while traveling around the circumference of the tooth and not stopping in any area.

8. The _____ pen grasp is the method of holding dental instruments.

9. Gentle irrigation of the sulcus flushes out trapped debris and _____ the intrasulcular fluids.

10. _____ should be taken to evaluate the dental and bony structures for periodontal bone loss, root canal disease, and other conditions.

8

Home-Care Instruction and Products

LEARNING OBJECTIVES

When you have completed this chapter, you will be able to:

- Discuss issues related to client education for dental care of their pets.
- Discuss methods used to acclimate patients to tooth brushing.
- Describe advantages and disadvantages of the various brushing devices available for use with dogs and cats.

- List and describe home-care products used for promoting oral health in dogs and cats.
- Explain the general rules for choosing toys and chews for dogs and cats.
- Describe the action of chlorhexidine and list products that contain chlorhexidine.
- Describe the use of fluoride-containing products in dental care of dogs and cats.

KEY TERMS

Chemical plaque control
Chlorhexidine
Coronal direction
Glucose oxidase

Lactoperoxidase
Mechanical plaque control
Monofluorophosphate fluoride
Periodontal disease

Stannous fluoride
Veterinary Oral Health Council
Xylitol
Zinc ascorbate

Client education should begin before the procedure is performed. In addition to informing the client about the procedure, client education is an important way to evaluate the client's willingness to perform home care and the patient's willingness to accept it. The decision to save a tooth or extract it depends on the client's desire and ability to comply with home-care instructions.

CLIENT EDUCATION

All members of the veterinary office staff play important roles in the promotion of pet oral health by home-care instruction. These efforts help bond the client to the practice. Staff members should review brushing and home-care techniques with clients. If possible, a "demonstrator" dog (or cat) should be used (Fig. 8.1). Otherwise, plastic or plaster dental models can be used to show brushing techniques. These models show pathologic as well as healthy conditions. However, skulls should not be used for demonstration because some clients respond negatively to them.

Demonstration

A circular or oval motion with emphasis on the coronal direction, away from the gumline, is recommended. Staff members who are properly trained in this area foster client rapport and increase the likelihood of successful therapy. Clients should be encouraged to return for further instruction as often as necessary.

Home-Care Products

The number of dental home-care products is increasing steadily, and all claim to be effective. Unfortunately, clients are going to the pet store and buying the wrong thing for the wrong reasons. "Natural, fresh, gluten free, healthier, whitening" may be a replacement for "scientifically proven" but it makes the client feel like they are doing something positive. In 1997 the American Veterinary Dental College (AVDC) formed the Veterinary Oral Health Council (VOHC). This organization was established to set testing protocol. If product testing is approved, the product is awarded the VOHC seal of approval (see Fig. 8.11). (See Figs. 8.12–8.14 for some examples of products that have been awarded the VOHC seal of approval.) As these products are constantly updated, the reader is recommended to periodically check the VOHC website at www.vohc.org.

Tips for Difficult Cases

For patients who resist attempts to brush, flavored material or toothpaste can be placed on the toothbrush. The patient is allowed to lick the brush, with no effort made to brush the teeth or restrain the patient in any way (Fig. 8.2). Once the patient begins to become comfortable with the process, the client can begin to swipe at the teeth. Eventually, full brushing can take place. Cats may respond positively to liquid drained out of water-packed tuna.

Advanced Techniques

Once the patient is accustomed to having its teeth brushed, a chew, or other prop may be placed in the mouth (Fig. 8.3). The mouth is held closed, and the teeth are brushed. When a VOHC-approved chew such as Purina Busy HeartyHide Chew Treats, Purina Pro Plan Veterinary Diets (PPVD) Dental Chewz Dog Treats,

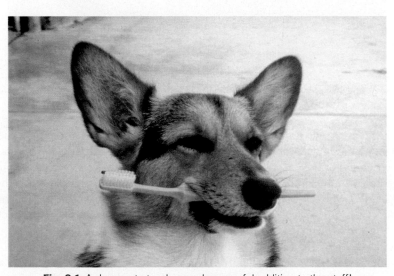

Fig. 8.1 A demonstrator dog can be a useful addition to the staff!

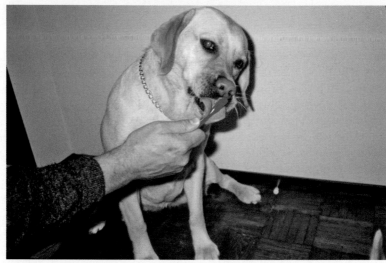

Fig. 8.2 To introduce brushing, start the patient with licking the toothpaste off the toothbrush.

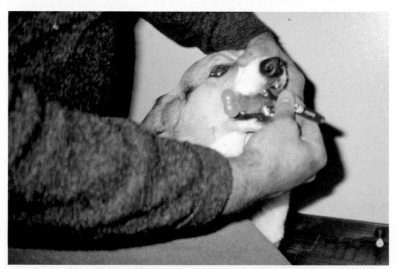

Fig. 8.3 A prop can be placed in the mouth to open the mouth and to brush the lingual and buccal sides of the mandible.

Tartar Shield Soft Rawhide Chews, Canine Greenies, Canine Greenies Weight Management, Canine Greenies Senior, Greenies Veterinary Formula Canine Dental Chews, Canine Greenies Canine Grain Free Dental Chews, HealthiDent, VetIQ Minties Medium Dental Treat, Bright Bites and Checkup Chews, Virbac CET VeggieDent Chews, Improved Milk-Bone Brushing Chews, Merial OraVet Dental Hygiene Chews, or Hill's Prescription Diet Canine Dental Care Chews, (Figure 3, Hills Dental Care Chews) is used, the patient can eat the prop as a reward. However, the client should be advised that all chews are "PG" (Parental Guidance!). A size appropriate for the patient should be fed and they should not be fed unattended as there is always the possibility of choking on the product or other complications if the patient swallows the product whole.

Visual Aids

Visual aids and client handouts are also beneficial in reinforcing the need for brushing and home care. Many manufacturers offer professionally designed handouts. Many clients feel reassured when they read or hear the same information from a variety of sources. Handouts are best displayed in the reception or examination rooms. Some commercial handouts leave spaces for the inclusion of the practice's name and phone number. The practitioner can also customize a handout specifically for the practice. Photographs of the dental area and equipment may increase client awareness of veterinary dentistry procedures performed in the hospital or clinic.

With the advent of computers, handouts can be customized to reflect each patient's specific condition. For example, a client whose pet has stage 1 periodontal disease (PD 1) requires different educational materials than a client whose pet has stage 4 periodontal disease (PD 4). These handouts can be linked to either diagnostic codes or service codes so that when a particular procedure is performed, the handout is generated automatically. Preprinted or computer-generated handouts provide information about periodontics, endodontics, orthodontics, and other dental diseases and treatments. Several companies make flip charts or wall charts that demonstrate various aspects of veterinary dentistry. Polaroid or digital photographs can be used to demonstrate each patient's pathologic condition and often are a key to client communication. Videotapes showing how to brush teeth are also available. Box 8.1 lists online videos that may be helpful. Take a look at them and choose the one that matches your "practice philosophy."

BOX 8.1 Online Videos

Some video sites that may be helpful:

For Brushing
Dr. Jo Banyard, DAVDC:
1. Dentistry for Pet Owners 101: Brushing your dog's teeth.
   https://www.youtube.com/watch?v=Wvmmc5DkJ4U
2. Dentistry for Pet Owners 101. Tooth brushing objectives -
   https://www.youtube.com/watch?v=k9AHc7IoEls&t=10s
3. Tooth brushing for puppies Dentistry for Pet Owners 101.
   https://www.youtube.com/watch?v=Ch8aIRfThWY
4. Brushing cat's teeth—Dentistry for Pet Owners 101.
   https://www.youtube.com/watch?v=Ch8aIRfThWY
5. Dentistry for Pet Owners 101. Tooth brushing objectives.
   https://www.youtube.com/watch?v=2n1V4VCtE0o
6. Dentistry for Pet Owners 101. Toothbrushes and Yummy Toothpastes.
   https://www.youtube.com/watch?v=KDZ-LKJv98c
   https://www.youtube.com/watch?v=BcRA9wf3cNA&list=PLgyMKAquGJOZHeMX7VmuAuCrujjBPPY1O
   Dr. Brett Beckman, DAVDC: veterinarydentistry.net/brushing-teeth-dogs-cats
   Dr. Dr J.C. Burcham via Dr. Susan Chowder, DAVDC: https://m.youtube.com/watch?v=nbi2Fsj95lk
   Dr. Helina Kuntsi: https://youtu.be/Jf6ldiOIPTE
   Dr. Norman Johnson, DAVDC: https://m.youtube.com/watch?v=xPvaXJ-Ki3M

Dr. Laura M. LeVan, DAVDC http://veterinarydentaleducationcenter.com/videos.php
Dr. Clarence Sitzman, DAVDC: https://www.youtube.com/watch?v=EAorj_C-20Q&t=19s
Dr. Keith Stein, DAVDC: https://youtu.be/_XyyBhm-cKg

For Applying OraVet
http://www.oravet.us.merial.com/oravet_homecare.html
   Veterinary Oral Health Council (VOHC) Statement on Obstructions as a Result of Chewing a Dental Chew or Treat. (http://www.vohc.org/chew.html September 14, 2017)
   VOHC occasionally hears of problems resulting from use of products on the VOHC Accepted list. One of the most serious problems is obstruction of the pharynx, esophagus, stomach, or intestines by chew treats, which may require endoscopic or surgical removal of the obstruction, and could cause death of the animal.
   Both the wild carnivore diet and manufactured chews for pet carnivores (dogs and cats) are not without risk. Wild carnivores are naturally chewers, given that their typical diet does not come in handy swallowable-sized pieces. VOHC understands that there is inevitably some risk for a product that relies on the animal obtaining the beneficial dental effect by chewing on the product, just as carnivores for millennia have chewed on cadavers, ripping and tearing off chunks.
   VOHC responds to reported issues regarding problems with use of products on its Accepted list initially by investigating the prevalence of the problem. VOHC contacts the company for additional information.

Continued

BOX 8.1   Online Videos—cont'd

Given the large sales volume of some chew products, if the problem appears to be a very infrequent, an isolated issue, or appears to have resulted from the owner feeding the wrong-sized product to the animal, VOHC takes no immediate action but monitors reports of any further problems with that particular product.

If it becomes evident that the issue is more wide-spread and is causing injury to a substantial number of animals, VOHC responds differently, by requiring the company to remove the VOHC Seal from the product packaging, and deleting the product from the VOHC Accepted list. VOHC has done this twice to date with particular dental chews, both of which are no longer marketed.

VOHC is not a regulatory body. In the USA, the Center for Veterinary Medicine of the Food and Drug Administration is the designated regulatory agency for pet products. The only action that VOHC can take when frequent serious problems are identified is to require the company to remove the VOHC Accepted Seal from packaging and advertisements, and to recommend that owners whose pets have been affected inform the FDA.

Although VOHC is not a regulatory body, VOHC requires applicants for the VOHC Accepted Seal to provide assurance that no major safety issues, such as toxicity, esophageal or gastro-intestinal obstruction or perforation, gross nutritional imbalance, or trauma to oral tissues such as fracture of teeth or laceration or penetration of oral mucosa, were identified during testing or since the product was first marketed. VOHC also requires assurance that all regulatory requirements have been met. In addition, VOHC requires the company to provide an annual report of any complaints or regulatory actions relating to the safety issues noted above.

Athough VOHC regrets any complication associated with using a dental chew, VOHC does not believe it is necessary to deny animals access to all chewable products with proven dental effectiveness, and thus deprive millions of dogs and cats the opportunity for a cleaner mouth, and perhaps fewer general anesthesia episodes for teeth scaling during their lifetime, in order to prevent an occasional obstruction, if the product complies with all current regulatory requirements.

Pet owners and veterinarians should be aware of two ways that obstructions from ingestion of dental chews can be significantly reduced:

Ensure that the right-sized product for the body weight of the dog is given.

Limit giving the treats to times when the owner is available to observe the dog chewing the treat.

Some companies have included these recommendations on the chew product package, and the VOHC encourages this notification.

PLAQUE CONTROL AND HOME CARE

The three methods of controlling plaque are the following: mechanical, chemical, and the combination of mechanical/chemical.

Toothbrushing

Clients frequently ask how often they should brush their pets' teeth. Because of the way plaque and calculus form, daily brushing is best. Plaque forms 6 to 8 hours after brushing. Bacteria attach to the tooth and aid in the formation of calculus in 3 to 5 days. The client advised to brush the teeth every other day may indeed do so. However, clients are susceptible to the human tendency of procrastination. Every other day stretches to every 3 days, and at that point calculus may form. One good tip is to advise the client to brush before feeding—use food as a reward! This is contrary to what most parents teach their children. However, in humans the primary concern is the accumulation of carbohydrate substances that may lead to cavities. Periodontal disease is caused by bacterial plaque, which is removed by conscientious brushing. Brushing daily is more important than the time of day that the brushing occurs.

Electric toothbrushes, such as those made by Braun or Crest, can be effective toothbrushes. It takes some conditioning for the patient to get used to the vibration and noise, but it can be done.

Brushing Devices

The most important strategy in the prevention of periodontal disease is plaque control. There are two major methods of plaque control: mechanical and chemical. The mechanical removal of plaque is particularly important in the control of periodontal disease. Many types of devices can be used. The use of a soft, child-size or preschool toothbrush is the most effective method. All

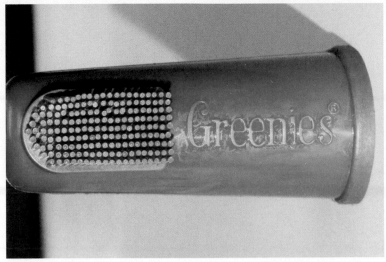

Fig. 8.4 A rubber fingerbrush may be used as a starter brush, but clients should be encouraged to use a child's preschool-sized toothbrush.

American Dental Association (ADA)-compliant soft-bristle, flat-head toothbrushes are VOHC approved. Rubber fingerbrushes are available and are easier for the client to adapt to their pet's teeth (Fig. 8.4). However, they may not be as effective as other toothbrushes and canine and feline toothbrushes (Figs. 8.5 and 8.6). A cotton-tipped applicator may be effective for some patients. Smaller brushes useful for brushing the interproximal and furcation areas are available at human pharmacies (Figs. 8.7–8.9).

Wipe

Wipes are also available that help introduce the concept of oral hygiene (Fig. 8.10).

Brushing Agents

Various chemical agents have been proposed for the removal and prevention of plaque in humans and animals. Unfortunately, a 100%-effective agent has yet to be developed; therefore, brushing is still the preferred method. Plain water or beef or chicken broth can be used initially to help the patient become accustomed to brushing. Sometimes, the addition of garlic powder to the water helps. The mechanical action of brushing or wiping is the important factor in plaque control, not the agent itself.

Plaque-Removing Chews

Despite the VOHC approval of dog and cat chew products, caution must be exercised in recommending all chew products. Foreign body obstructions have been reported from dogs swallowing large particles of dog chews (Fig. 8.11). See the VOHC statement on product safety.

Most chew products move by mechanical means; they "scrub" plaque and sometimes calculus off the tooth surface and sulcus. There are some exceptions:
- OraVet works by mechanical and chemical mechanisms to prevent bacterial attachment. The mechanical action of chewing loosens and dislodges plaque to remove it from teeth. Delmopinol is present to disrupt the plaque matrix and also forms a barrier that prevents bacteria from adhering to the teeth.
- Tartar Shield Soft Rawhide Chews contains malic acid, a chemical that combines with calcium present in dental plaque, thus preventing calculus formation.

The following three rules should be explained to the client in choosing toys and chews:
1. The item must bend or break easily when flexed.
2. If the item is hit on your knee cap and it hurts, it should not be fed.
3. If you mentally think "I'm going to chew this item" and you grimace, it should not be given.

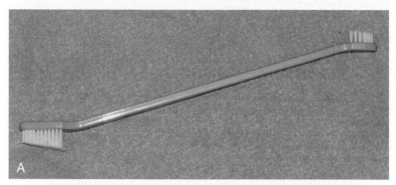

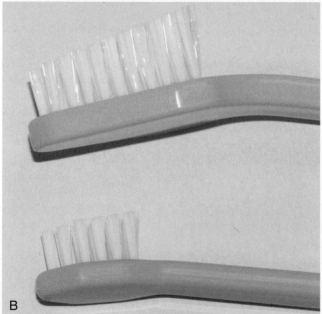

Fig. 8.5 A and B, Canine toothbrush.

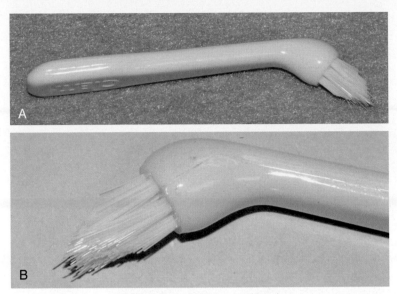

Fig. 8.6 A and B, Feline toothbrush.

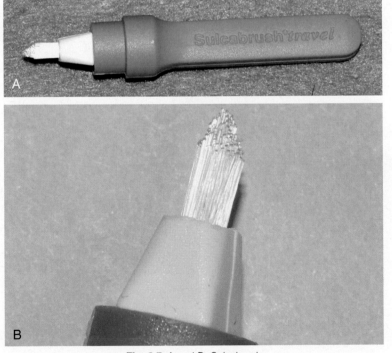

Fig. 8.7 A and B, Sulcabrush.

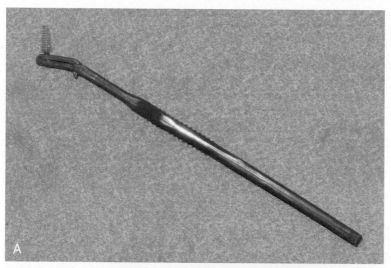

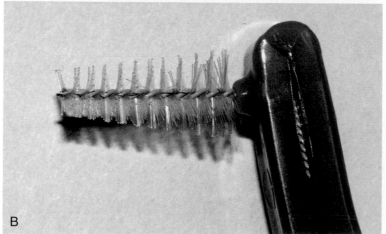

Fig. 8.8 A and B, Proxabrush.

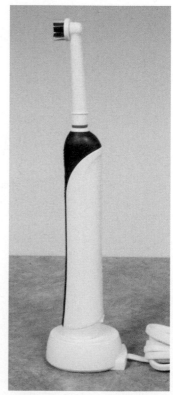

Fig. 8.9 Electric toothbrush.

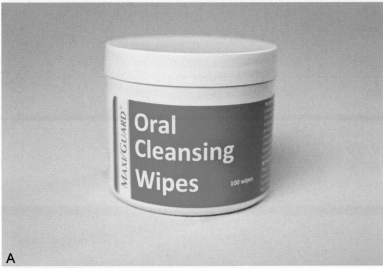

A

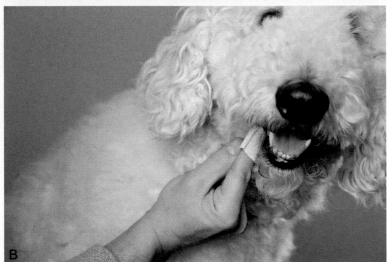

B

Fig. 8.10 A, Wipe jar product shot. B, Wipe with Frankie; It is wrapped around the finger.

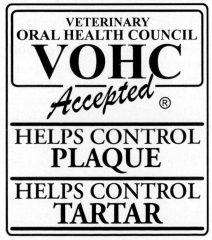

Fig. 8.11 Veterinary Oral Health Council seal of approval.

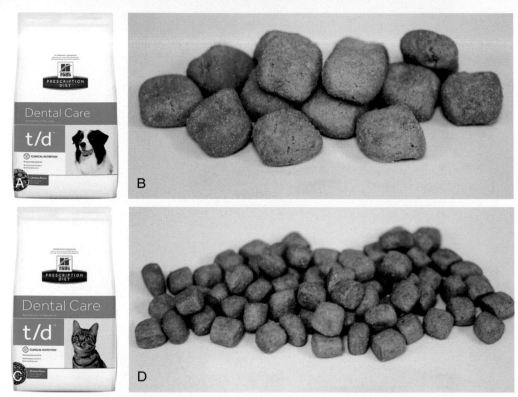

Fig. 8.12 A, Prescription Diet Canine t/d: Original Bites and Small Bites—Plaque and Tartar. B, Prescription Diet Canine t/d: Original Bites. C, Prescription Diet Feline t/d—Plaque and Tartar. D, Prescription Diet Feline t/d—Plaque and Tartar. (New and Improved Prescription Diet Feline t/d—Plaque and Tartar is also VOHC-approved.)

Figs. 8.12–8.19 show some great plaque-removing toys and chews.

Water Additives

Water additives are approved by the VOHC. Although not as effective as brushing, they are helpful as an adjunct to brushing and for those patients who will not accept brushing (Fig. 8.20). The following HealthyMouth products are VOHC approved as of the date of this printing:
Dog: ESSENTIAL HealthyMouth antiplaque water additive
Cat: ESSENTIAL HealthyMouth antiplaque water additive

Dog and Cat Foods

The products shown in Fig. 8.21 may be effective, but as of the date of publication, they do not have the VOHC seal of approval.

Enzyme Toothpastes

Canine enzymatic toothpaste (C.E.T.) reportedly enhances and activates the natural defense mechanisms of the mouth by providing key catalysts and antiplaque chemicals (Fig. 8.22). In addition to abrasive materials, glucose oxidase and lactoperoxidase are chemicals that combine to produce the hypothiocyanite ion, which is the same ion produced naturally in saliva to help inhibit bacterial growth.

Text continued on page 196

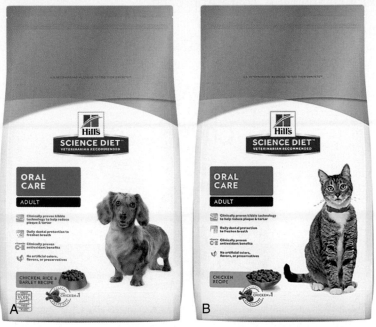

Fig. 8.13 A, Science Diet Oral Care Diet for Dogs—Plaque and Tartar. B, Science Diet Oral Care Diet for Cats—Plaque and Tartar.

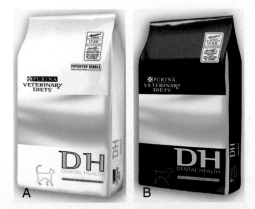

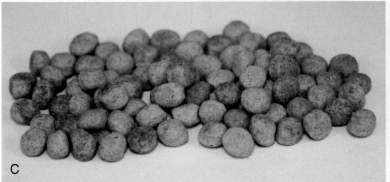

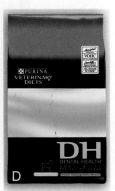

Fig. 8.14 A, Purina Veterinary Diets DH Dental Health brand Feline Formula—Plaque and Tartar. B, Purina Veterinary Diets DH Dental Health brand Canine Formula—Tartar. C, Purina Veterinary Diets DH Dental Health brand Canine Formula. D, Purina Veterinary Diets DH Dental Health brand Small Bites Canine Formula—Tartar.

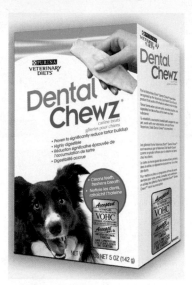

Fig. 8.15 Purina Veterinary Diets Dental Chewz brand Canine Treats—Tartar.

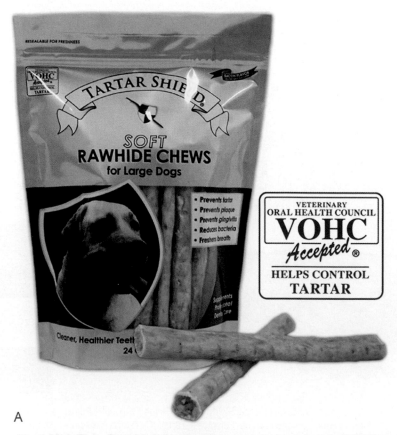

A

Fig. 8.16 A, Tartar Shield Soft Rawhide Chews bag for large dogs and VOHC seal of approval.

Continued

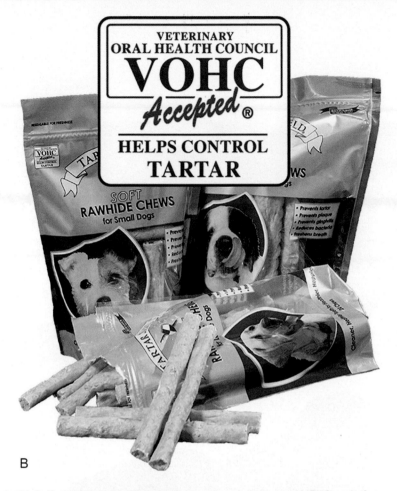

B

Fig. 8.16, cont'd B, Tartar Shield Rawhide Chews bag for small dogs and VOHC seal of approval. (Courtesy Therametric Technologies, Inc.). Tartar Shield comes in a variety of sizes. It is very important that the directions on the package be followed for the size of the dog for all products.

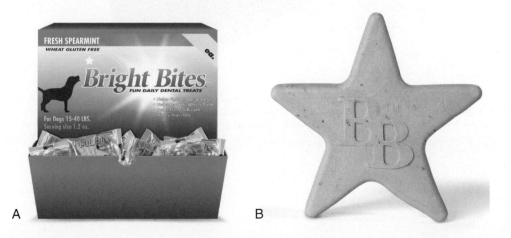

A   B

Fig. 8.17 A, Bright Bites and Checkup Chews for Dogs. B, Bright Bites and Checkup Chews for Dogs, all sizes—for plaque and tartar.

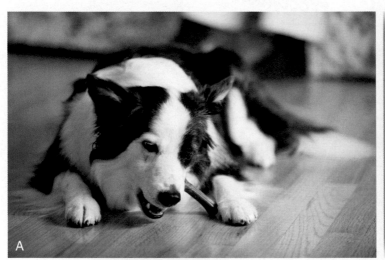
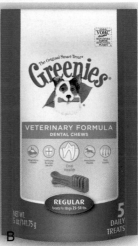
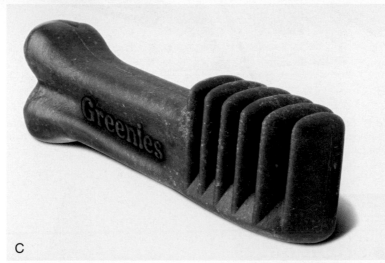

Fig. 8.18 A, Chew products. B, Greenies Veterinary Formula. C, Close-up of Greenies Veterinary Formula. (Other great Greenies products include Canine Greenies, all sizes—for plaque and tartar, Canine Greenies Lite, all sizes—for plaque and tartar, Canine Greenies Senior, all sizes—for plaque and tartar.) (Courtesy Greenies.)

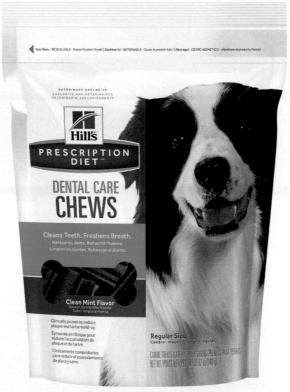

Fig. 8.19 Hill's Dental Care Chews.

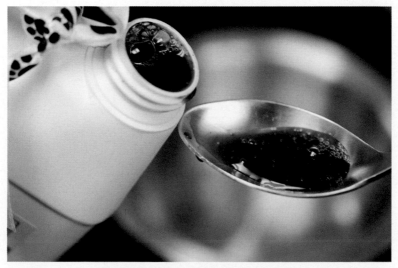

Fig. 8.20 Adding HealthyMouth to water.

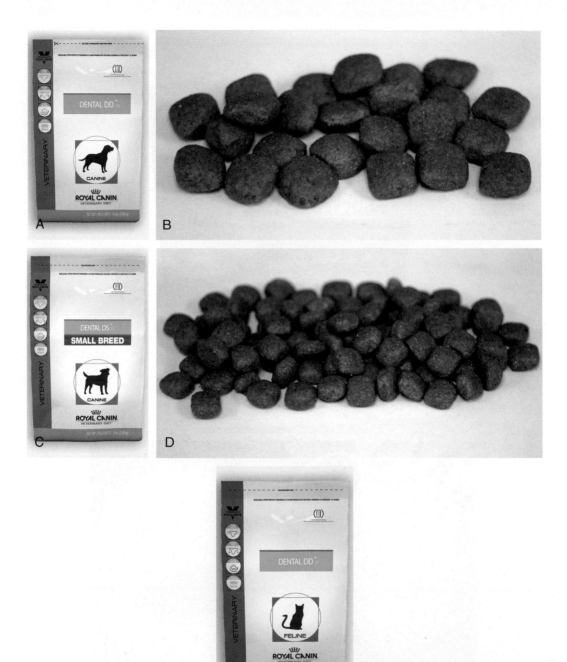

Fig. 8.21 A, Royal Canin Large Breed. B, Royal Canin Large Breed. C, Royal Canin Small Breed. D, Royal Canin Small Breed. E, Royal Canin Feline.

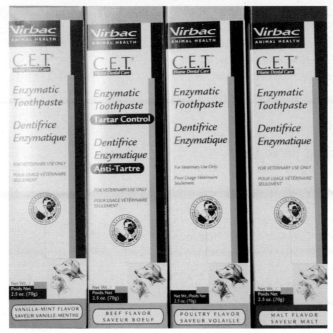

Fig. 8.22 C.E.T. toothpastes.

Antibacterial and Anticalculus Products
Rinses/Brushing Agents

Chlorhexidine. An increasing number of products contain chlorhexidine. The advantage of chlorhexidine is its substantivity, or its ability to adhere to oral tissues and release its agents slowly. The active ingredient in C.E.T. Oral Hygiene Rinse is chlorhexidine gluconate (Fig. 8.23). Novadent contains chlorhexidine acetate.

Water additives. C.E.T. AquaDent uses a low dose of xylitol, an ingredient commonly used in chewing gum for plaque control. Although xylitol can be toxic to dogs at higher doses, studies have shown that at the dosage used it is not toxic (Fig. 8.24).

Zinc. Zinc ascorbate (MaxiGuard) is effective in the elimination of plaque and the stimulation of healing. MaxiGuard contains vitamin C and zinc sulfate, which are reported to clean the mouth and help decrease inflammation. MaxiGuard may be used before or after surgery (Fig. 8.25). For routine brushing, the manufacturer recommends the use of MaxiGuard OraZn. Both of these products are applied by brushing, spraying, or wiping.

Fluoride gels. Several types of fluoride are available. Stannous fluoride, the most bactericidal agent, is stable

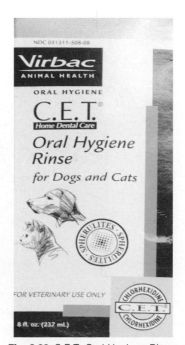

Fig. 8.23 C.E.T. Oral Hygiene Rinse.

at a pH of 6.5. The 0.4% strength should be used. Fluoride has been shown to aid in plaque prevention when deposited on the surface of the enamel. Although it is unlikely to cause toxicity at this strength, the client should be cautioned to use the product sparingly. Any food in the stomach at the time of ingestion will likely neutralize the fluoride. Table 8.1 summarizes the various home-care products available.

Selecting the Appropriate Home-Care Product

The type of dental product recommended depends on the severity of the pathologic condition. The only way to thoroughly judge oral health is by periodontal probing and intraoral radiographs. The need for oral hygiene can be prescribed only after knowing these parameters. There have been cases where clients have diligently brushed teeth with severe periodontal disease. The result was a delay of appropriate treatment.

For those patients whose oral health is good (e.g., stage 1), the priority is to begin the brushing procedure.

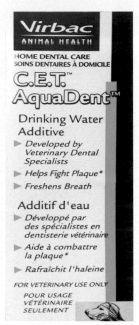

Fig. 8.24 C.E.T. AquaDent.

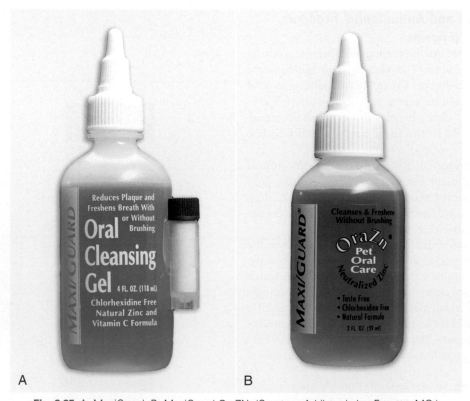

Fig. 8.25 A, MaxiGuard. B, MaxiGuard OraZN. (Courtesy Addison Labs, Fayette, MO.)

TABLE 8.1 Tooth-Brushing Agents

Product	Manufacturer	Active Ingredients
Cat::ESSENTIAL HealthyMouth anti-plaque gel	HealthyMouth	Yucca, clove, cinnamon, papain, pomegranate, blueberry, zinc gluconate, ascorbic acid, riboflavin, chlorophyll, xanthan gum, sorbic acid, glycerine, salmon oil
C.E.T. Mint, Malt, and Poultry Flavor	Virbac Corporation	Glucose oxidase, lactoperoxidase
C.E.T. Forte (canine)	Virbac Corporation	Glucose oxidase, lactoperoxidase
C.E.T. Forte (feline)	Virbac Corporation	Glucose oxidase, lactoperoxidase
Novadent solution	Fort Dodge	Chlorhexidine acetate
Dog::Essential HealthyMouth anti-plaque Gel	HealthyMouth	Yucca, clove, cinnamon, papain, pomegranate, blueberry, zinc gluconate, ascorbic acid, riboflavin, chlorophyll, xanthan gum, sorbic acid, glycerine
Dog::ESSENTIAL HealthyMouth anti-plaque spray	HealthyMouth	Yucca, clove, cinnamon, papain, pomegranate, blueberry, zinc gluconate, ascorbic acid, riboflavin, chlorophyll, xanthan gum, sorbic acid, glycerine
Dog::ESSENTIAL HealthyMouth anti-plaque water additive–Mobility Formulation	HealthyMouth	Yucca, clove, cinnamon, papain, pomegranate, blueberry, zinc gluconate, ascorbic acid, riboflavin, chlorophyll, xanthan gum, sorbic acid, glycerine
Dog::ESSENTIAL HealthyMouth anti-plaque Gel and Brush Combination	HealthyMouth	Yucca, clove, cinnamon, papain, pomegranate, blueberry, zinc gluconate, ascorbic acid, riboflavin, chlorophyll, xanthan gum, sorbic acid, glycerine
Gel-Kam	Colgate	Stannous fluoride
Pettura Oral Care Gel	Lifes2Good	Caprylic acid, whey protein isolate
MaxiGuard (canine)	Addison Labs	Vitamin C, zinc sulfate
MaxiGuard OraZn	Addison Labs	Vitamin C, zinc sulfate
MaxiGuard (feline)	Addison Labs	Vitamin C, zinc sulfate, taurine

C.E.T., Canine enzymatic toothpaste.

For these patients, starting out with flavored animal toothpastes, such as VRx C.E.T., or VOHC-approved products such as ESSENTIAL HealthyMouth Gel, Petsmile by Supersmile toothpaste, or Pettura Oral Care Gel, establishes the routine. For patients with stage 2 or 3 periodontal disease, the introduction of a fluoride product for plaque control becomes more important. The use of flavored animal toothpastes to establish the routine interjected with twice-weekly treatments with stannous fluoride to help inhibit plaque formation is advised. Patients with stage 4 periodontal disease need more help at home; coating the mouth with chlorhexidine gel and rinsing the mouth with a chlorhexidine solution twice daily for 2 weeks may be beneficial. At the end of the 2-week period, a stannous fluoride gel is substituted for the chlorhexidine for continued use.

OTHER HOME-CARE AIDS
Plaque-Removing Chew Toys
Clients frequently ask veterinary staff to recommend chew toys. Objects such as pig ears and hooves, bones, and other animal parts are simply too hard and will fracture teeth. Toss-n-Tug, Booda Bones, Kong toys, or "Pull" or "Pool" toys are all acceptable products (Fig. 8.26). However, the client must be reminded that all toys should be used under proper supervision.

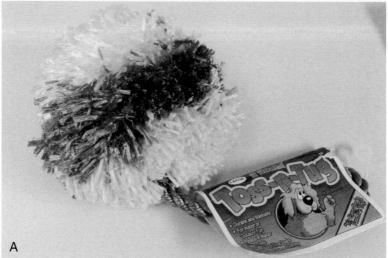

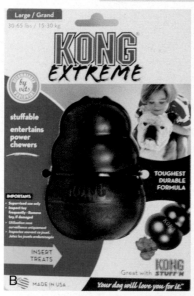

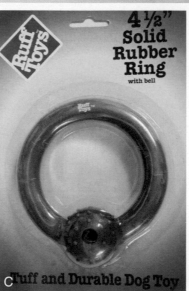

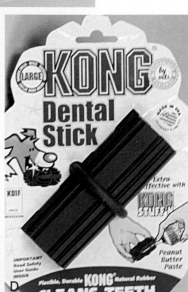

Fig. 8.26 A, Toss-n-Tug. B, Kong toy. C, Pull toy. D, Dental stick.

CHAPTER 8 WORKSHEET

1. Client education should begin _____ the procedure is performed.
2. If possible, a "_____" dog (or cat) should be used to demonstrate tooth brushing to the client.
3. A circular motion with emphasis on the _____ stroke is recommended to demonstrate tooth brushing to the client.
4. _____ _____ and _____ _____ are also beneficial in reinforcing the need for brushing and home care.

5. The most important strategy in the prevention of periodontal disease is _____ _____.
6. In 1997 the American Veterinary Dental College formed the _____ _____ _____ _____.
7. The advantage of _____ is its substantivity.
8. The client must be reminded that all toys should be used under _____ _____.
9. _____ brushing is advised.
10. Plaque forms _____ to _____ hours after brushing.

Periodontal Therapy

LEARNING OBJECTIVES

When you have completed this chapter, you will be able to:

- Describe the purpose and procedure for performing root planing.
- Explain the purpose and result of periodontal debridement.
- Define cementum and discuss its role in periodontal disease.
- List various ultrasonic scaler tips available for use in veterinary dentistry.
- Describe the use of ultrasonic scalers in periodontal therapy.
- Discuss the use of local antibiotic therapy with veterinary dental patients.

KEY TERMS

Antibiotic therapy
Cementum
Mucocitis
Periodontal pockets
Periodontal debridement
Root planing

The primary objective of periodontal therapy is the treatment of periodontal disease. The difference between preventive dentistry and dentistry for the treatment of disease is important. As discussed in Chapter 7, a prophylaxis, or prophy, is performed on patients with stage 1 (early gingivitis) to prevent periodontal disease. Periodontal therapy, which is nonsurgical, is used in the treatment of patients with stage 2 (early periodontitis), stage 3 (established periodontitis), and stage 4 (advanced periodontitis) periodontal disease. Root planing, the traditional method of treatment, differs from scaling and the newer form of treatment, periodontal debridement. The patient in Fig. 9.1 is not a candidate for a "prophy"! It is a candidate for further evaluation and possible periodontal therapy or exodontia. The term "COAPT" (Complete Oral Health Assessment and Prevention or Treatment) may be the most appropriate acronym as it covers assessment (clinical examination, probing,

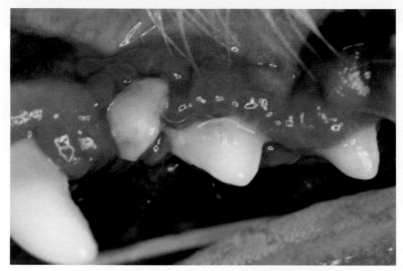

Fig. 9.1 This patient is not a candidate for a "prophy."

and radiographs) and/or prophy (preventative dentistry) or treatment (periodontal therapy, periodontal surgery. or extraction).

SCALING

Scaling is the mechanical removal of plaque, calculus, and stains from the crown and root surfaces. The act of scaling does not necessarily treat periodontal disease. It only removes the surface irritants. The technique for scaling is discussed in Chapter 7 in the section that deals with gross calculus removal.

ROOT PLANING

Root planing is more definitive than scaling. The objective of root planing is the removal of calculus and cementum from the root surface and the creation of a clean, smooth, glasslike root surface. In this treatment, everything, including cementum, is removed from the root surface.

Root Planing: Technique

A routine, systematic approach should be used on each quadrant and each tooth. The blade of the curette is positioned against the root surface. Root planing is performed using a curette with overlapping strokes in

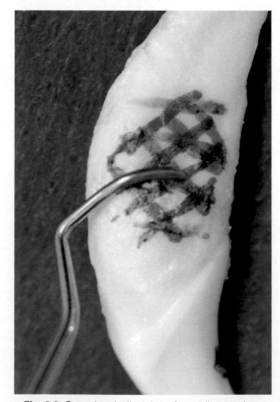

Fig. 9.2 Cross-hatch directions for scaling strokes.

horizontal, vertical, and oblique directions (Fig. 9.2). This cross-hatch planing creates an optimally smooth surface and maintains root anatomy.

PERIODONTAL DEBRIDEMENT

Periodontal debridement is the treatment of gingival and periodontal inflammation. Its goal is the mechanical removal of surface irritants while maintaining soft tissue and allowing it to return to a healthy, noninflamed state.

Changes in Instrumentation Theory

Theories have changed with regard to root-planing techniques and instruments. Most experts no longer recommend the complete stripping of the dentin surface. This change in theory came about with the increased availability of higher-frequency ultrasonic scalers and thinner tips. Unlike the wider tips used in ultrasonic scaling for gross calculus removal, the newer tips are thinner and can enter the periodontal pocket with less distention of the gingiva and less risk of harm to the tissues, which sometimes occurs with curettes. A periodontal pocket is an area of diseased gingival attachment, characterized by loss of attachment and eventual damage to the tooth's supporting bone. Proper use of the new ultrasonic instruments is much easier. In addition, newer antimicrobials and antibiotics are available for use in treatment.

Cementum Removal

Cementum is the substance that attaches the periodontal ligament to the tooth. In the past, experts believed that calculus and toxins from bacteria were embedded in the cementum; therefore, removal of the cementum was necessary. Newer research has shown that bacterial plaque is loosely bound and molecular growth factors are contained within the cementum, aiding in the reattachment of the periodontal ligament to the root surface. Now, only the removal of plaque and calculus is mandatory.

Benefits of Ultrasonic Periodontal Therapy

When properly used, ultrasonic scalers remove the least amount of cementum, as compared with sonic scalers or hand instruments. In addition, the ultrasonic scalers provide water lavage that allows better visualization of the tissues and flushes or removes debris from the pocket. Because they irrigate the tissues, ultrasonic scalers also improve cleanliness and wound healing.

Ultrasonic scalers are able to clean the root surface more efficiently than hand instruments. The result is less time on treatment and less time when the patient is under anesthesia. Moreover, the sonic waves produced have a cavitation effect, disrupting the bacterial cell wall.

Ultrasonic periodontal therapy has several advantages over traditional ultrasonic therapy, in which a curette is used. Because the ultrasonic tip creates less distention of the gingival tissues than a curette, less trauma occurs and healing is faster. No sharpening of the instrument is required. Because there are no cutting edges, the risk of gingival laceration is reduced, making ultrasonic periodontal therapy safer.

Ultrasonic Tips

Several companies (e.g., Dentsply, Parkell, Hu-Friedy) manufacture various types of ultrasonic tips, including the metal stack–type ultrasonic tip (Table 9.1). Generally, the use of shorter tips for shallow pockets and longer tips for deeper pockets is recommended. Some tips have corkscrew-type angles. These are designed to advance around crowns and into furcations (Fig. 9.3).

LOCAL ANTIBIOTIC THERAPY

Antibiotics may be applied directly into periodontal pockets after root planing or periodontal debridement. In addition to the antibacterial action, there can also be anticollagenase activity.

Doxirobe

Antibiotic therapy can be used with periodontal debridement techniques. One product is Pfizer's Doxirobe gel (doxycycline hyclate), which delivers doxycycline directly to the periodontal pockets. The medication provides local delivery of an antibiotic to afford local control of the microorganisms responsible for periodontal disease. According to the manufacturer, the gel reduces periodontal pocket depth, increases attachment levels, and reduces gingival inflammation. The two-syringe system necessitates mixing before use. Syringe A contains the polymer delivery system, and syringe B contains the active ingredient (doxycycline) (Fig. 9.4). A blunted needle is used for delivery (Fig. 9.4C).

The A and B syringes should be connected to each other (Fig. 9.5A). The material is transferred back and forth 100 times (Fig. 9.5B). The material is transferred into the "A" syringe for the final mix and placed on edge

TABLE 9.1	Ultrasonic Scaler Tips		
Use/Type	Parkell	Cavitron	Hu-Friedy
Supragingival "beavertail"	DBI25, DBI30	TFI-3, TFI-9	UI325K, UI330K
Supragingival "universal"	External water: DUE25, DUE30 Internal water: DUI25, DUI30	External water: 25KP-10, 30KP-10	External water: UI1025K, UI1030K or UI25KP10, UI30KP10
Subgingival straight	Internal water: DPI25, DPI30 External water: DPE25, DPE30	Internal water: "Slimline" 25K or 35K SLI10S	"Streamline" Internal water: UI25K100S, UK30K100S, or "After Five" External water: UI25KSL10S, UI30KSL10S "After Five Plus": UI25KSF10S, UI30KSF10S
Subgingival curved	Internal water: left DPL25, DPL30 or right DPR25, DPR30	Internal water: "Slimline" left 25K or 30K SLI10L, right 25K or 30K SLI10R	"After Five" External water: left UI25KSL10L, UI30KSL10L, right UI25KSL10R, UI30KSL10R "After Five Plus": left UI25KSF10L, UI30KSF10L or right UI25KSF10R, UI30KSF10R

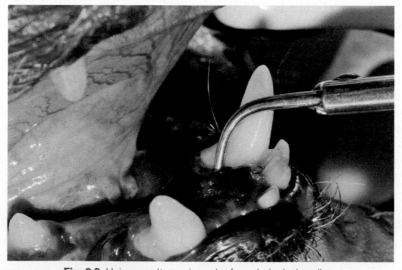

Fig. 9.3 Using an ultrasonic scaler for subgingival scaling.

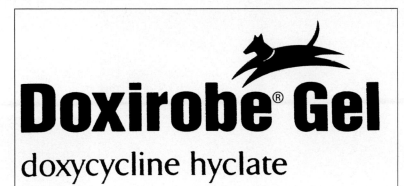

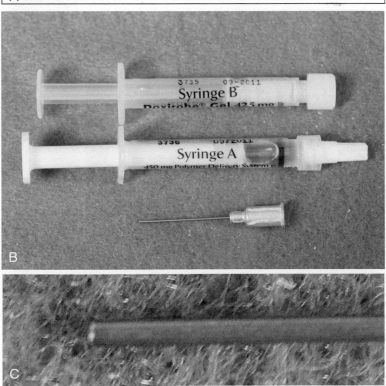

Fig. 9.4 A, Doxirobe label. B, Doxirobe contents. C, Close-up of tip of a Doxirobe needle.

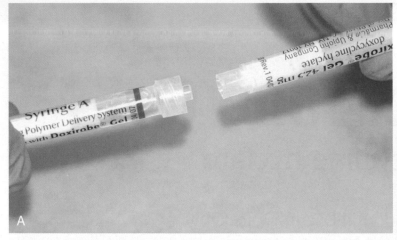

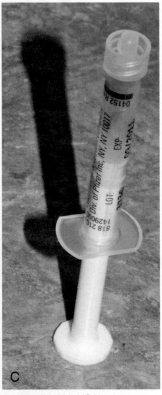

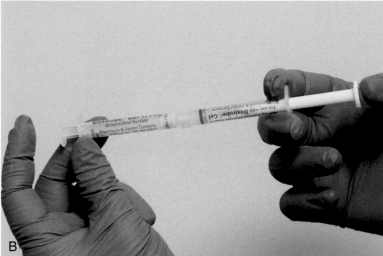

Fig. 9.5 A, Connecting Doxirobe. B, Mixing Doxirobe. C, Settling Doxirobe (Zoetis, NJ, USA).

and allowed to sit for a few minutes to allow the material to settle so that air can be expressed (Fig. 9.5C). The material is inserted into a pocket with the provided cannula (Fig. 9.6A). The gel hardens when exposed to water. The hardened material is packed into the pocket with a plastic working instrument (Fig. 9.6B).

Doxirobe gel is indicated for the treatment and control of periodontal disease in dogs. Depths greater than or equal to 4 mm in the periodontal pockets are evidence of disease that may respond to treatment with Doxirobe gel. As a medical treatment, this procedure should be performed by the veterinarian.

Arestin

Arestin (minocycline hydrochloride) is a sustained-release, locally applied antibiotic that targets the *Porphyromonas* and other bacteria that cause periodontal disease. Like Doxirobe, Arestin is indicated along with periodontal debridement. Arestin is a powder that is applied with a syringe (Fig. 9.7).

Clindoral

Clindoral (Clindoral, AL, USA) is a sol-to-gel liquid of clindamycin hydrochloride that is slowly released from the sol-to-gel matrix slowly over 7 to 10 days to fight

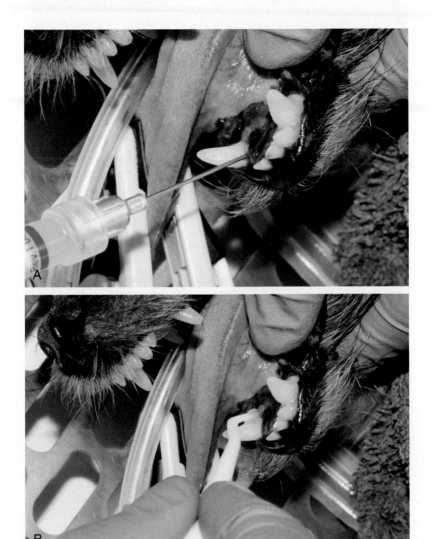

Fig. 9.6 A, Placing Doxirobe. B, Plastic working instrument.

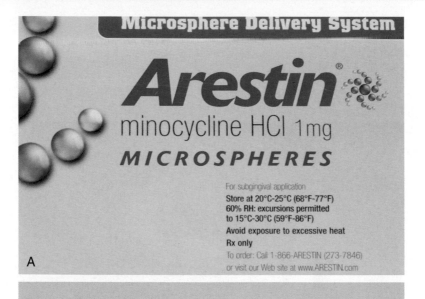

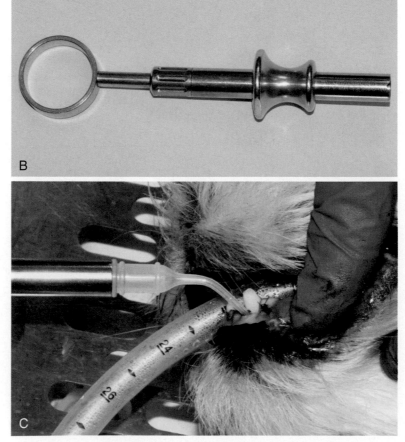

Fig. 9.7 A, Arestin label. B, Arestin syringe. C, Arestin application (http://arestinprofessional.com).

periodontal pathogens by inhibiting protein synthesis in the bacterial cell. A syringe and blunt-tipped applicator are used to infuse periodontal pockets.

MUCOSITIS IN DOGS

Oral mucositis, also referred to as chronic ulcerative paradental stomatitis (CUPS), in dogs is similar to chronic gingivostomatitis found in cats. It is believed that patients with this condition have developed intolerance to the indigenous microbial constituents of their oral cavity. The result is the development of painful ulcers of the mucosa that is in intimate contact with the accumulations of plaque on the surfaces of the teeth. Normally, microbes are present in the form of a biofilm that attaches to all oral surfaces, including the surface of the cheeks, tongue, lips, tonsils, and palate. The epithelium covering those soft tissue structures is continuously sloughed and swallowed. The bacterial community is in a constant state of flux involving attachment to epithelium and teeth and multiplication and sheading of the epithelium and biofilm. In contrast, the teeth are non-shedding surfaces, so the microbial biofilm accumulates, forms calculus and another layer of biofilm, and is not shed. The teeth may, or may not, have dental disease; in fact, mucositis can develop even in the presence of perfectly healthy teeth. However, dental disease such as periodontitis and endodontic disease will exacerbate the mucositis.

Treatment is thorough and complete professional hygiene followed by thorough home care or exodontia. Extraction works by removing the nonshedding surface. The bacterial intolerance remains present, but the contact ulcers disappear once the teeth are removed. Except for initial "rescue therapy," antibiotics, corticosteroids, oral rinses, pain medications, dental diets, and so forth, without home care or extraction, have no place in the management of this disease.

CHAPTER 9 WORKSHEET

1. The primary objective of periodontal therapy is to _____ _____ _____.
2. Periodontal therapy is performed on patients with stage _____, stage _____, or stage _____ periodontal disease.
3. _____ is the mechanical removal of plaque, calculus, and stains from the crown and root surfaces.
4. The objective of _____ _____ is to create a clean, smooth, glasslike root surface.
5. Root planing is performed using a curette with overlapping strokes in _____, _____, and _____ directions.
6. _____ _____ is the treatment of gingival and periodontal inflammation.
7. Newer research has shown that it is no longer necessary to remove _____.
8. The sonic waves produced by ultrasonic scalers have a cavitation effect, _____ the bacterial cell wall.
9. Doxirobe gel and Arestin deliver _____ directly to the periodontal pocket.
10. Doxirobe gel should be mixed _____ times before use.

Feline Dentistry

LEARNING OBJECTIVES

When you have completed this chapter, you will be able to:

- Differentiate between stomatitis, gingivitis, and periodontitis.
- Differentiate between type 1 and type 2 feline chronic gingivostomatitis.
- List the diagnostic testing used for evaluation of patients with suspected feline chronic gingivostomatitis.
- Describe the management of patients with feline chronic gingivostomatitis.
- Describe the classification scheme used to stage tooth resorption.
- List possible causes for feline orofacial pain syndrome.
- Describe alveolar osteitis.

KEY TERMS

Association of American Feed
   Control Officials
Caudal stomatitis
Calicivirus

Feline chronic gingivostomatitis
Feline orofacial pain syndrome
Hyperglobulinemia
Hyperproteinemia

Mucositis
Pasteurella species
Stomatitis
Tooth resorption

Cats have most of the conditions discussed in the other chapters. However, four conditions of the oral cavity are more common in cats than they are in other species. This chapter focuses on these conditions, but does not intend to minimize the importance of other diseases previously discussed with regard to all species. One condition associated with cats is feline chronic gingivostomatitis (FCGS). The second condition discussed is tooth resorption (TR), most recently called *feline odontoclastic resorptive lesion* (FORL), which afflicts many cats and is challenging to prevent. A third condition is alveolar osteitis and a fourth condition that is even less frequent but more difficult to treat is the feline oral pain syndrome (FOPS).

FELINE CHRONIC GINGIVOSTOMATITIS

Cause

Stomatitis is defined as "inflammation of the mucous lining of any of the structures in the mouth." It has been previously called stomatitis, faucitis, feline chronic ulcerative gingivostomatis, plasma cell stomatitis-pharyngitis, and lymphocytic-plasmacytic gingivitis-stomatitis. In clinical use the term should be reserved to describe widespread oral inflammation beyond gingivitis and periodontitis. When it extends into the mucosal tissues, it is known as *mucositis*. When it extends into the tissues of the lateral palatine folds, it may be termed *caudal stomatitis*. In other words, gingivitis and periodontitis do not constitute stomatitis unless they are part of a broader inflammation involving the mucosal tissues in the mouth.

Feline chronic gingivostomatitis is frustrating and can be difficult to manage. It is a painful, often debilitating, condition in cats with long-standing oral inflammation that typically has been present months to years before treatment is sought. Type 1 cases involve only alveolar and labial/buccal mucositis/stomatitis, and type 2 cases include caudal mucositis/stomatitis (with or without alveolar and labial/buccal mucositis/stomatitis). Type 1 cases may be manageable and teeth can be maintained, whereas type 2 cases tend to be less so (Fig. 10.1).

FCGS can be thought of as an individual, inappropriate immunologic response from the cat to a variety of antigenic triggers. The trigger factors probably include periodontal disease, tooth resorption, *Pasteurella* species, *Pseudomonas* species, *Tannerella forsythia, Chlamydophila felis,* plaque bacteria, *Bartonella* species, calicivirus, and herpesvirus in combination together or with other factors. Factors that can complicate management owing to their contribution to overall inflammation and/or immunomodulation are feline immunodeficiency virus (FIV), feline leukemia virus (FeLV), and dietary antigens. Some evidence suggests that this disease is immune-mediated or some type of aberrant immune response to one or more infectious agents and/or environmental stimuli. From the onset, the client should be advised that initial treatment is extensive and long term, therapies have potentially dangerous side effects, and some drugs used have not been approved for use in cats. An important concept in the treatment of FCGS is that whole-mouth extraction may be necessary and even with that 30% of cases will require continued medical management, and some may not respond to any treatment.

Diagnostics should go beyond a brief physical examination; however, clinical appearance and clinical signs may be enough for a diagnosis. They should include testing for calicivirus, FeLV, and FIV. They should also include a blood biochemistry profile and a complete blood count (CBC) in light of future treatment options involving anesthesia and the use of pain relief. Although these tests are often negative, they may reveal information about the cause of the individual patient's

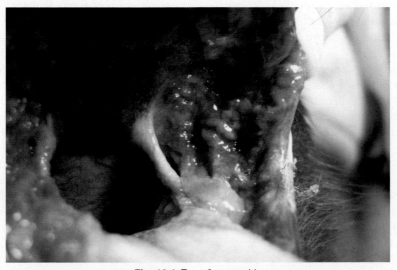

Fig. 10.1 Type 2 stomatitis.

stomatitis. Most cats with classic stomatitis have elevated blood protein (hyperproteinemia) and elevated globulin (hyperglobulinemia). A full-mouth examination under general anesthesia must include intraoral dental radiographs and periodontal charting. Good-quality photographs also aid the ability to make comparisons and gauge treatment success. Diagnosis begins with a history and a complete physical examination of the mouth, which may require chemical restraint. The examination should include observation of the buccal mucosa, tongue, gingiva, teeth, pharynx, tonsillar region, and the hard and soft palates. All surfaces should be examined for color, shape, size, consistency, surface texture, ease of bleeding, and response to pain. Gingival bleeding is one of the earliest signs that may be noted. Inflamed gingiva and mucosa may appear swollen, cobblestone-textured, bright red, or raspberry-like, which is often symptomatic of stomatitis. Light touching of the gingiva of the patient can result in spontaneous hemorrhage.

A biopsy of unusual-appearing or unilateral different-appearing tissue will rule out conditions such as eosinophilic granuloma or squamous cell carcinoma. Careful harvesting technique avoids inaccurate results.

One of the difficult diagnostic challenges is to determine whether the FCGS is an allergic reaction to an additive in commercial pet foods. Colorants, preservatives, binders, and other chemicals are added to commercial pet foods to make them more attractive to the cat and owner. If the client is cooperative, food-related causes should be investigated. Some holistic practitioners have made claims of resolution with "raw diets." There have been no studies to prove or disprove these theories.

Currently there are no approved evaluation standards, treatments, or outcome reporting standards specifically for this condition. Perhaps this is because this is a syndrome rather than one disease. Despite ongoing research, the exact etiology or etiologies have not been discovered.

Management practices come in the following four stages:

Stage 1: Complete oral health assessment and treatment (COHAT) and intraoral radiographs are mandatory. Teeth affected by resorption or periodontitis must be extracted. Retained tooth root tips must be extracted. If the client is unwilling or unable to provide this care, extraction of all caudal teeth may be a more appropriate option. Antibiotics, corticosteroids, nonsteroidal antiinflammatory drugs (NSAIDs), and pain medications are prescribed as indicated for "rescue therapy."

Corticosteroids have been the mainstay of medical management of FCGS. Their actions are complex and basically suppress the immune system, suppressing both white cells and antibody synthesis. In addition, a positive side effect is increased appetite, which is often helpful in these cats. Less desirable side effects include skin and hair coat changes, muscle wasting, insulin resistance leading to diabetes mellitus, and decreasing efficacy over time. Owing to these negative attributes, long-term use of corticosteroids is discouraged for cats with FCGS.

Stage 2: When the client cannot perform home care, extraction of all teeth caudal to the canines may be helpful. The canines and incisors can be spared if (1) the gingiva and bone are in perfect health, (2) the client is willing and able to brush the remaining teeth daily, (3) the client realizes that COHAT of the remaining teeth will be necessary every 4 to 12 months, and (4) the client accepts that quite often the canines and incisors need to be removed some time in the future. After this treatment, rescue therapy is provided again as appropriate.

Stage 3: For those cats that still do not respond, the next step may be extraction of all teeth. This is still controversial, with several studies giving contradicting results for partial mouth extraction (PME) versus full mouth extraction (FME).

As an alternative to FME, omega interferon, which may be administered by local injection and followed by daily oral dosing has shown promise in some studies. At this time, omega interferon must be imported from Europe; does not have United States Department of Agriculture (USDA) approval and must be handled very carefully to maintain potency.

Stage 4: For those cats that still do not respond, long-term antibiotic and steroid therapy is used to control the patient's condition. This treatment will need to be continuous and adapted to each patient.

Additional therapies that have worked on individual—but not all—patients include diet modification, azithromycin, cyclosporine, bovine lactoferrin, mesenchymal stem cells, and vitamin supplementation.

TOOTH RESORPTION

Cause

Another condition common in cats is tooth resorption (TR), which has had a number of names: feline odonto-clastic resorptive lesion (FORL), neck lesions, cervical line lesions, and cat cavities ("catvities"). The incidence of TR varies according to the study, but most research suggests that a little less than one-half of the cat population is clinically affected. Intraoral radiographs may increase this number to 75%. The effects of TR include resorption of the tooth and proliferation of the gingiva or pulp to cover the resulting lesion. The signs of TR are essentially those of pain. Because all patients react to pain differently, the signs may be difficult to interpret. The patient's behavior might change; some cats become aggressive or start hiding. Appetite decreases, and the animal may drop food or even hiss at it.

Many theories regarding the cause of TR have been proposed since the lesions were first reported. An early hypothesis was that they were caused by acids regurgitated with hairballs; the effect on the teeth was compared with that of humans suffering from bulimia. However, in humans the lesions tend to be on lingual surfaces, whereas in cats they occur on either side. Some researchers have suggested that the acids produced by bacteria associated with periodontal disease are responsible. However, studies have shown that periodontal disease usually follows TR. Current research indicates that TR may be caused by nutritional problems aggravated by unknown genetic factors. Excess vitamin D has been proven to cause TR in rats. However, there are conflicting studies regarding correlation between the amount of vitamin D in blood and the incidence of TR in the cat.

Diagnosis

The clinical sign of inflamed gums may initially lead the clinician to suspect that TR lesions are present. Some lesions are immediately apparent, and others are covered by hyperplastic gingiva. In most cases, the extent of the lesion is impossible to determine by visual clinical examination alone. Dental radiographs are necessary to diagnose and treat TR accurately.

AVDC Stages

The American Veterinary Dental College (AVDC) has created a system of classifying TR by stages. There is some controversy regarding this system because it is not known whether the disease progresses in stages. Also, staging assumes one cause, which may not necessarily be so.

Stage 1 (TR 1): Mild dental hard tissue loss (cementum or cementum and enamel) (Fig. 10.2).

Stage 2 (TR 2): Moderate dental hard tissue loss (cementum or cementum and enamel with loss of dentin that does not extend to the pulp cavity) (Fig. 10.3).

Stage 3 (TR 3): Deep dental hard tissue loss (cementum or cementum and enamel with loss of dentin that extends to the pulp cavity); most of the tooth retains its integrity (Fig. 10.4).

Stage 4 (TR 4): Extensive dental hard tissue loss (cementum or cementum and enamel with loss of dentin that extends to the pulp cavity); most of the tooth has lost its integrity. In Fig. 10.5, the crown and root are equally affected. Fig. 10.6 shows the crown more severely affected than the root. In Fig. 10.7, the root is more severely affected than the crown.

Stage 5 (TR 5): Remnants of dental hard tissue are visible only as irregular radiopacities, and gingival covering is complete (Fig. 10.8).

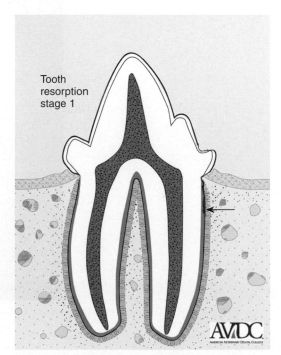

Fig. 10.2 Tooth resorption, stage 1: Enamel or cementum loss *(arrow).* (Copyright AVDC, with permission.)

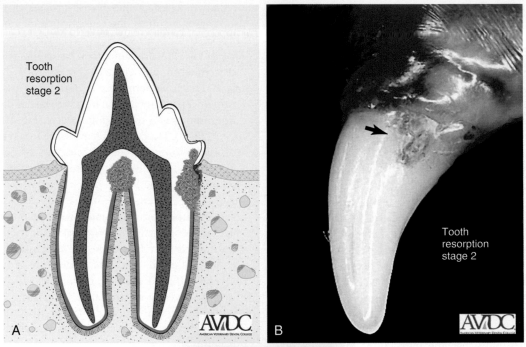

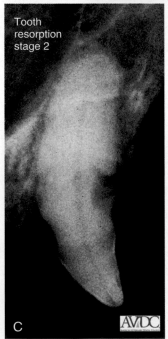

Fig. 10.3 A to C, Tooth resorption, stage 2: Deeper than stage 1 but not into pulp. (Copyright AVDC, with permission.)

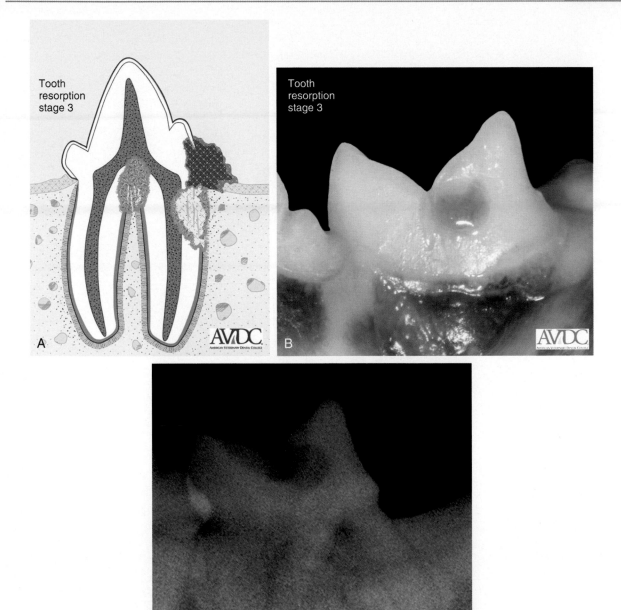

Fig. 10.4 A to C, Tooth resorption, stage 3: Into pulp but tooth maintains integrity. (Copyright AVDC, with permission.)

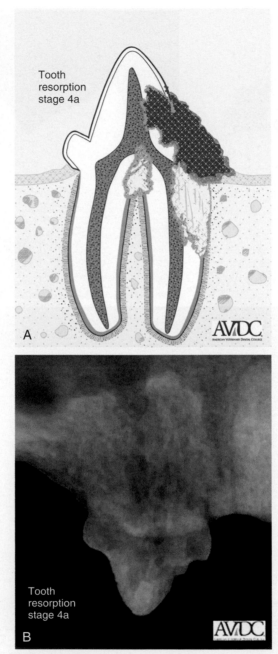

Fig. 10.5 A and B, Tooth resorption, stage 4a: Extensive tooth destruction of crown and root. (Copyright AVDC, with permission.)

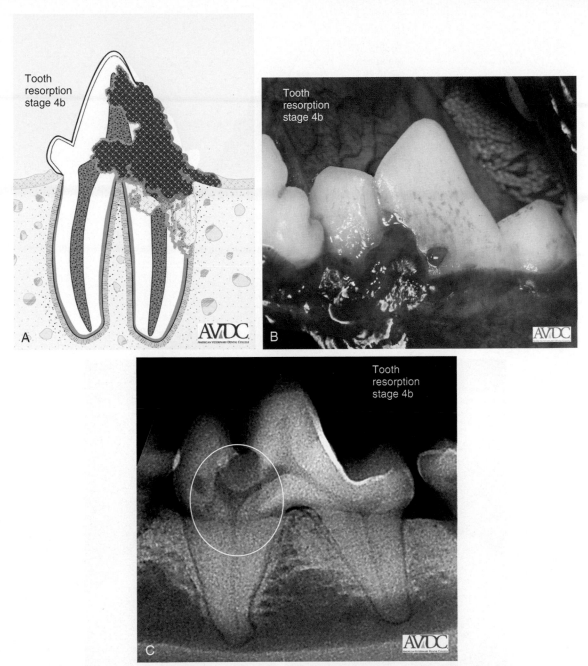

Fig. 10.6 A to C, Tooth resorption, stage 4b: Extensive tooth destruction, crown worse. (Copyright AVDC, with permission.)

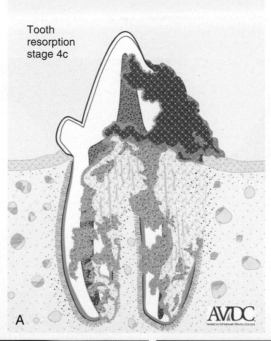

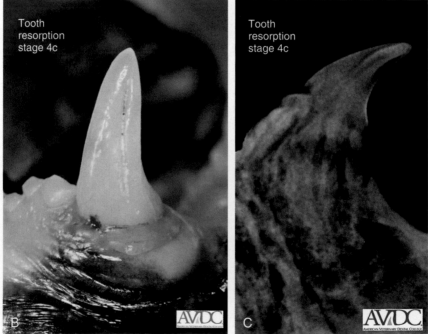

Fig. 10.7 A to C, Tooth resorption, stage 4c: Extensive tooth destruction, root worse. (Copyright AVDC, with permission.)

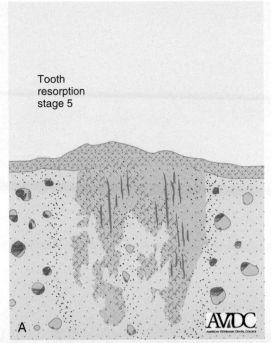

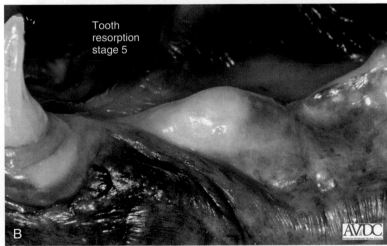

Fig. 10.8 A to C, Tooth resorption, stage 5: End stage. (Copyright AVDC, with permission.)

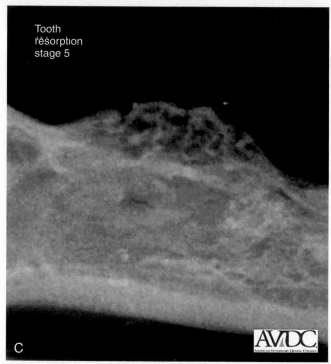

Tooth
resorption
stage 5

C

Fig. 10.8, cont'd

Treatment of Tooth Resorption

After radiographic evaluation, TR is treated by extracting teeth with stage 2 to stage 4 lesions. Stage 1 lesions usually do not cause pain, and stage 5 lesions, unless there is gingival inflammation, do not require treatment.

Prevention of Tooth Resorption

At this point, little known about prevention of TR. Although it is not known for sure, the reduction of vitamin D in the diet may have some benefit. The Association of American Feed Control Officials (AAFCO) placed upper limits of vitamin D in foods. Prior to this, there were no upper limits and many cat food manufacturers had placed more than the required amounts of vitamin D in cat foods. The AAFCO is a voluntary membership association of local, state, and federal agencies charged by law to regulate the sale and distribution of animal feeds and animal drug remedies. However, there is no requirement that cat foods follow AAFCO standards. Therefore, the client should look for an AAFCO statement on the package label.

Alveolar Osteitis

The cat often expresses canine periodontal disease or tooth resorption by a process called alveolar or buccal bone expansion or alveolar osteitis. It is commonly associated with advanced periodontal disease. Early cases can be treated by periodontal debridement and the placement of a perioceutic such as Doxirobe or Arestin. Advanced cases need extraction (Fig. 10.9).

FELINE OROFACIAL PAIN SYNDROME

Feline orofacial pain syndrome is a pain disorder of cats with behavioral signs of oral discomfort and tongue mutilation. It occurs mainly in Burmese cats. FOPS is thought to be caused by damage to nerves of the peripheral nervous system, possibly involving central and/or

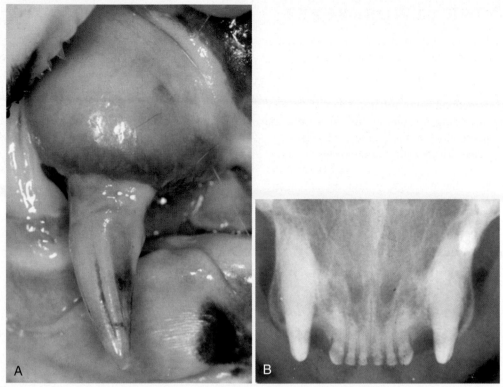

Fig. 10.9 A, Alveolar osteitis: clinical. B, Alveolar osteitis: radiograph. This patient has alveolar osteitis caused by periodontal disease and tooth resorption. The radiograph shows a deep pocket between the tooth root and bone. (Photo courtesy Dr. Jan Bellows.)

ganglion processing of sensory trigeminal information. There appears to be sensitization of trigeminal nerve endings as a consequence of oral disease such as TR or even eruption of adult teeth. The predominance within the Burmese cat breed suggests that it is an inherited disorder. Patients will have sporadic one-sided discomfort, followed by pain-free intervals. Mouth movements trigger discomfort. The disease is often recurrent and, with time, may become constant. It can be resistant to traditional pain medication but responds to anticonvulsants with an analgesic effect. Clients should establish diaries with regard to dates and times, the activity before the attack, and description of the attack. Video recording is also very useful, and video taken by a cell phone can be sufficient to make the diagnosis.

Other differential diagnoses for FOPS are retained root fragments, small intestinal lymphoma, or inflammatory bowel disease. They all may cause the same signs of grinding teeth and pawing at the mouth.

CHAPTER 10 WORKSHEET

1. Three conditions of the oral cavity more common in cats than they are in other species are _____ _____ _____, _____ _____, and _____ _____ _____ _____.

2. _____ is defined as an inflammation of the oral mucosa, including the buccal and labial mucosa, palate, tongue, floor of the mouth, and gingiva.

3. _____ cells activate immune responses.

4. _____ _____ _____ _____ is a pain disorder of cats with behavioral signs of oral discomfort and tongue mutilation.

5. In the treatment of stomatitis, _____, _____, _____, and _____ _____ are prescribed as indicated for "rescue therapy."

6. About _____ % of the domestic cat population has TR.

7. The lesions of TR cause _____ of the tooth.

8. Stage _____ lesions involve the enamel only.

9. The most common treatment for TR is _____.

10. _____ _____ are necessary to diagnose and treat TR accurately.

Intraoral Imaging

OUTLINE

LEARNING OBJECTIVES

When you have completed this chapter, you will be able to:

- List and describe the indications and contraindications for performing intraoral radiography.
- Differentiate between AC and DC dental radiographic units and describe criteria for choosing a dental radiographic unit.
- Describe the structure of intraoral radiographic film.
- List and describe the components of digital veterinary dental radiology systems.
- Differentiate between parallel and bisecting-angle dental radiographic techniques and describe when each would be used.

- List and describe the views needed for a complete intraoral radiographic study.
- Describe common complications in dental radiology related to improper exposure, positioning, and developing.
- Describe the technique for chairside processing of dental radiographic film.
- Describe normal radiographic anatomy of dogs and cats and common abnormalities that may be seen with radiographic evaluation.
- Understand the fundamentals of cone beam tomography (CBT)

KEY TERMS

Alternating current
Apex
Bisecting-angle technique
Computerized radiology (CR) phosphorous plate
Cone beam tomography
Dental radiographic film
Dental x-ray machine
Dentine
Digital veterinary dental radiology

Digital x-ray system
Digital radiology (DR) sensor
Dilaceration
Direct current
Edentulous
Embedded tooth
Exodontics
Fistula
Impacted tooth
Interproximal

Intraoral film
Kilovoltage peak
Lamina dura
Lamina lucida
Lucency
Milliamperage
Odontoblasts
Parallel technique
Pulse
SLOB rule

"I can't take dental radiographs; it costs too much to buy the dental x-ray unit and digital sensor." This is a statement commonly made by general practitioners. Yet, one cannot really practice veterinary dentistry without it. Also, if properly charged for, veterinary dentistry can help pay for other equipment in the veterinary practice that does not pay for itself. In reality, practices that do not offer intraoral radiographic services are cheating their patients, their clients, and themselves. Dental radiography may be used in all veterinary offices. Although dental radiography is surrounded by a great deal of mystique, it is not extremely difficult to master, given time and practice.

INDICATIONS FOR DENTAL RADIOGRAPHY

Dental radiographs may be used to document and study the progress of therapeutic programs in the treatment of all types of dental and oral diseases. When neoplasia or metabolic disease is suspected, radiographs may be used to evaluate the involvement of teeth and bone; in cases of oral trauma, radiographs are helpful in the evaluation of the mandible and maxilla.

Unerupted or Impacted Teeth

In young patients, radiographs help the practitioner determine whether unerupted or impacted teeth are present (Fig. 11.1). An impacted tooth is an unerupted or partially erupted tooth that is prevented from erupting further by any structure. Dental radiographs are taken in all patients to evaluate the status of root and tooth when the tooth is missing or partly erupted. The practitioner may discover that the patient is edentulous or has a dilacerated or an embedded tooth. Edentulous is the absence of teeth. A dilaceration is an abnormally shaped root resulting from trauma during tooth development (see Fig. 2.18). An embedded tooth is a tooth that is usually covered in bone, has not erupted into the oral cavity, and is not likely to erupt.

Periodontal Disease

During prophylactic or therapeutic teeth cleaning, radiographs can be used to determine the extent of periodontal disease. Dental radiographs allow the practitioner to evaluate bone loss and select an appropriate method of treatment. In patients with oral stomas (fistulas), radiographs can also be used as a diagnostic tool.

Endodontics

Radiographs allow the practitioner to evaluate the effectiveness of endodontic therapy and to study radicular

health and size before, during, and after endodontic therapy (Fig. 11.2). Chapter 13 has illustrations of endodontic before and after treatment.

Exodontics

Dental radiographs are indicated before extractions for diagnosis and evaluation of possible complications. Dental radiographs are obtained during the procedure to determine the presence of retained roots and other complications. Radiographs are indicated after extraction to ensure completeness of the procedure. Fig. 11.3 shows a preoperative radiograph of a persistent deciduous tooth. The entire root must be extracted. Fig. 11.4 shows multiple retained deciduous teeth. The canine tooth will require elevation to extract. The second, third, and fourth premolar roots have resorbed and are being held in place by attached gingiva. They should be removed for the patient's comfort.

Routine Dental Procedures

Routine dental radiographs on all patients undergoing anesthesia will result in findings that were undetected during clinical examination 25% of the time in dogs and 40% of the time in cats. This is a very high diagnostic yield.

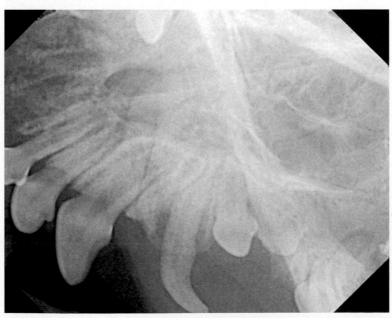

Fig. 11.1 Missing adult canine.

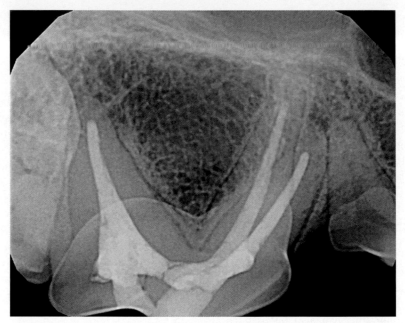

Fig. 11.2 After root canal therapy.

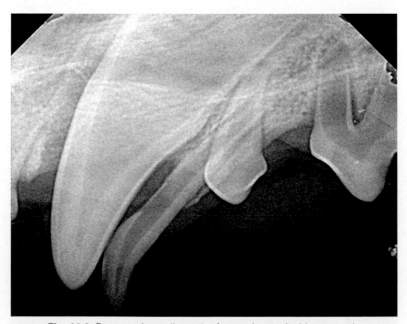

Fig. 11.3 Preoperative radiograph of a persistent deciduous tooth.

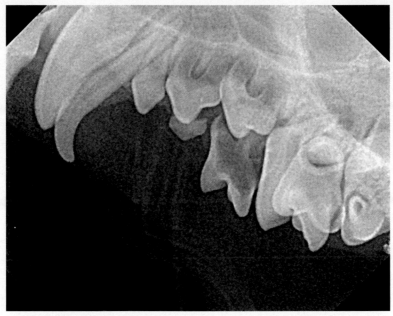

Fig. 11.4 Radiograph of multiple retained deciduous teeth.

CONTRAINDICATION FOR DENTAL RADIOLOGY

Dental radiology is contraindicated in critical patients that may have difficulty undergoing anesthesia, which is necessary to allow proper patient positioning. Dental radiology may be used in diagnosis, documentation of progress, and referral consultation.

DENTAL RADIOGRAPHIC EQUIPMENT AND MATERIALS

Veterinary Medical Machines

Dental radiographs can be taken using veterinary medical radiographic units. However, these require considerable effort in positioning the patient. With the stationary radiographic unit, the patient must be moved several times to reorient the head.

Dental Machines

The advantage of the dental radiographic unit is its fairly flexible radiographic head and jointed extension arm. The unit can be angled, which minimizes the need for patient repositioning. Human nature being as it is, practitioners tend to take more radiographs when the unit is easy to use. The greater the number of radiographs, the greater the amount of diagnostic information.

There are two types of current that can be input into dental x-ray machine heads: alternating current (AC) and direct current (DC). In most dental machines, the amount of voltage applied to the tube determines the power of the x-ray. An AC unit (that produces a sine wave) produces impulses of x-rays. In the United States, the rate is 60 pulses every second; in some parts of the world, the rate is 50 pulses per second. The amount is measured at its kilovoltage peak (kVp). DC units are actually more like very high-frequency AC units—they produce a wave in the 70,000 cycles per second range. Thus, the high pulse is not perceived and is expressed as kilovolt (kV) and the power is more consistent. Therefore, a DC unit is used with less kV than an AC unit's kVp. Milliamperage (mA) is often fixed in AC dental x-ray units—most typically at 7 mA, but it can be 6 or 8 mA; mA is usually variable in DC x-ray units—typically in a range of 4 to 8 mA.

There are two important criteria in choosing an x-ray unit. First, the stability of the arm is important, especially if there is a long reach from where the x-ray unit is mounted and the patient. Good arms hardly wobble after they are positioned. The second criterion is the focal spot size inside the x-ray head—the smaller the spot, the sharper the image: a 0.4-mm spot will be much sharper than a 0.7-mm spot.

The kVp in most dental radiographic units is fixed and usually does not need to be adjusted. Likewise, the mA is fixed for most units. Time, however, is a variable that may require adjustment according to the thickness of the area to be studied. Some units measure time in portions of a second and others set time in impulses—one impulse equals one-sixtieth of a second; thus, 30 impulses would equal 0.5 second.

Dental x-ray units may be mounted on the wall (Fig. 11.5A), on stands (Fig. 11.5B and C), or handheld (Fig. 11.5D). The advantage of a wall-mounted unit is that it has a smaller footprint than stand-mounted units. However, wall-mounted units cannot be moved from room to room. Stand-mounted units take space in the dental operatory but can be moved around to different rooms or tables. Handheld units tend to be less powerful than stand-mounted (floor-mounted) units.

Intraoral Film

Intraoral radiographic film is inexpensive, small, and flexible. It fits neatly into the oral cavity and conforms to the area in which it is placed. Intraoral film is non-screen film, which provides greater detail than the screen films used in most veterinary situations. Intraoral film can be processed in 1 to 2 minutes in rapid developer and fixer solutions, with minimal loss of detail. This film allows small areas of interest to be isolated.

Description

Most intraoral film is composed of a series of layers. A plastic coating covers the external portion. Between the plastic coating and the radiographic film is a layer of paper. The next layer is the radiographic film, sandwiched by another layer of paper. Finally, a layer of lead is followed by another layer of paper that can be peeled from the plastic coating. Some manufacturers have combined the lead and paper layers (Fig. 11.6).

Dental Radiographic Film Sizes

Dental radiographic film is available in a number of sizes. DF-58, which is size 2 film, is the most common film used in human dentistry. It is also called *periapical film*. In veterinary dentistry, this type of film is suitable for small patients. DF-50, or size 4 film, is also called *occlusal film* and is appropriate for larger patients. For cats, size 0 may be useful for radiographic evaluation of the mandible.

Digital Radiology

Digital veterinary dental radiology (DVDR) for veterinary dentistry has made intraoral radiology possible in all practices. Although it is very easy to learn, there is a learning curve to the process. This learning curve can be cut short by proper training.

The two basic components to DVDR are (1) the dental x-ray machine and (2) the digital x-ray system. These components are independent and can be purchased from different manufacturers. The dental x-ray machine consists of a control unit, a tube head that produces radiation, a collimator that aims and confines the radiation, and a timer that turns the unit on.

One digital x-ray system, which is known as direct or digital radiology (DR), uses a sensor (Fig. 11.7) to capture the image. DR sensors have almost unlimited uses, unless one does bad things to them, such as drop them, soak them, or allow animals to bite them. Another digital system has a phosphorous plate (Fig. 11.8A) and processing unit (Fig. 11.8B); this system is known as indirect or computerized radiology (CR). In either case, a laptop or desktop computer is used to process and read the image on a computer screen. Although there are differences in appearance, the function is very similar for either of these systems. One of the most important components to the whole system is the computer that is being used to read the image. Both the graphics card and monitor must be high quality and capable of image reproduction.

A unique dental unit is a combination dental table, x-ray generator, and digital sensor (Fig. 11.9).

Prior to taking any intraoral radiographs, it is important to be concerned with radiation safety. Individual and area radiation monitors should be used. The patient and dental x-ray machine should always be positioned so that radiation is never aimed directly at coworkers. Shields and protective devices should always be used if there is any chance of exposure.

The equipment also must be protected, because it is very fragile and subject to damage from being dropped or bitten or from water getting inside. Protective covers should be placed on the unit and secured (Fig. 11.10). Another way to be safer is to use Velcro to attach a wire from the sensor to the x-ray arm. Some units come with the sensor attached to the radiographic machine arm (Fig. 11.11).

Text continued on page 231

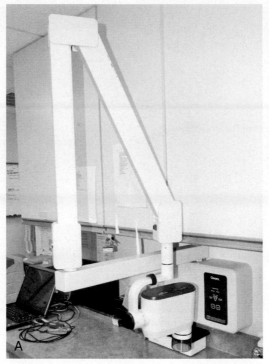

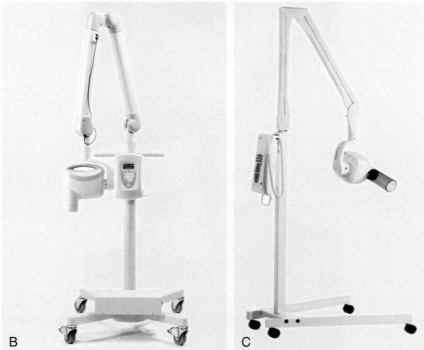

Fig. 11.5 A, Wall-mounted x-ray unit. B and C, Stand x-ray units.

Continued

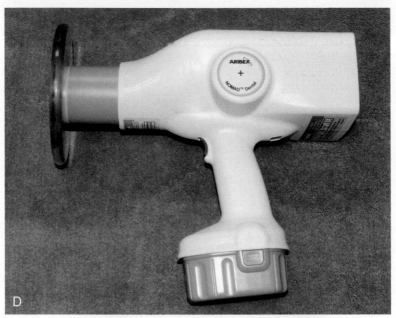

Fig. 11.5, cont'd D, Handheld x-ray unit.

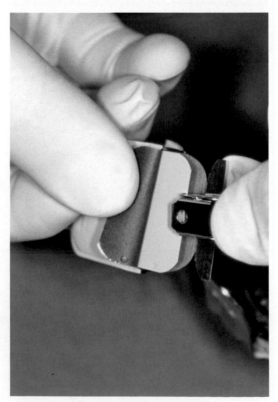

Fig. 11.6 Inside intraoral film.

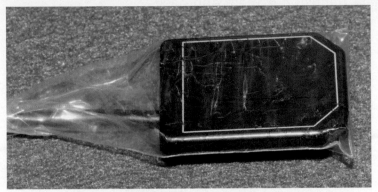

Fig. 11.7 Digital sensor for digital or direct radiology.

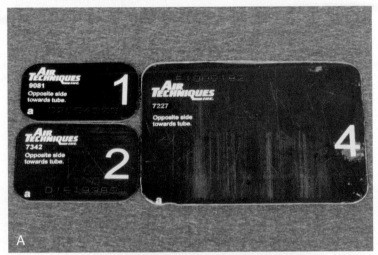

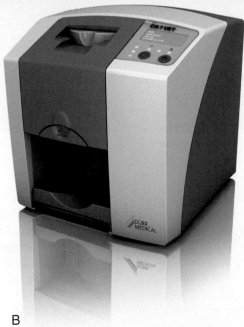

Fig. 11.8 Plates (A) and processing unit (B) for computerized radiography.

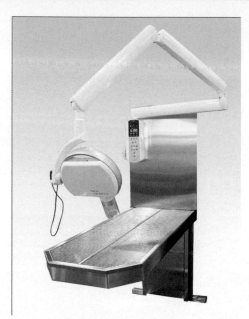

Fig. 11.9 X-mind unity on vet table. A dental unit that combines work table, x-ray generator, and sensor in one unit. (Photo courtesy Dental Focus.)

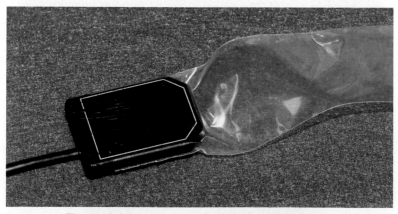

Fig. 11.10 Protective covers should be used at all times.

The protective cover will not protect the sensor from animal bites. The patient must be completely anesthetized. Even the slightest flexing may damage a sensor (Fig. 11.12).

It is important to understand how both the dental x-ray machine and digital x-ray system work. Most dental x-ray machines have fixed kVp and mA. The user only sets the time. Two types of timers measure portions of seconds and pulses. Some timers are in units of 1/100th of a second. Other timers use a "pulse," which is 1/60th of a second; thus, 6 pulses equals 1/10th of a second. The third type of timer uses a chart, which graphically represents areas of the mouth. In this type of timer, the user must select dog or cat, select digital, and indicate which tooth is being radiographed. Also, some units have a sensitivity setting, which must be set to digital.

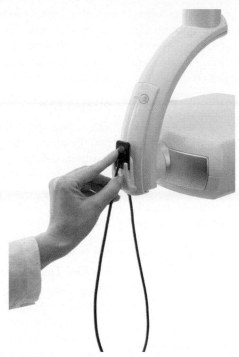

Fig. 11.11 This unit has the direct radiology sensor cord running through the arm with storage on the arm, making it difficult to damage if dropped. (Courtesy Dental Focus.)

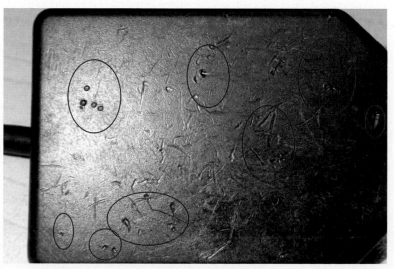

Fig. 11.12 This sensor damage on the outside *(red circles)* may destroy the electronics inside.

Because radiation is invisible, practitioners often have a difficult time in understanding positioning. Visual aids can make this easier. A flashlight can be used to visualize the direction of radiation. An extracted tooth or model tooth can be positioned to visualize a shadow on a white card to represent the image cast by radiation.

When it comes to actual application, a live patient is not the place to practice taking radiographs. Skulls (see www.skullsunlimited.com) should be used to perfect the technique. Although children's play dough is not used in clinical practice, it can be used to position the skull and sensor. In practice, a clean washcloth, laparotomy pad, or gauze can be used to position the sensor.

Protective Measures

Personnel should protect themselves by wearing lead safety aprons and using screens. They should also maintain a safe distance from the beam of radiation emitted by the radiographic unit. A variety of devices may be used to hold the film in place. Placing the film in holders, resting the film against the endotracheal tube, and securing the film with gauze sponges are a few common methods.

Radiographic Technique

In general, the following tips are helpful to obtain the best technique in setting up for exposure. The distance of the x-ray machine head from the patient should be kept as short as possible. On most radiographic units, the lower mA (e.g., 50 mA) settings use the smaller focal spots. The smaller the focal spot, the sharper the image. The beam of the x-ray unit should be collimated to include only the area of the subject needed.

The following technique is used: First, the radiographic unit control panel is set for the appropriate mA, kVp, and time. Optimal image is created with a proper balance between kVp and mA. This image will provide a full range of tones from white to black. The practitioner should determine the proper balance. When kVp is low, the result is low density and high contrast. When the kVp is high, the result is high density with very little contrast. The patient is positioned appropriately for the radiograph to be taken. The intraoral film is placed in the proper position. As an aid in positioning the film, a mouth gag, film wedge,

or other object can be placed behind the film. The head of the x-ray machine is placed 8 to 12 inches or as close as possible from the structure being evaluated and positioned for the study. The film is exposed and then developed.

Placing Film

The radiographic film should be placed in the mouth so that the plastic side is facing toward the subject and head (position-indicating device) of the radiographic unit. Most radiographic film is printed with a message such as "opposite side toward radiographic unit." A maximal amount of root and supporting bone should be included in the film. Placing the radiographic film in such a way that most of the film is not over tooth and bone is ineffective.

Parallel Technique

The parallel technique for oral radiographs is indicated to evaluate the caudal mandibular teeth and nasal cavity. The x-ray film packet is placed parallel to the structure to be radiographed. In the posterior mandible (for mandibular premolar and molar teeth), the x-ray film packet or sensor is inserted between the tongue and mandible (Figs. 11.13 and 11.14).

In many areas of the mouth, the parallel technique cannot be used. Other structures in the mouth are superimposed on the x-ray film on exposure or prevent the film from being placed parallel to the subject. Examples are the rostral and caudal maxilla, where the hard and soft palates are in the way, and the rostral mandible, where the mandible prevents placing the film parallel to the teeth.

Bisecting-Angle Technique

In areas where the parallel technique cannot be used, the bisecting angle should be used. The bisecting angle is obtained by visualizing an imaginary line that bisects the angle formed by the x-ray film and the structure being radiographed (Fig. 11.15). If the x-ray beam is aimed at the tooth, the image on the finished film will be distorted by elongation (Fig. 11.16). If the x-ray beam is aimed at the film, the image will also be distorted, this time by foreshortening (Fig. 11.17). To obtain a proper radiograph, the x-ray machine head is positioned so that the beam of the x-ray will be perpendicular to the imaginary bisecting-angle line. When first learning this technique, some technicians find it helpful to use

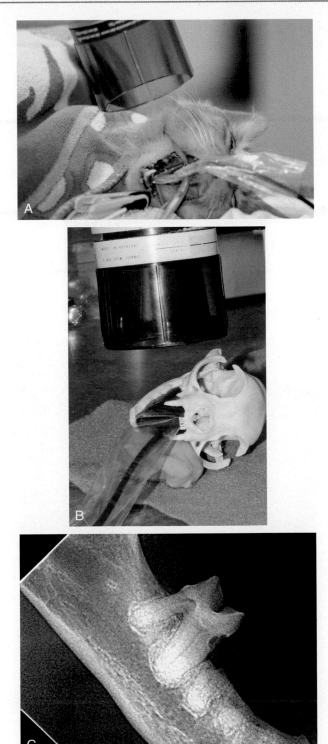

Fig. 11.13 A, Mandibular caudal cat photograph. B, Mandibular caudal cat skull. C, Mandibular caudal x-ray of a cat.

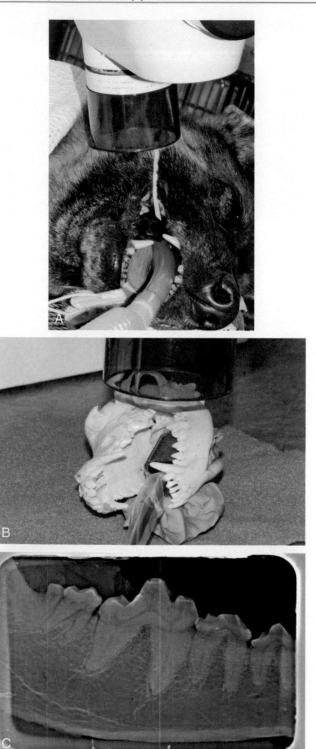

Fig. 11.14 A, Mandibular caudal dog photograph. B, Mandibular caudal dog skull. C, Mandibular caudal x-ray of a dog.

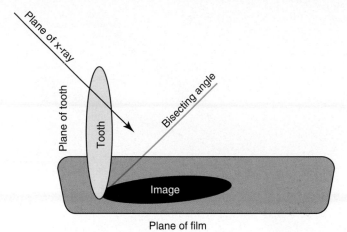

Fig. 11.15 The plane of the tooth is at a 90-degree angle to the film. The bisecting angle is therefore 45 degrees. The radiographic cone is aimed at this imaginary line. As a result, the image is recorded with slight magnification.

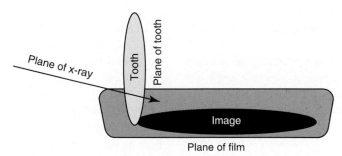

Fig. 11.16 Elongation caused by aiming the radiographic cone at the tooth rather than the bisecting angle.

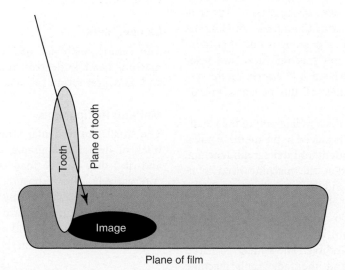

Fig. 11.17 Foreshortening caused by aiming the radiographic cone toward the film.

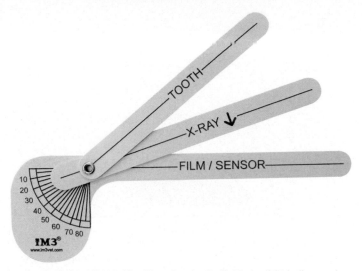

Fig. 11.18 Bisecting Angle Guide X8000. The Bisecting Angle Guide by iM3 indicates the angle to be aimed.

props, such as sticks (cotton-tipped applicators), to help visualize the bisecting angle.

Spending a lot of time with a protractor to measure all the angles and find the perfect bisecting angle is a waste of effort. Instead, it is easier to follow some simple rules. However, there are some devices that can make it easier (Fig. 11.18).

Maxillary caudal. For the maxillary caudal teeth (premolars and molars), the film is simply placed across the maxilla parallel to the hard palate. The film is placed so that it does not favor the left or right side; rather, it has an equal margin on both sides of the maxilla. The long end of the film is parallel with the muzzle. Angling the film as close to the tooth as possible is not important. The patient and radiograph machine head are positioned so that the machine head is 45 degrees off the vertical and horizontal planes of the patient's muzzle (Figs.11.19 and 11.20).

Maxillary rostral. To take a radiograph of the maxillary rostral teeth, the film is placed in the mouth parallel to the hard palate. The patient and radiograph machine head are positioned so that the machine head is 45 degrees off the vertical and horizontal planes of the patient's muzzle (Figs. 11.21 and 11.22).

Mandibular rostral. To take a radiograph of the mandibular anterior teeth, the film is placed in the mouth parallel to the mandible. The patient is placed in dorsal recumbency, and the radiograph machine head is positioned so that it is 20 degrees off the vertical plane of the anterior mandible or 70 degrees off the horizontal plane of the anterior mandible (Figs. 11.23 and 11.24).

Complete Study

The complete radiographic study can be obtained in as little as six views: right and left posterior maxilla, right and left posterior mandible, anterior maxilla, and anterior mandible. Larger patients require additional films to cover all the teeth.

Canine Teeth

The canine teeth are best evaluated by placing the machine head 45 degrees from the front of the patient and 45 degrees from the side of the patient.

Marking Radiographs

The small size of dental x-ray film can make keeping track of dental radiographs difficult. Once developed and dry, they can be inadvertently shuffled and lost. Alternatively, after exposure, the film may be written on with radiographic marking pens. The developed films can also be fixed in cardboard or plastic film mounts on which the film, patient, and owner information is written. The dimple on the film should be on the right side of

Text continued on page 242

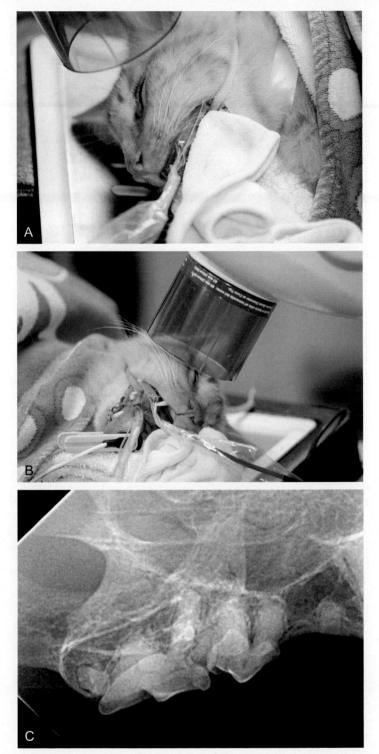

Fig. 11.19 A and B, Maxillary caudal photographs of a cat (different views). C, Maxillary caudal x-ray of a cat.

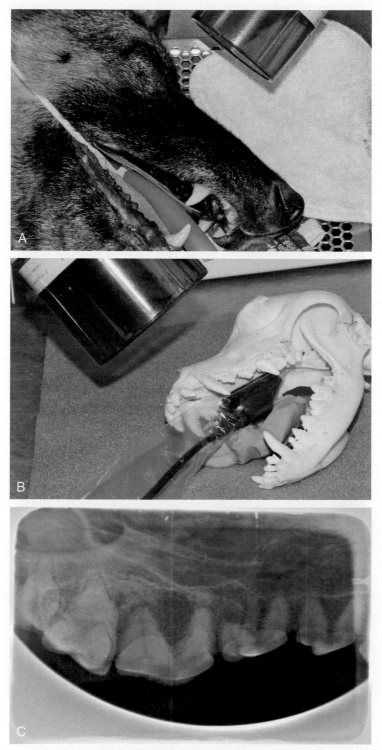

Fig. 11.20 A, Maxillary caudal photograph of a dog. B, Maxillary caudal dog skull. C, Maxillary caudal x-ray of a dog.

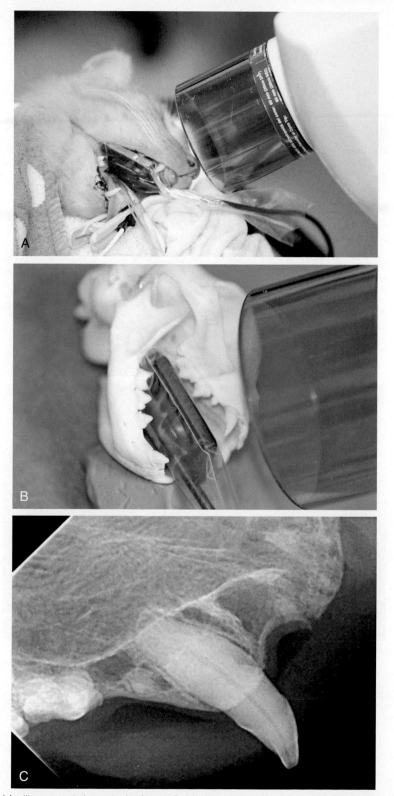

Fig. 11.21 A, Maxillary rostral photograph of a cat. B, Maxillary rostral cat skull. C, Maxillary rostral x-ray of a cat.

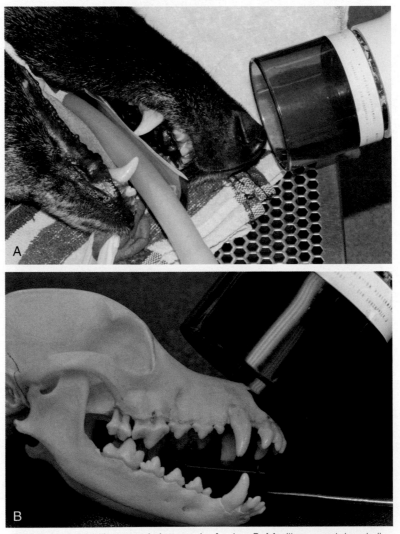

Fig. 11.22 A, Maxillary rostral photograph of a dog. B, Maxillary rostral dog skull.

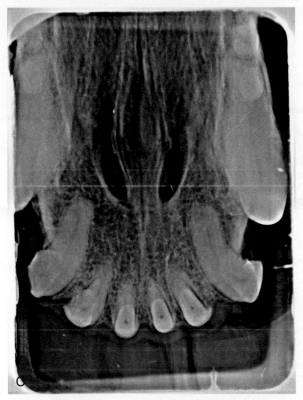

Fig. 11.22, cont'd C, Maxillary rostral x-ray of a dog.

the mouth or upper on the right mandible and lower on the left mandible. In this way the dimple (or number placed next to the dimple) will be "in the air" on the right side and "in the bone" on the left.

The advantage of DR is that the image can be marked as it is exposed.

Positioning Guides

iM3 has developed an x-ray positioning kit with the aim of making it easier to position the plate. The system consists of the positioning kit, size 2, 4, and 5 plate protector; 30-, 45-, and 55-degree angle guides; and positioning diagrams for dogs and cats. In addition, size 2, 4, and 5 image plates are required for cats and dogs developed by iM3 for use in the iM3 CR7 VET x-ray processor. The CR image plate is put into the bite protector and the angle guide is placed in the edge of the bite protector

in the center. The angle guide gives the bisecting angle to aim for and the distance from the CR plate, and the center of the CR plate (Fig. 11.25). For example, for a dogs's maxillary lateral view, use the 45-degree angle guide and a size 4 image plate (Fig. 11.26).

Trouble Spots

Maxillary fourth premolar. The maxillary fourth premolar has three roots. Most of the time it is impossible to evaluate all three roots with a single radiograph. Multiple radiographs need to be taken by keeping the sensor in the same position and moving the radiographic cone rostral or caudal. The SLOB (**s**ame **l**ingual, **o**pposite **b**uccal) rule describes what to do when the mesiobuccal and palatal roots are lining up together. When the machine cone is moved forward, the root on the image that appears to move forward is the

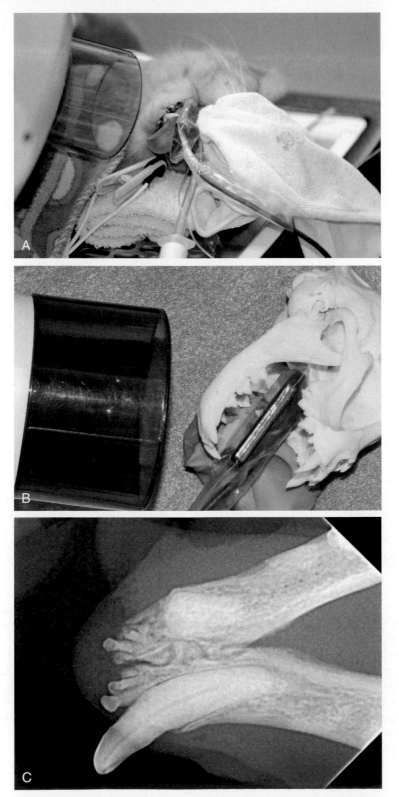

Fig. 11.23 A, Mandibular rostral photograph of a cat. B, Mandibular rostral cat skull. C, Mandibular rostral x-ray of a cat.

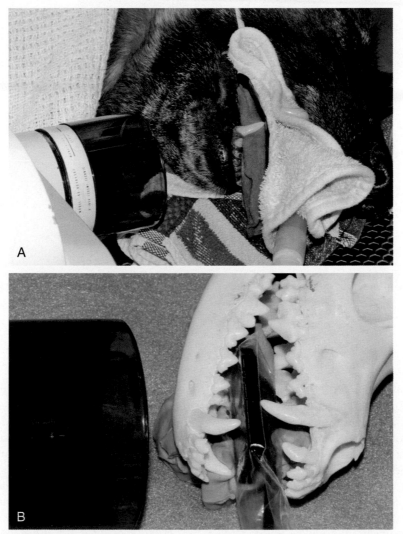

Fig. 11.24 A, Mandibular rostral photograph of a dog. B, Mandibular rostral dog skull.
Continued

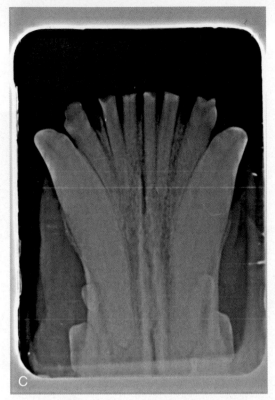

Fig. 11.24, cont'd C, Mandibular rostral x-ray of a dog.

lingual (palatal) root. The mesial root moves in the opposite direction. One trick to learn this is to use your fingers. For the right maxillary fourth premolar use your right hand. Hold up the thumb to represent the distal root, the index finger to represent the mesiobuccal root, and the middle finger to represent the palatal root. Holding the index and middle fingers so they line up would represent an overlap of the mesiobuccal and palatal roots. If the observer's head is tilted to the left without moving the fingers, the middle finger, representing the palatal (lingual) root, will move in the same direction (right or forward) as the tilting head (Fig. 11.27).

Maxillary second molar. Because of the thickness of the sensor, it is often difficult to get the sensor back far enough in the mouth to reach the maxillary second

molar. The solution is to place it as far back as possible, then move the machine head further caudal and aim it more rostral.

Mandibular third molar. Because of the thickness of the sensor and the musculature and angle of the jaw, it may be difficult to position the sensor back far enough to reach the mandibular third molar. The solution is to move the machine head further caudal and aim it more rostral.

Maxillary canine. Because of the location of the maxillary canine, the best bisecting angle may be angled midway between the front and side of the muzzle and midway from the plane of the tooth and plane of the sensor.

Feline caudal maxillary teeth. Owing to the shape of the head and zygomatic arch, many times the zygomatic arch will obscure visualization of the roots of the third

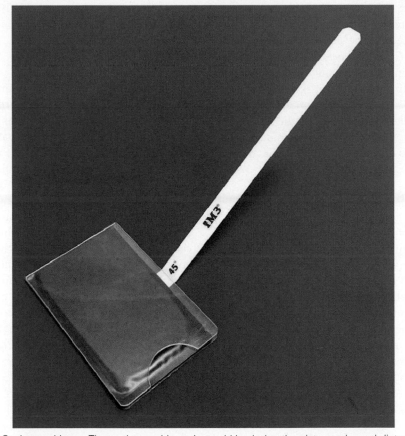

Fig. 11.25 Canine positioner. The canine positioner is an aid in placing the plate, angle, and distance.

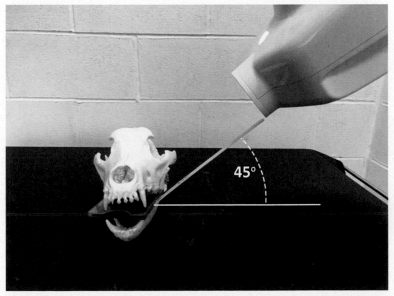

Fig. 11.26 Dog maxilla 45. With plate inserted, the positioner is placed in the mouth; using the guide, the x-ray generator can be aimed at the patient at the proper angle and distance.

and fourth premolar. Two techniques are used to overcome this. The extraoral technique places the sensor directly on the tabletop. The patient's head is placed on the sensor, with mouth opened about 1½ inches and mandibular canines tipped about 1 inch off the table. The x-ray beam is directed so that it skylines the palate (Fig. 11.28).

The almost parallel technique places the film on the opposite side of the mouth that is being studied. The radiographic beam is directed so that it skylines the palate (Fig. 11.29).

Dolichocephalics, Brachycephalics, and Toy Breeds

Anything off the "normal" head is going to require practice, practice, and practice! The big advantage to the digital sensor in this situation is that most of the time it is the machine head that requires moving. Radical deviations in the position of the cone head are often necessary. The radiograph can be taken after a slight or major adjustment to the machine cone.

By taking the time to train staff to take radiographs, DVDR can greatly add to patient and user benefit. Depending on the size of the patient and number of radiographs taken, a typical DVDR series can be performed in 10 to 15 minutes.

Efficient Radiology

One common complaint about intraoral radiology is that it takes too long. The process requires being as efficient as possible. It can be beneficial to use the restaurant server analogy. There are some that are extremely efficient and quick and others that are inefficient and slow. The ones that are efficient and quick have a pattern— they never go anywhere empty-handed. A repetitive pattern must be established when taking radiographs. Back-and-forth trips between the computer, the patient, and the radiographic unit must be minimized. A pattern that can work well is position patient (the author prefers lateral recumbency), set-up computer, position sensor, position x-ray machine head, set-up dental radiographic machine, step away, and warn that a radiograph is about to be taken. Then expose, review, correct or set-up next, and repeat. The key is to be systematic, taking the radiographs in the order of the dental chart if selecting your own radiographs, or to follow template order if

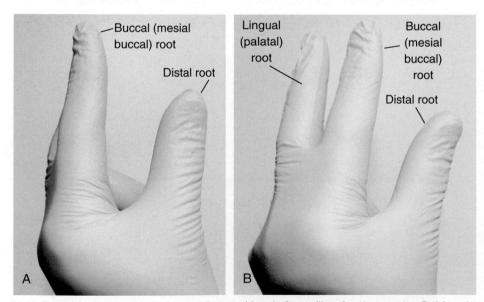

Fig. 11.27 Example of using fingers. A, Lined-up position. Left maxillary fourth premolar. B, Moved to left positioning.

Continued

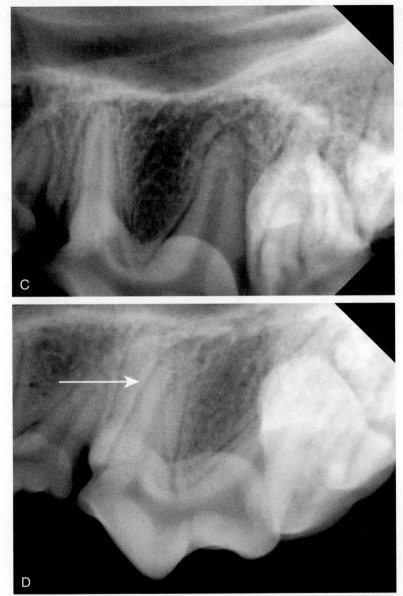

Fig. 11.27, cont'd C, Lined-up radiograph. D, Machine head moved to left radiograph, lingual (palatal) root *(arrow).*

following template. The following order has worked well for the author, using a cat as the example:

1. Caudal maxilla, sensor parallel with palate, tip of sensor on tip of cusp of fourth premolar, machine head at 45-degree angle. This should take a radiograph of the second, third, and fourth premolars and the first molar.
2. Without moving the sensor, move the machine head to 45-degree angle from side, 45 degrees from front. This should take a radiograph of the incisors, canines, and second premolars. If the zygoma obscures

visibility, it may be necessary to note this and take either extraoral or almost parallel radiographs.

3. Move the sensor to caudal mandible, between mandible and tongue. This should take a radiograph of the third and fourth premolars and first molar.
4. Move the sensor parallel with the mandible, sensor at tip of canine cusp, aim x-ray head to 45 degrees from side, 70 degrees from front. This should take a radiograph of the incisors, canines, and premolars.

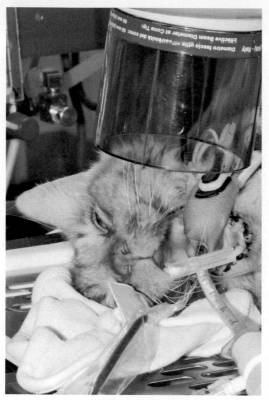

Fig. 11.28 Extraoral technique.

COMPLICATIONS IN DENTAL RADIOLOGY

Complications in dental radiology occur because of improper exposure, positioning, and developing. Table 11.1 is a troubleshooting guide.

Failure to Position Film Sensor Properly

There is a tendency to attempt to get as close to the tooth as possible. This may result in the film or sensor's "real estate" being wasted (Fig. 11.30).

Blurred or Double Images

Movement of either the patient or the x-ray machine head causes blurred or double images. If the movement continues throughout the exposure, the image will be blurred. When the film is in one position for part of the exposure and then moved to a second position for the remainder of the exposure, a double image results. Tongue movement in lightly sedated patients may also cause the film to move.

Elongation of Image

If the image appears elongated, the radiographic cone head was probably aimed too directly at the subject as opposed to bisecting the angle between the subject

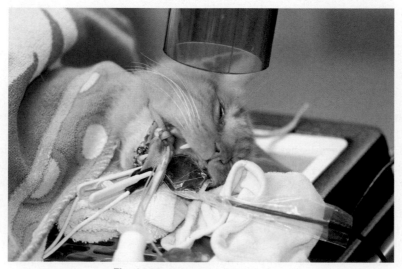

Fig. 11.29 Almost parallel technique.

TABLE 11.1 **Troubleshooting Guide for Dental Radiology**

Error	Correction
Backside of sensor electronics or no image	Turn over the sensor
Missing tooth	Reposition sensor or machine cone
Elongation	Reposition machine cone to aim more at film
Foreshortening	Reposition machine cone to aim more at the sensor
Blurring	Make sure patient is not moving Make sure radiographic unit is not swinging
Underexposure	Increase exposure time or decrease distance
Overexposure	Decrease exposure time or add distance
Cervical burnout	Take multiple exposures at multiple timings
Out of dynamic range	Take multiple exposures
No exposure	Was button held down long enough? Lights on? Make sure the unit is plugged in Check fuses Check digital sensor (is it backward?) Reboot computer

and film or sensor. Another possibility is that the film was placed incorrectly (Fig. 11.31). To correct, first check film placement and, if this was correct, aim the machine head more toward the film.

Foreshortening of Image

If the image appears foreshortened, the radiographic cone head may have been aimed too directly at the radiographic film or sensor as opposed to the bisecting angle. Another cause is improper positioning of the film (Fig. 11.32).

Overlapping Dental Structures

To determine the identity of three-dimensional structures seen on a two-dimensional plane, particularly in the evaluation of maxillary fourth premolar palatal and mesiobuccal roots, a second film is taken, with the x-ray beam moved either anterior or posterior to the previous position of the radiographic cone head. The structure that is more lingual (the palatal root) will be shadowed on the film in the same direction as the x-ray beam. The structure that is more buccal (the mesiobuccal root) will be shadowed in the opposite direction as the x-ray beam. This phenomenon may be remembered by the SLOB rule. When successive radiographs are taken, the most lingual (palatal) root will move in the same direction on the radiograph as the cone head was repositioned. If the cone is moved forward, the lingual root will be the root that moves forward.

RADIOGRAPHIC FILM PROCESSING

With the standard hand-tank developing method, the same procedure is used as for other x-ray film. Specialized racks or holders may be used to hold the film(s) during the developing process. The advantage of this technique is that additional equipment and material are not required. The most significant disadvantage is the slow developing time. Automatic processors establish constant developing and fixing, eliminating human error and decreasing operator time. Unless the processor is designed to transport small films, this method will present difficulties. Automatic dental film processors are expensive. The use of "leaders" and large film processors is impractical and therefore discouraged. The two-step rapid processing technique is recommended. Solutions designed for rapid developing and fixing of dental film are used in small dip tanks. One tank is for the developer, one or two tanks for the water rinse, and one for the fixer. Small dip tanks may be bought for this purpose or empty, clean medicine jars may be used. The dip tanks may be housed in a darkroom or in a "chairside darkroom." A chairside darkroom is a plastic box that allows the developing of radiographs at chairside. The box has two holes for the operator's hands and a Plexiglas shield that does not allow the radiograph to be exposed to light but still allows the operator to see the processing.

Technique

The solutions are stirred to mix. In a dark environment the film is opened and attached to a film clip. The film clip must be dry and not contaminated with solution from previous developing radiographs. The paper must be completely removed from the radiographic film or

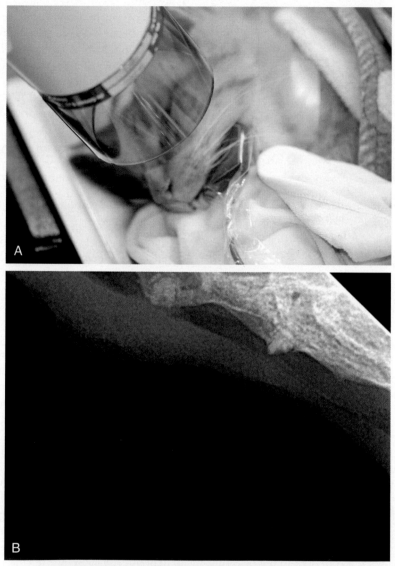

Fig. 11.30 A, Too much air positioning. B, Too much air radiograph.

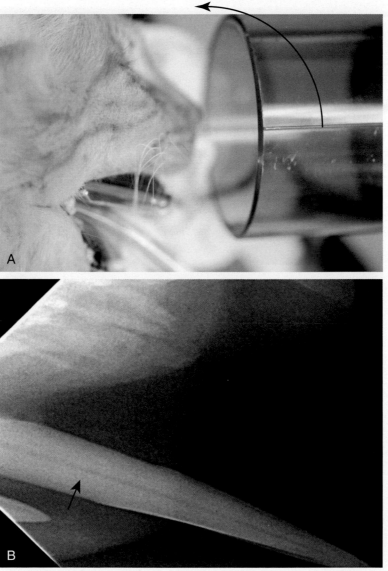

Fig. 11.31 A, Elongated incorrect positioning. B, Extremely elongated radiograph of canine tooth *(arrow)*.

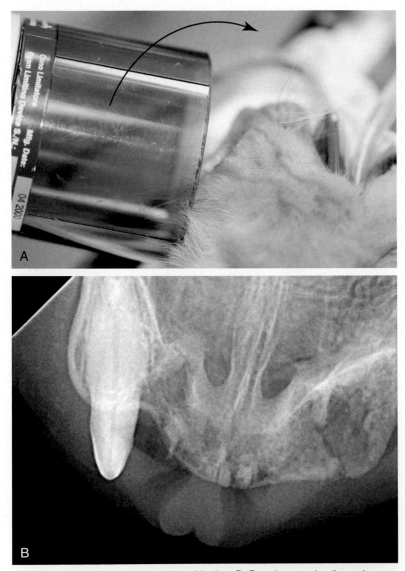

Fig. 11.32 A, Foreshortened positioning. B, Foreshortened radiograph.

the developer and fixer will not penetrate the paper, and the radiograph will have to be retaken. Placing the film in water for approximately 5 seconds softens the emulsion and ensures equal penetration of the developer into the film.

The film is then immersed in the developer and briefly agitated to remove any bubbles. The time that the film is left in the developer depends on the solution and the temperature; the manufacturer's recommendations should always be followed. The film is removed from the developer with minimal drip-back into the developing tank. The film is placed into the water rinse and dipped five times. The film is then transferred to the fixer and intermittently agitated during its fixing. The fixing is usually twice the developing time.

After the time prescribed by the manufacturer, the film is transferred into the final rinse. The fixer is allowed to drip back into the fixing tank. The film may be read at any time, but it should be returned for a minimum of 10 minutes to a fresh water rinse. (A longer rinse time ensures that all fixer has been removed from the emulsion.)

Developing Complications

Once the film is removed from the protective packet, processing should begin as soon as possible. Following are some complications that can occur during developing.

Clear Film

If the film is clear, it has not been exposed to x-ray beams (Fig. 11.33). Failure to turn the radiograph machine on, a burned-out machine tube, and aiming the radiograph machine head incorrectly all can cause this complication.

Light Film With Poor Contrast

If the film is light with poor contrast and other developing problems are eliminated, the film could have been underexposed. Underexposure may be caused by a time setting that was too short, mA setting that was too low, or kVp that was too low. Also, the focal-film distance may have been too great. Finally, the exposure button may have been released prematurely before a full exposure was obtained. Use of old developer causes a washed-out background and fogs the film. If the developing time is too short, a film with low contrast and density will result.

Light Film With Markings

If cross hatches appear on the film or the image is barely visible and all other aspects of the technique were correct, the problem may be the result of placing the film in the mouth with the wrong side toward the tube head.

Black Film

Excessively dark film may be caused by overexposure of the film (Fig. 11.34). Another cause may be a light leak in the darkroom or chairside darkroom. Prolonged viewing

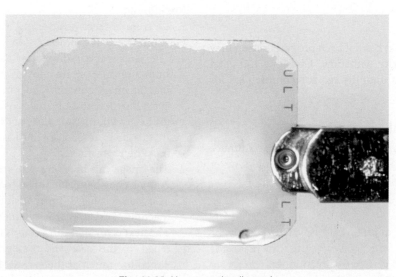

Fig. 11.33 Unexposed radiograph.

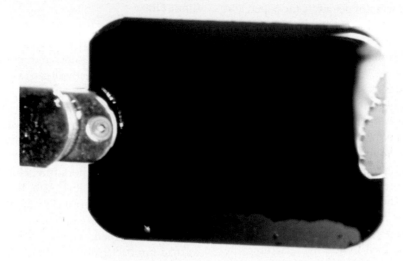

Fig. 11.34 Overexposed radiograph.

of the film between the developing and fixing stage is discouraged; doing so results in an overall grayness of the film.

If Ektaspeed (EP) film is used or the unit is below a bright light source, a red filter should be placed on the amber filter to prevent overexposure. If the film is overdeveloped, excessive density and low contrast will result.

Brown Tint

If the film is not rinsed sufficiently, it will turn brown with age.

Green Tint

Radiographic film that has not been properly rinsed may turn green or splotchy with time. Checking film that was processed several months ago is recommended for quality control.

Solution Disposal

Processing solutions must be discarded in accordance with federal and state guidelines. They should never be poured down the drain.

Film Storage

Envelopes or film mounts can be attached to the patient's medical record. However, this can make the medical record bulky. Often, practitioners prefer to store the radiographs separately, either with the larger radiographs taken for other veterinary medical procedures or in a separate file for dental films only.

Four Simple Rules for Positioning

- Make sure you are aiming at the subject and sensor.
- Do not take a radiograph of air.
- If the image is elongated, aim at the sensor.
- If the image is foreshortened, aim at the subject.

Radiographic Errors
Positioning

Aside from correct positioning, the three results from positioning are as follows:

1. The sensor and radiographs can miss the intended subject or not contain enough subject. It is important that the image contains 2 to 3 mm of bone around the apex. Most commonly, the sensor is placed very close to the crown, missing the root and imaging only air. In this case, the sensor and radiograph cone head must be repositioned.

2. The image can be elongated. In this case, the radiographic cone has been aimed too much at the subject. The correction is to reposition the radiographic machine head so that it is aimed more at the sensor. The next error that can occur is the image is foreshortened. In this case, the radiographic cone has been aimed too much at the sensor. In this case, the cone should redirected so that it aims more at the tooth.

3. Although the positioning may be correct, other errors may occur. Blurring can be caused by patient motion or machine head motion. The image can be overexposed or underexposed. One weakness of DR is dynamic range. Dynamic range is the difference between the least and most amount of radiation that can be recorded on the sensor. When the dynamic range is exceeded, one part of the image is overexposed and another is underexposed. The neck region of the tooth is one area in which this may cause a misdiagnosis. If overexposed, it may appear that there are tooth resorption (TR) lesions, yet this overexposure may be necessary to evaluate the root structure.

Maintenance of Computerized Radiographic Equipment
Units (CR7 or ScanX)

CR systems are very low maintenance. They should be turned off and the power cord disconnected from the wall outlet before cleaning. The outside of the units can be wiped with a soft paper towel dampened with a disinfectant solution such as chlorhexidine or nonabrasive household cleaner. Liquids should not be sprayed or dripped into the system. Allow to air dry before plugging in or turning back on.

Cleaning Phosphorous Plates

Phosphorous plates should be handled carefully. Take care not to scratch, dust, or soil the plates. If the plates become dirty, the following procedures should be used:

1. Using lint-free, 100% cotton gauze. gently wipe over the dry plate surface. Wipe back and forth and then in a circular motion.
2. To clean any remaining stains, dampen the gauze in anhydrous ethanol or anhydrous isopropyl alcohol and wipe using the same motion as above.
3. Completely dry the surface by wiping with another piece of cotton gauze. Ensure that the phosphorous plate is completely dry before use.

If routinely using a cover, there is no reason to routinely disinfect the phosphorus plate unless it has been contaminated. If the phosphorous plate has touched a contaminated surface, unless otherwise recommended by the plate manufacturer, it may be immersed briefly in a cold sterilant such as a 2% glutaraldehyde solution.

After disinfection, the plate should be cleaned and dried with a dust-free gauze. However, if there is any evidence of deep scratches in the surface of the plate or nicks in the edges of the plate, do not immerse the plate.

RADIOGRAPHIC FINDINGS

Radiographic findings can be recorded in the medical record, dental chart, or a radiology notes chart. See Figs. 11.35 and 11.36 for sample canine and feline radiographic notes that can be copied and reused.

Radiographic Anatomy

The important landmarks in reviewing an individual tooth are enamel, dentin, pulp chamber, periodontal ligament space, and alveolar bone. Each of these areas should be recognized and evaluated (Fig. 11.37).

Normal Young Patient

In the young patient the dentinal wall is thin and the pulp chamber is large. As the tooth develops, odontoblasts that line the pulp chamber produce dentin. Dentin thickens the dentinal wall and reduces the size of the pulp canal. The apex may be open, depending on the age of the patient. In the young patient the dense cortical alveolar bone forming the wall of the socket appears radiographically as a distinct, opaque, uninterrupted, white line parallel to the tooth root (Fig. 11.38). This line is known as the *lamina dura*. Lamina dura is a radiographic term referring to the dense cortical bone forming the wall of the alveolus. The lamina dura appears radiographically as a bony white line next to the dark line of the periodontal space. The radiolucent image between the lamina dura and tooth is the periodontal space; it is known as the *lamina lucida*. It is occupied by the periodontal ligament. The trabecular pattern of interdental bone should also be studied.

Normal Older Patient

The dental radiograph of a healthy adult shows a decreased canal size and increased dentinal wall thickness. Generally, the *lamina lucida* becomes narrower with age until it disappears. Although an apex is present, the apical delta or apical foramen is usually not seen. Thinning of the alveolar crest may occur.

Radiographic Notes - Canine

Right Maxilla	Findings	Left Maxilla	Findings
101		201	
102		202	
103		203	
104		204	
105		205	
106		206	
107		207	
108		208	
109		209	
110		210	
Right Mandible		Left Mandible	
301		401	
302		402	
303		403	
304		404	
305		405	
306		406	
307		407	
308		408	
309		409	
310		410	
311		411	

Fig. 11.35 Canine radiographic notes.

Periodontal Disease

Radiographic signs of periodontal disease include rounding and loss of the alveolar crest. These signs are particularly visible between teeth in the interproximal space, as well as in the furcations. The interproximal space is the area between adjacent surfaces of adjoining teeth. Periodontal disease may also be noted as horizontal bone loss. If vertical bone loss has occurred, increased periodontal ligament space will be evident. Subgingival calculus and an oronasal fistula may be noted (Fig. 11.39). See also Chapter 6 for additional radiographs of periodontal disease.

Endodontic Disease

Signs of endodontic disease include lucency around the apex of the tooth root, resorption of the tooth root internally, or resorption of the tooth root externally (Fig. 11.40). Fractures may be noted above or below the gumline. Bacteria enter the pulp chamber, then root canal, and progress into the periapical tissue. This is

Radiographic Notes - Feline

Right Maxilla	Findings	Left Maxilla	Findings
101		201	
102		202	
103		203	
104		204	
106		206	
107		207	
108		208	
109		209	
Right Mandible		Left Mandible	
301		401	
302		402	
303		403	
304		404	
307		407	
308		408	
309		409	

Fig. 11.36 Feline radiographic notes.

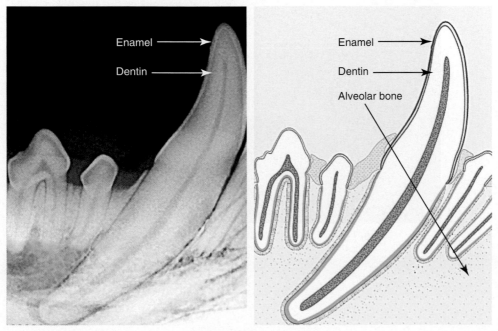

Enamel
Dentin

Enamel
Dentin
Alveolar bone

Fig. 11.37 A tooth.

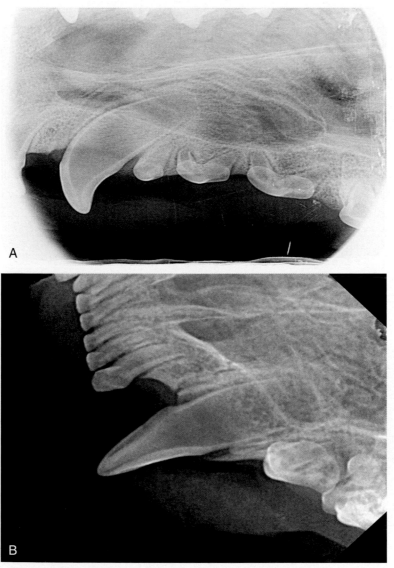

Fig. 11.38 A, Normal young dog. B, Normal young cat.

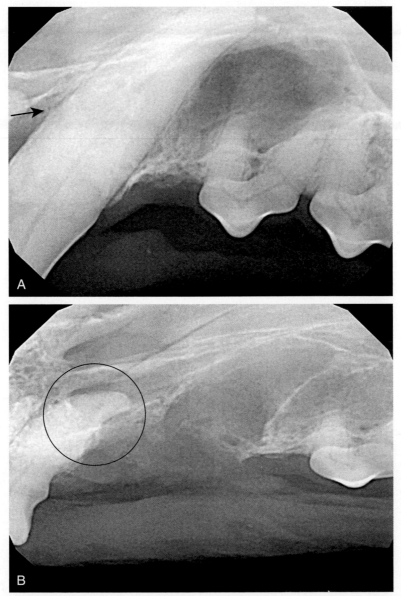

Fig. 11.39 A, Radiograph with subgingival calculus *(arrow)*. B, The oronasal fistula is easily visualized after extraction *(circle)*.

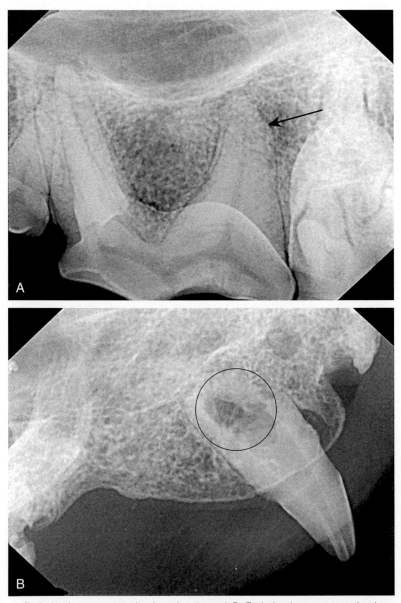

Fig. 11.40 A, Endodontic root resorption in a dog *(arrow)*. B, Endodontic root resorption in a cat *(circle)*.

known as periapical lucency or apical periodontitis. Apical periodontitis is an inflammatory process of the periapical tissues in response to endodontic infection.

Tooth Resorption

Radiographic signs of a TR lesion range from a barely visible coronal lucency to resorption of the entire root. See Chapter 10 for further description of TR.

Retained Roots

Radiographs may be taken, both diagnostically and intraoperatively, to evaluate retained roots. The presence of lucency around the root may indicate disease that needs to be treated. The radiograph should be evaluated to determine whether other oral structures have been compromised.

Neoplasia

The proliferation of bone, missing bone, and/or displacement of teeth are the hallmark radiographic signs of neoplasia

Maxillary Multilobular Osteochondroma

The combination of matrices production and the radiographic appearance most likely classifies this tumor as a multilobular tumor of bone.

Common Radiographic Interpretation Questions

Normal Chevron Sign versus Pathologic Apical Periodontitis

Distinguishing the chevron sign around the apex from pathology is a very common problem for the practitioner.

The chevron sign tends to be fairly distinct with sharp demarcation between the chevron sign, which represents the area that vessels and nerve are entering the apex, and bone (Fig. 11.41).

Pathologic apical periodontitis, also called periapical lucency or periapical abscess, is less distinct. A patient had a chronically complicated fractured right first molar. Radiographs were taken before endodontic therapy was performed, right after endodontic therapy, 6 months

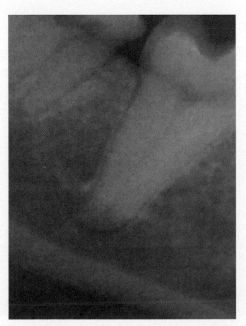

Fig. 11.41 Right mandible. A normal chevron sign in a nondiseased tooth.

postoperative, and 1 year postoperative. Bone has filled in, indicating a successful procedure (Figs. 11.42–11.46). Although bone density may never be "normal," there is resolution of the periapical periodontitis.

Feline Mandibular Symphysis

The mandible in the cat (and dog) is actually a joint that calcifies in some patients, but not in others. In addition, the blood vessels in the area penetrate through foramina that can be pathologic, but cause concern in interpretation (Figs. 11.47 to 11.49).

Canine Tooth Resorption—Is There a Fracture?

With the increased number of whole mouth intraoral radiographs that are being taken comes an increased recognition that TR occurs in the canine as well. These often appear as fractured roots at the intersection of the resorption and normal root (Fig. 11.50).

Cone Beam Computed Tomography

Computers have allowed progression of cone beam computed tomography (CBCT). CBT can be rolled in

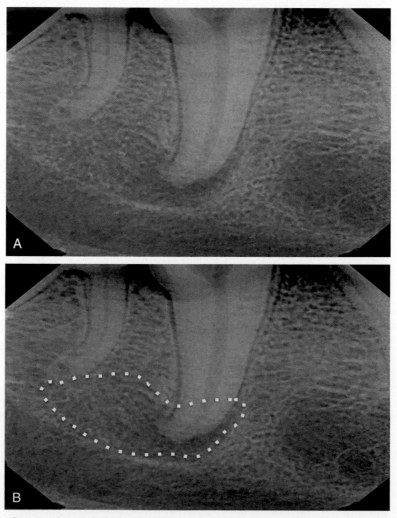

Fig. 11.42 A, Preoperative periapical periodontitis. Radiograph upon presentation and before treatment. B, Periapical periodontitis outlined. The area of lucent bone has been outlined in yellow.

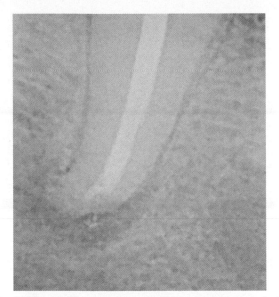

Fig. 11.43 409 Postoperative endodontic therapy: Endodontic therapy has been performed on the tooth. Note the slight "puff" of sealer in the periapical region, indicating filling of the apical delta.

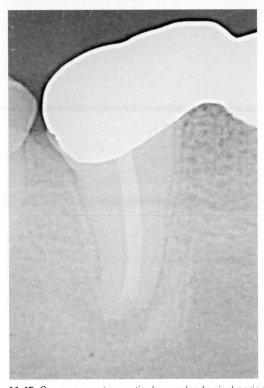

Fig. 11.45 One-year post operatively, resolved apical periodontitis. Bone continues to fill in.

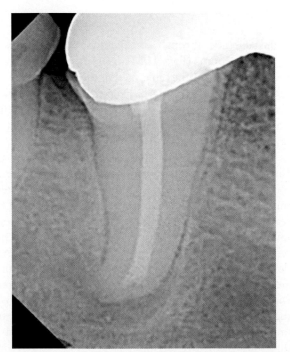

Fig. 11.44 Six months resolved apical periodontitis. The bone density is becoming more uniform as the periodontitis resolves. A metal crown has been placed on the tooth and is radiodense.

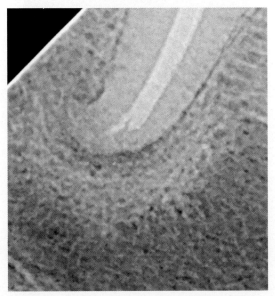

Fig. 11.46 A 2.5 years pathologic apical (PA) post. Bone has filled in nicely.

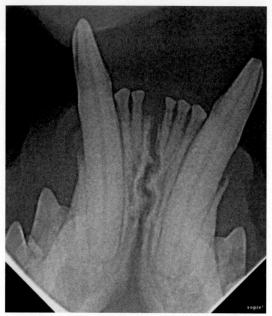

Fig. 11.47 Mandibular symphysis 1. While irregular, this symphysis is not pathologic and should not be treated. (Courtesy Dr. Christopher Garg.)

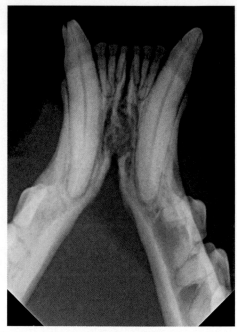

Fig. 11.49 Mandibular lucency symphysis. (Image courtesy Dr. Alex Erickson.)

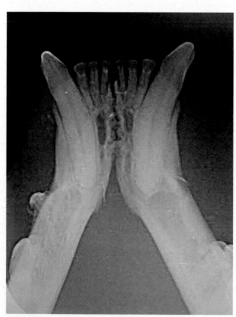

Fig. 11.48 Mandibular mental foramen. Enlarged mandibular mental foramen from which blood vessels and nerves enter and exit. (Courtesy Dr. Laura Thiel.)

to the table, goes through a regular door, and can be used in multiple rooms (Figs. 11.51 and 11.52). An extension must be placed on the table, so that there is no metal in the field. The patient must be anesthetized and it takes about 20 to 30 seconds to acquire x-rays and make the image. An x-ray generator is on one side and a detector on the other side that rotates around the patient.

Repeated radiographs taken in a patient are used to construct a three-dimensional view. As the x-ray beam traverses the anatomy and is repeatedly captured, rotated images are formed. The slices of radiographs are used to read the image. It takes time to get used to reading these images, but using the lines and bearings with the 3D rendering, the image can be read. Sagittal (Fig. 11.53A), dorsal (Fig. 11.53B), and transverse (Fig. 11.53C) planes are obtained. This is in contrast to a radiograph taken with an intraoral sensor that shows abnormal bone above the first molar (Fig. 11.53D) and a clinical image of multilobular osteochondrosarcoma (Fig. 11.53E), and a three-dimensional rendering (Fig. 11.53F).

The field of view is the portion of anatomy being imaged. Veterinary units have a larger field of view than

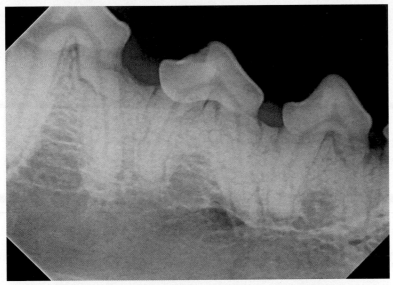

Fig. 11.50 Canine tooth resorption (TR). The interface between the normal root and portion of the root with TR gives the appearance of a fracture.

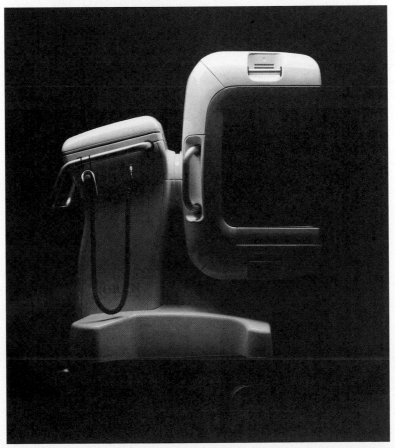

Fig. 11.51 Cone beam computed tomography. This unit can be rolled into position over the patient's head for scanning. (Photo courtesy Dental Focus.)

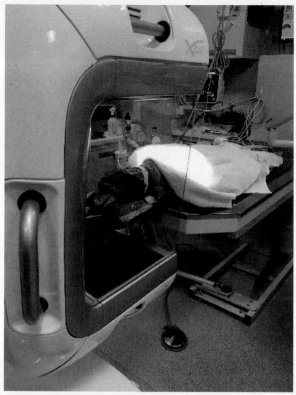

Fig. 11.52 An anesthetized patient in position so that its head is in the CBCT unit. (Photo courtesy Dental Focus.)

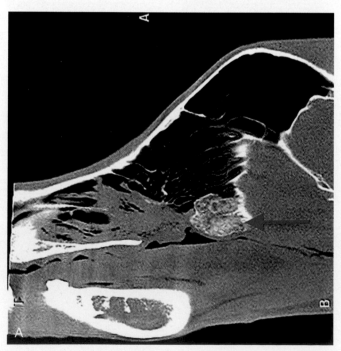

Fig. 11.53 A multilobular osteochondrosarcoma *(red arrow)* was diagnosed by biopsy in this patient. A, Sagittal plane. (Photos courtesy Dr.Kate Knutson and Pet Crossing Animal Hospital and Dental Clinic.)

Continued

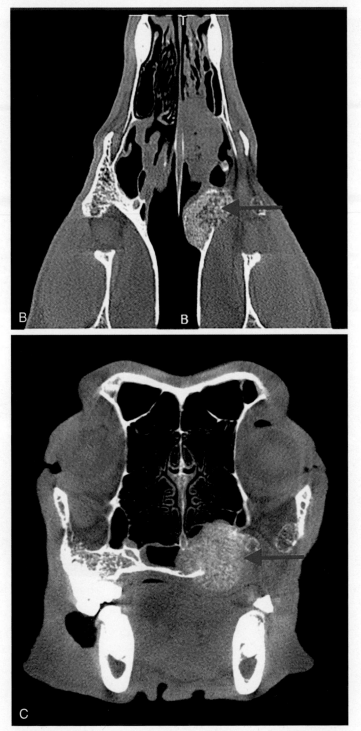

Fig. 11.53, cont'd B, Dorsal plane. C, Transverse plane. (Photos courtesy Dr.Kate Knutson and Pet Crossing Animal Hospital and Dental Clinic).

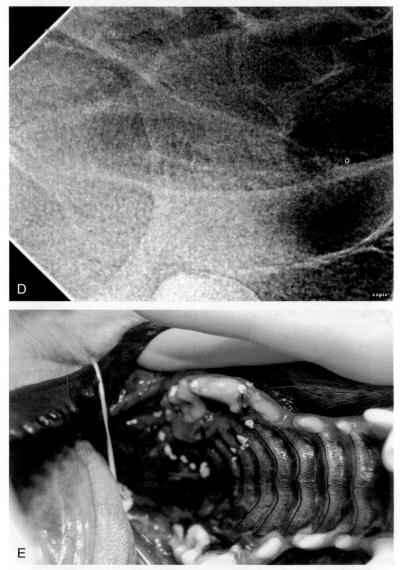

Fig. 11.53, cont'd D, Radiograph of the bone above the first molar. E, Clinical image. (Photos courtesy Dr.Kate Knutson and Pet Crossing Animal Hospital and Dental Clinic.)

Continued

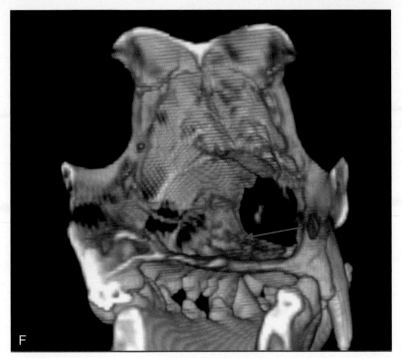

Fig. 11.53, cont'd F, Three-dimensional rendering of the nasal side of the mass. (Photos courtesy Dr. Kate Knutson and Pet Crossing Animal Hospital and Dental Clinic.)

human applications. Cone beam less contrast than conventional radiology in general, but software can enhance. The three-dimensional rendering can often demonstrate pathology that is not visible clinically (Fig. 11.54).

Cone beam tomography is useful in evaluating periodontal and endodontic disease, neoplasia, and trauma. The widening of the periodontal ligament (PDL) can be seen and one can truly see bone level and bone thickness around teeth, evaluating the thickness of bone and periodontal ligament. The normal periodontal ligament will appear thicker in CBT than in conventional radiology (Fig. 11.55).

Soft tissue versus fluids can be seen well because fluids will show a waterline inside the soft tissue. However, this can be difficult if the fluids are in areas such as the nose.

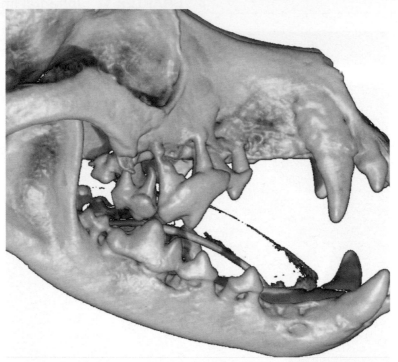

Fig. 11.54 Interradicular bone loss. A cone beam computed tomography rendering of a patient with severe periodontal disease showing extensive bone loss.

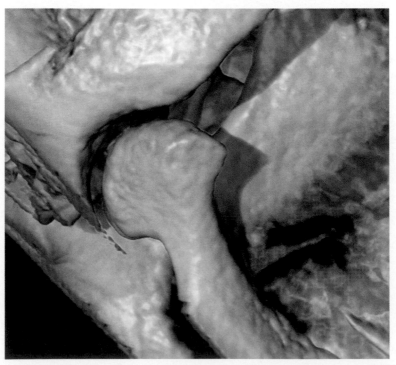

Fig. 11.55 Temporomandibular joint (TMJ) computed tomography. This is an image of a normal TMJ using cone beam computed tomography.

CHAPTER 11 WORKSHEET

1. Most intraoral film is a series of layers. A _____ coating covers the external portion.
2. Between the plastic and the radiographic film itself is a _____ _____ _____.
3. Personnel should be protected by use of _____, _____, and/or safe _____.
4. A maximal amount of _____ and supporting bone should be included in the sensor or film.
5. The parallel technique is indicated for radiographs to evaluate _____ _____ _____ and _____ _____.
6. The _____ _____ _____ is used when parallel projections cannot be made.
7. If the radiographic machine is aimed at the tooth, the x-rays may miss the sensor or film. If anything shows up on the image, it will be distorted by _____.
8. If the radiographic machine is aimed at the sensor or film, the x-rays may miss the tooth. A distorted tooth by _____ is the complication with this approach.
9. To take a radiograph of the maxillary posterior teeth, the sensor or film is placed in the mouth _____ to the hard palate.
10. To take a radiograph of the maxillary posterior teeth, the radiographic machine head is positioned so that it is _____ degrees off the vertical or horizontal plane of the palate and radiographic sensor or film.
11. The complete radiographic study can be obtained in as little as _____ views.
12. The canine teeth are best evaluated by placing the x-ray generator head _____ degrees from the front of the patient and _____ degrees from the side of the patient.
13. Blurred or double images are caused by _____ of either the patient or the x-ray machine head.
14. _____ film is film that has been overexposed, overdeveloped, or exposed to light during processing.
15. Old _____ gives a washed-out background and fogs the film.
16. Processing solutions should never be poured down the _____.
17. AC units produce _____, whereas DC units do not produce _____.
18. Make sure you aim at the _____ and _____.
19. Do not take a radiograph of _____.
20. If the image is elongated, aim at the _____.
21. If the image is foreshortened, aim at the _____.

Exodontics (Extractions)

LEARNING OBJECTIVES

When you have completed this chapter, you will be able to:

- Define exodontic and describe indications for this type of treatment.
- Discuss legal concerns related to performance of tooth extractions by veterinary technicians.
- List the instruments used for performing dental extractions and describe the function of each.
- Describe the procedure for removal of a single-rooted tooth.
- Describe the procedure for removal of a multirooted tooth.
- List and describe potential complications to tooth extraction.

KEY TERMS

Autoclaving
American Veterinary Dental College
Bone augmentation
Bone necrosis
Curettage

Dental elevator
Dental luxator
Exodontics
Extraction forceps
Force technique

Free gingiva
Irrigation
Surgical flaps
Suturing

Although the object in veterinary dentistry is to save teeth, extraction often becomes necessary. Exodontics (exodontia) is the branch of dentistry that involves the extraction of teeth. This chapter's intent is to familiarize the reader with indications, equipment, and techniques for exodontics. It is not a substitute for proper hands-on training given by experts to those legally authorized to do so.

INDICATIONS FOR EXODONTICS

Exodontics is indicated when the tooth cannot be salvaged or the client is unable or unwilling to perform home care. The client should be consulted for authorization before any teeth are extracted. In addition to becoming upset with the extra fees, clients may respond emotionally to their pet's loss of teeth. Alternative types of treatment should always be discussed. Staff members must always remember that extraction is final.

Preliminary to Exodontics

In addition to authorization, preanesthetic blood analysis, including a complete blood count (CBC) and platelet analysis, should be performed (Fig. 12.1).

THE TECHNICIAN AND EXTRACTIONS

With regard to extraction, laws vary from state to state. In all states, if extraction by someone other than a veterinarian is permitted, the extraction must be performed under a veterinarian's supervision. Some state regulations are contradictory. For example, in some states, registered veterinary technicians are permitted to perform extractions. However, the law forbids registered veterinary technicians from performing surgery. Many extractions are surgical (e.g., when teeth are split or flaps performed). This presents a conflict for the technician. Further, there may be insurance issues concerning whether the veterinarian can allow unauthorized individuals to perform procedures for which they are not authorized by law or regulation to do. The safe position, if allowed by state law and the veterinarian, is for the technician to perform only nonsurgical extractions such as removal of extremely mobile teeth.

The American Veterinary Dental College (AVDC), which represents board-certified veterinary dental specialists throughout the world, has evaluated the duties of the veterinarian, registered veterinary technician, and nonlicensed individuals in practice. As a result, the AVDC developed a position statement stipulating that only veterinarians should provide extraction services (Box 12.1).

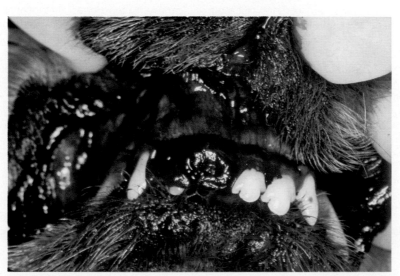

Fig. 12.1 Hemorrhage from coagulation defect. This defect is detected in preoperative blood testing.

BOX 12.1   American Veterinary Dental College (AVDC) Position Statement Regarding Veterinary Dental Healthcare Providers

The American Veterinary Dental College (AVDC) developed this position statement as a means to safeguard the veterinary dental patient and to ensure the qualifications of persons performing veterinary dental procedures.

Primary Responsibility for Veterinary Dental Care

The AVDC defines veterinary dentistry as the art and practice of oral health care in animals other than man. It is a discipline of veterinary medicine and surgery. The diagnosis, treatment, and management of veterinary oral health care is to be provided and supervised by licensed veterinarians or by veterinarians working within a university or industry.

Who May Provide Veterinarian-Supervised Dental Care

The AVDC accepts that the following health care workers may assist the responsible veterinarian in dental procedures or actually perform dental prophylactic services while under direct, in the room supervision by a veterinarian if permitted by local law: licensed, certified or registered veterinary technician or a veterinary assistant with advanced dental training, dentist, or registered dental hygienist.

Operative Dentistry and Oral Surgery

The AVDC considers operative dentistry to be any dental procedure which invades the hard or soft oral tissue including, but not limited to, a procedure that alters the structure of one or more teeth or repairs damaged and diseased teeth. A veterinarian should perform operative dentistry and oral surgery.

Extraction of Teeth

The AVDC considers the extraction of teeth to be included in the practice of veterinary dentistry. Decision making is the responsibility of the veterinarian, with the consent of the pet owner, when electing to extract teeth. Only veterinarians shall determine which teeth are to be extracted and perform extraction procedures.

Dental Tasks Performed by Veterinary Technicians

The AVDC considers it appropriate for a veterinarian to delegate maintenance dental care and certain dental tasks to a veterinary technician. Tasks appropriately performed by a technician include dental prophylaxis and certain procedures that do not result in altering the shape, structure, or positional location of teeth in the dental arch. The veterinarian may direct an appropriately trained technician to perform these tasks providing that the veterinarian is physically present and supervising the treatment.

Veterinary Technician Dental Training

The AVDC supports the advanced training of veterinary technicians to perform additional ancillary dental services: taking impressions, making models, charting veterinary dental pathology, taking and developing dental radiographs, performing non surgical subgingival root scaling and debridement, providing that they do not alter the structure of the tooth.

Tasks that May Be Performed by Veterinary Assistants (Not Registered, Certified, or Licensed)

The AVDC supports the appropriate training of veterinary assistants to perform the following dental services: supragingival scaling and polishing, taking and developing dental radiographs, making impressions and making models.

Tasks that May Be Performed by Dentists, Registered Dental Hygienists, and Other Dental Healthcare Providers

The AVDC recognizes that dentists, registered dental hygienists and other dental health care providers in good standing may perform those procedures for which they have been qualified under the direct supervision of the veterinarian. The supervising veterinarian will be responsible for the welfare of the patient and any treatment performed on the patient.

The AVDC understands that individual states have regulations that govern the practice of veterinary medicine. This position statement is intended to be a model for veterinary dental practice and does not replace existing law.

Adopted by the Board of Directors April 1998; revised October 1999 and September 2006. Courtesy American Veterinary Dental College (AVDC) at www.AVDC.org/.

INSTRUMENTS FOR EXODONTICS

A variety of instruments are used for extractions (Box 12.2). Dental elevators are used to engage teeth and raise them from the root socket. Extraction forceps grasp the tooth and remove it from the socket. Spring-loaded forceps are recommended (Fig. 12.2). Another useful forceps is a root removal forceps (Fig. 12.3).

Luxators, Elevators, Root Tip Picks, and Periosteal Elevators

Luxator

A luxator is for cutting the periodontal ligament and expanding the alveolus (tooth socket). It is not used for elevation or for leverage. Luxators have a fairly thin flat blade as compared to the curved thicker blade of the elevator. Luxators can be flat or curved (Fig. 12.4). Elevators have curved blades to be wrapped around the tooth being extracted. Root tip picks are thin and pointed for retrieving root fragments. All of these

instruments can be manufactured with different handles. The handle should be comfortable for the surgeon to hold.

Because teeth vary in size, a variety of sizes of dental luxators and elevators are necessary (Figs. 12.5 and 12.6).

To add to the confusion, different manufacturers use different names and numbering systems to identify their instruments.

Elevators

The 301, 301S, and 301SS types are fine elevators. The 301S elevator is especially useful in extracting feline teeth. The 301SS elevator is even smaller. All the elevators in the 301 series have been modified by notching the back side of the instrument, creating a fork to assist in preventing the instrument from sliding off alveolar crests. Fig. 12.7 is an example of a notched elevator. The 301SS elevators are effective in elevating small teeth in cats. The 301S elevators are effective in elevating primary canine teeth in dogs and premolars in cats.

BOX 12.2   Instruments for Exodontics

Surgical extraction: Scalpel handle with blade (11 blade, 15 c Blade)
Periosteal elevator: Molt No. 2 (small patient) or Molt No. 4 (large patient)
Burs: Tapered crosscut bur, No. 701L for sectioning multi-rooted teeth
Dental elevators: 301SS, 301S, 301, 34
Winged elevators: 1–6 (7–10 are available for larger patients)
Root tip picks: Miltex 76, HB 11, Heidbrink

Irrigation solution: Sterile saline, dilute chlorhexidine solution
Periodontal scissors to release flap
Needle holder
Thumb forceps
Resorbable suture with swaged needle
Suture scissors
Bone implant material: Consil (Nutramax Laboratories, Edgewood, MD)
Dental radiographic material

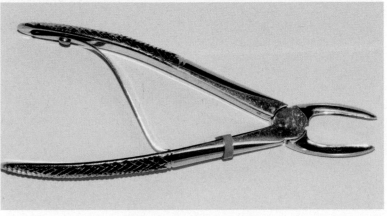

Fig. 12.2 Extraction forceps.

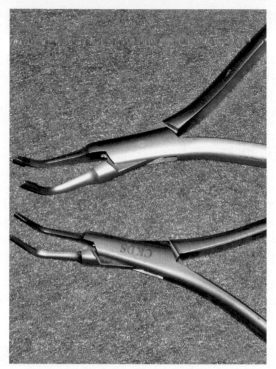

Fig. 12.3 Root removal forceps.

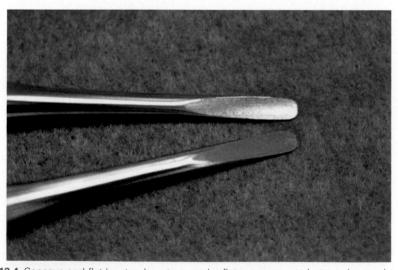

Fig. 12.4 Concave and flat luxator. Luxators can be flat or concave to better adapt to the root.

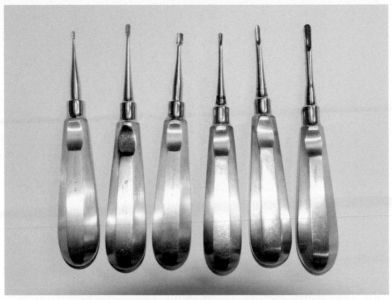

Fig. 12.5 The practice should have a variety of elevator sizes. Elevators are used to rotate and elevate.

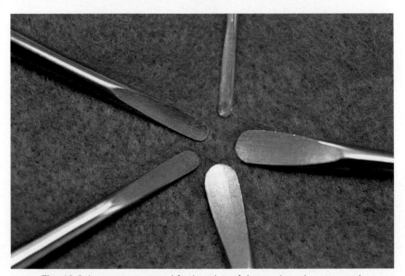

Fig. 12.6 Luxators are used for luxation of the tooth and not rotated.

The 301 elevators are effective in elevating canine teeth in cats and incisors and premolars in dogs. Medium-sized elevators are used for elevating larger premolar roots and moderate-sized canine teeth in dogs. Large elevators are used for extracting larger canine teeth in dogs (Fig. 12.8).

Dr. Robert Wiggs developed winged elevators that have the advantage of wedging out teeth with the shaft side of the wing.

Root Tip Picks

The Heidbrink root tip pick, HB10/11, and Miltex 76 are useful in elevating and extracting retained root tips. Root tip picks are used to loosen, then tease root fragments, from the alveolus. They can be used with a second root tip pick or hypodermic needle to "chopstick" root tips to pick up root fragments. They also can be used to cut the gingival attachment from the tooth before elevation with dental elevators (Fig. 12.9).

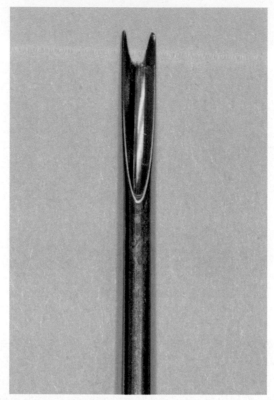

Fig. 12.7 Notched elevators may prevent slippage of the instrument.

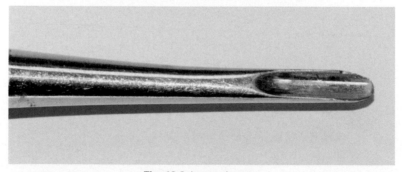

Fig. 12.8 Large elevator.

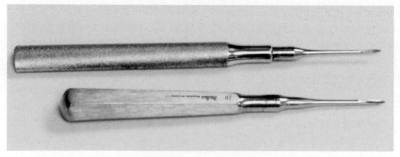

Fig. 12.9 Root tip picks.

Periosteal Elevators

Periosteal elevators are heavy instruments used to elevate the gingiva and periosteum from the bone in periodontal surgery and procedures such as oronasal flap repair (Fig. 12.10).

Vet-Tome Powertome

The Vet-Tome is a solenoid-driven periotome with foot pedal operation that causes minimal or no alveolar bone loss and less trauma. Replaceable ultra-thin stainless steel blades are attached to the handpiece and a mechanical in-and-out action cuts the periodontal ligament similar to a luxator. A thin blade is inserted into the periodontal ligament (PDL) between the tooth and alveolus. The instrument is turned on and the blade driven into the space. After advancing a few millimeters, the foot peddle is released and a side-to-side movement by the operator is made, cutting the adjacent PDL. Once the blade is freed up, the instrument is turned on again and the blade advanced in similar fashion.

The Vet-Tome will not go through bone and hard tissues, so it may not work for PDLs that are mineralized. It is not a replacement for good extraction technique, but it makes extractions easier (Fig. 12.11).

Magnification and Lighting

One frustrating aspect of root extraction is limited access and visibility. This problem may be decreased by the use of magnification and head lamps. (See Chapter 3, Equipment for more information.)

SHARPENING EQUIPMENT

Elevators are sharpened with either a flat stone or Rx Honing Machine. The bevel (convex) side is positioned on the stone and sharpened in a back-and-forth motion as the tip is in a rotational movement.

To sharpen with the Rx Honing Machine, the instrument is held at the proper angle and rotated as the disk spins. The angle should follow the manufacturer's edge (Fig. 12.12).

STERILIZATION OF EQUIPMENT

Because extraction is a surgical procedure and the instrument enters tissue, sterile instruments should always be used (Fig. 12.13). Although most often the tissue around the tooth is already infected, use of a nonsterile instrument could introduce a different species of bacteria to the infection. Chemical disinfectants

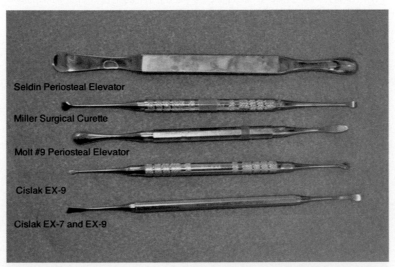

Fig. 12.10 A variety of periosteal elevators are available; the best one to use is up to the practitioner performing the procedure.

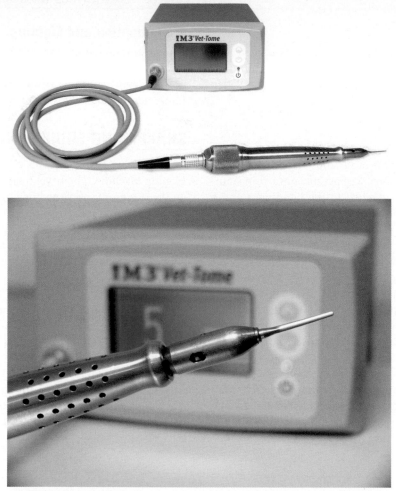

Fig. 12.11 The Vet-Tome Powertome is a mechanical periotome that assists in cutting the periodontal ligament. (Photo courtesy iM3 Inc., WA, USA.)

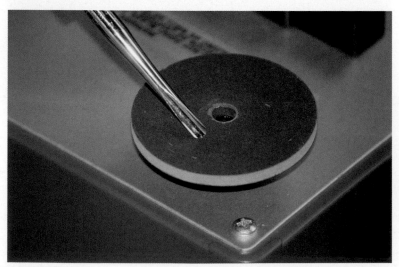

Fig. 12.12 A Rx Honing Machine is used to sharpen the elevator by rotating as the wheel spins. (Photo courtesy Rx Honing Machine Corp., IN, USA)

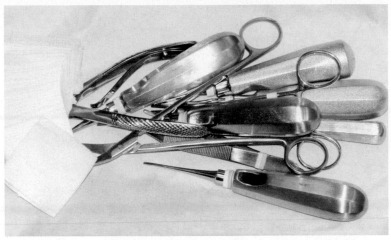

Fig. 12.13 Opened pack.

may be effective, but they take time to work and necessitate complete cleaning of the instrument before use. Moreover, chemical sterilization can dull sharp instruments and weaken some metals. Gas sterilization techniques do not cause as much damage to the instruments. However, the gases must be properly used to prevent health hazards. Autoclaving techniques use a combination of pressure and steam heat to sterilize instruments.

Sterilization Monitoring

Sterilization must be monitored, either with chemical strips that turn color when the proper sterile conditions have been achieved or with biologic monitors in which bacterial growth is observed after sterilization.

EXODONTIC PRINCIPLES

The tooth may be removed from the socket in two ways. The force technique breaks bone (and tooth root) and causes more trauma than necessary; its use is therefore discouraged. The best approach is to stretch and tear the periodontal ligament fibers. The use of elevators to fracture bone by excessive force is not recommended. Often, both bone and root are fractured, which causes excessive trauma. A rotational motion (rather than a "seesaw" motion) should be used. The tooth should be eased out of the socket rather than forced. The key to this approach is patience.

Root Removal

All of the root should be removed, except in the rare instance when more root retrieval would cause more damage. With any extraction procedure, dental radiographs help ensure that all the root tissue has been removed.

Exodontic Technique

A step-by-step approach in the exodontic technique is important. Practitioners must always remember that the object is to remove the tooth with as little trauma as possible. Use of each of these techniques may not be necessary for every extraction, nor is the order of steps necessarily followed each time. Combinations of vertical and horizontal extraction may be used.

Single-Root Extraction

Single-rooted teeth in the dog are the incisors, canines, first premolars, and mandibular third molar; in the cat, they are the incisors, canines, and maxillary second premolar. The cat's maxillary first molar may be treated as a single-rooted tooth even though it has more than one root. The first step in tooth extraction is to sever the gingival attachment (Fig. 12.14). A root tip pick or dental elevator is most commonly used. The practitioner should work all the way around the tooth and remember to be patient.

Occasionally, use of a round or pear-shaped bur on a high-speed handpiece may be helpful in separating the

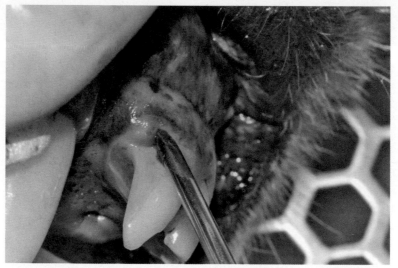

Fig. 12.14 Severed gingival attachment.

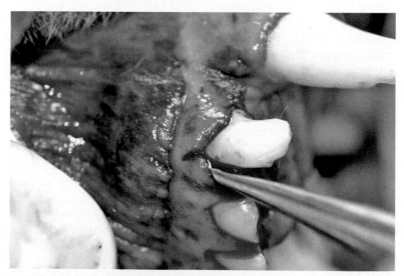

Fig. 12.15 Vertical rotation.

ligament. Plenty of water should be used to keep the tissues cool; otherwise, bone necrosis could result from excessive heating of the bone.

Vertical rotation. In vertical rotation the elevator is used parallel to the root (Fig. 12.15). Once the attached gingiva, which is the portion of the gingiva directly attached to the tooth, has been severed, the practitioner should begin to work an elevator, whose curve approximates the tooth, into the space between the tooth

and the alveolus. Placing slow, gentle, steady pressure on the tooth rather than quick, rocking motions is helpful. The slow, steady pressure (holding the pressure on each side 5 to 15 seconds may be necessary) will break down the periodontal ligament so that the tooth exfoliates easily.

Horizontal rotation. In horizontal rotation the elevator is placed perpendicular to the crown and tooth root. Pressure is applied to the coronal aspect of the tooth to be

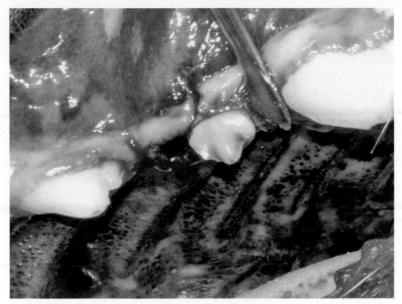

Fig. 12.16 Horizontal rotation.

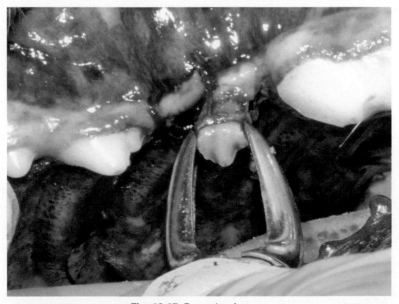

Fig. 12.17 Extraction forceps.

extracted. Care should be taken not to luxate the tooth that is acting as a fulcrum (Fig. 12.16). When the periodontal ligament breaks down, the tooth is held with extraction forceps for easy removal (Fig. 12.17).

To increase the speed of healing, the socket and associated gingiva should be cleaned by curettage and irrigation.

Bone augmentation. Although not always indicated, a synthetic material (Consil, Nutramax Laboratories

Consumer Care Inc., MD, USA) is available to fill in the socket after the tooth is extracted.

Suturing. Finally, the gingiva is sutured using 3-0 or 4-0 synthetic suture material. Monocryl is recommended because it dissolves or becomes untied and falls out in several weeks. A variety of suture patterns may be employed. The most commonly used is the simple interrupted (Fig. 12.18A). It has the advantage of multiple knots, so that if one fails the entire suture line does not fail. Cross-pattern mattress sutures have the advantage of speed (Fig. 12.18B), but the disadvantage is the larger suture mass as compared to a continuous interlocking pattern. A continuous interlocking pattern has the advantage of speed and less suture mass in the extraction sites (Fig. 12.18C). Also, there may be less irritation to the patient from multiple knots. The disadvantage is that if one knot fails, the entire suture line can dehisce (fall apart).

Multirooted Teeth

Splitting multirooted teeth before extracting them is almost always the easiest method. After the teeth are split, each section should be removed as if it were a single-rooted tooth (Fig. 12.19).

Premolar Extraction

All premolars, except the first (one root) and the maxillary fourth, should be split by using a high-speed bur to cut between the furcation and the tip of the crown (Fig. 12.20).

Maxillary Fourth Premolar

The maxillary fourth premolar should be separated between the furcations and the crown of each of the three roots. The first cut is made between the cusps over the mesiobuccal and distal roots (Fig. 12.21A). The second cut is made to separate the mesiobuccal and palatal roots (Fig. 12.21B).

Maxillary First and Second Molars

In dogs, a T-shaped cut can be made on the maxillary first and second molars. This T should first split off the mesial and distal roots from the palatine root and then separate the mesial and distal roots. Once the crown has been split, each individual root is treated as a separate tooth and extracted. The only difference with this technique is that adjoining roots may be used as fulcrums for the extraction before and after the root has been elevated.

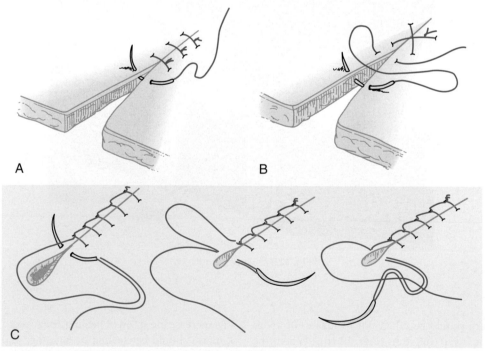

Fig. 12.18 Suture patterns. A, Simple interrupted. B, Cruciate pattern mattress. C, Continuous interlock. (Adapted from Fossum TW: *Small Animal Surgery,* ed 3, St. Louis, MO: Mosby, 2007.)

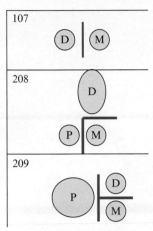

Fig. 12.19 Sectioning. Two rooted teeth are split between the mesial and distal root. The maxillary fourth premolar is split between the mesial root and distal root and then between the mesiobuccal and palatal root. The maxillary first molar is split between the buccal and palatal roots, and then between the mesiobuccal and distobuccal roots.

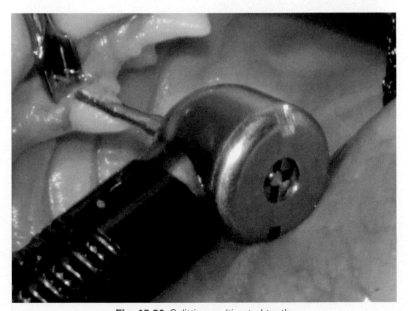

Fig. 12.20 Splitting multirooted teeth.

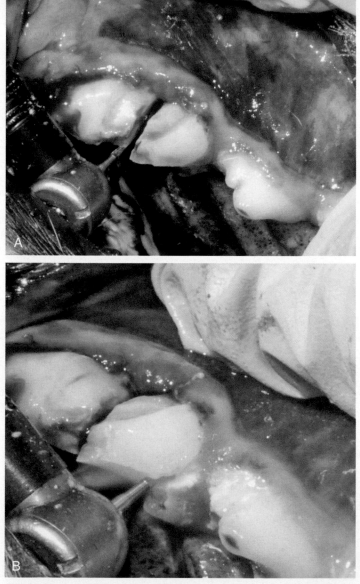

Fig. 12.21 A, Splitting mesiobuccal roots. B, Splitting buccal-palatal roots.

COMPLICATIONS OF EXTRACTIONS

Complications of extractions include trauma from teeth at the location of the extraction, hemorrhage, and instrument slippage.

In addition to the loss of function of the extracted tooth and possibly the tooth it occludes with, exodontia can also lead to complications such as lip and tongue biting. The maxillary canine tooth acts as a guide to keep the upper lip away from the canine tooth. Some patients may have severe trauma to the upper lip if this tooth is extracted (Fig. 12.22). The lower canine tooth acts as a guide for the tongue, and the tongue may hang out on the extracted side if this tooth is extracted.

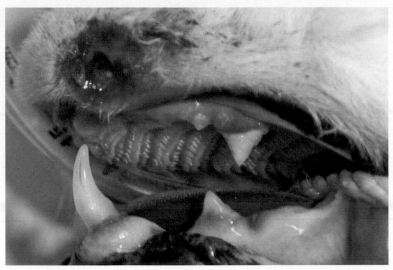

Fig. 12.22 Lip trauma.

The first step in controlling hemorrhage is to apply pressure with a gauze sponge. When applying pressure, the gauze sponge should be rolled onto the wound. After 1 to 2 minutes of pressure, the gauze sponge should be carefully rolled off. This rolling action is continued until the bleeding stops. If a hemostat is necessary to control hemorrhage, it is applied, then pressure with a gauze sponge should be rolled, or applied onto the wound, and hemorrhage checked in similar fashion (Fig. 12.23).

Products such as HemaBlock, Gelfoam, Vetigel, and Vetspon can be used to control hemorrhage (Table 12.1).

Damage from slippage of the instrument is prevented by holding the instrument as close to the tip as possible so that if there is slippage, the finger will act as a stop, preventing further damage. This is called the "shortstop grip" (Fig. 12.24).

Loss of Root Into the Mandibular Canal

Surgical flaps may be necessary to extract root fragments that have ended up in the mandibular canal (Fig. 12.25).

Flap Surgery

Releasing incisions are made on the mesiobuccal and distobuccal line angles of adjacent teeth. These releasing incisions are joined by an intrasulcular incision that follows the gingival margin. The gingiva is stripped from

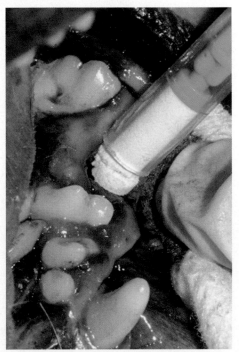

Fig. 12.23 HemaBlock is applied to this extraction site to control hemorrhage. (Photo courtesy Dr. Jan Bellows.)

the bone with a periosteal elevator. The buccal plate of bone over the tooth is removed with a high-speed handpiece and irrigation. The root is removed, and the flap is closed.

TABLE 12.1   Products to Aid in Hemostasis

Product	Manufacturer	Source	Bio-Absorbable	Time to Hemostasis	Mode of Action
Floseal	Baxter	Thrombin in a gelatin matrix	6–8 weeks	–3 minutes	Converts fibrinogen to fibrin and mechanical
Gelfoam	Pfizer	Porcine collagen	4–6 weeks	5 minutes	Incorporated into clot and swell
HemaBlock	HemaBlock	Potatoes and cotton Microporous polysaccharide bead technology	< 1 week	1–2 minutes	Molecular sleeve
Vetigel	Cresilon	Plant-based polysaccharide polymer	1–2 minutes	1–2 minutes	Mechanical barrier
Vetspon	Novartis	Porcine collagen	4–6 weeks	5 minutes	Incorporated into clot and swell

Hemorrhage also can be controlled by ligation, electrosurgery, radiosurgery, and lasers.

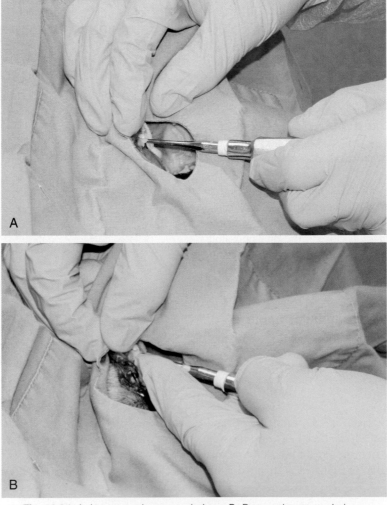

Fig. 12.24 A, Improper elevator technique. B, Proper elevator technique.

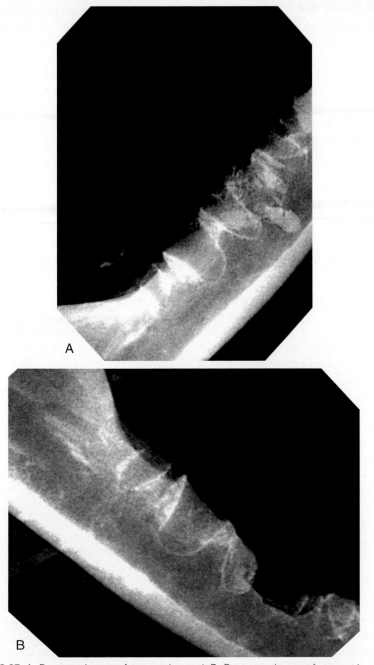

Fig. 12.25 A, Preoperative root fragment in canal. B, Postoperative root fragment in canal.

Keys to Successful Exodontia

1. Hands-on training: Without hands-on training, it is impossible to expect any veterinarian to know how to extract teeth successfully. The patient is not the place to learn how attendance of wet labs is encouraged!

2. Have proper equipment: Using the correct, properly maintained equipment is essential in any act of veterinary surgery. Sterile instruments should stored in dental pouches, cassettes or trays ready for use.

3. Anatomy: A sound knowledge of anatomy is essential. Dental anatomy should be reviewed and understood before extraction attempts.

4. Regional anesthesia: The use of dental local or regional anesthesia (dental nerve blocks) should begin prior to the extraction procedure. This may reduce the amount of general anesthesia necessary and aid in a pain-free recovery.

5. Intraoral dental radiography: Intraoral dental radiographs must be taken before the procedure. Radiographs guide treatment options, demonstrate anatomic abnormalities, and ensure complete extraction. A skull film, while sometimes important, is not a substitute for intraoral radiographs with the proper intraoral equipment.

6. Remember Halsted's Tenants of Surgery: Particularly, gentle handling of tissue, meticulous hemostasis, preservation of blood supply, minimum tension on tissues, and accurate tissue apposition. Two of the principles of strict aseptic technique and obliteration of all dead space may be difficult to follow. As the mouth is not sterile to begin with, too strict aseptic technique is difficult to follow, but attempts should be made not to introduce contamination to the greatest extent possible. Likewise, obliteration of dead space in the socket may suffice by allowing a blood clot to form.

7. Remove little bone as needed to extract the tooth, but do not hesitate to remove as much bone as needed to extract. And never compromise adjacent teeth unless extraction of those teeth is planned as part of the procedure.

8. If you can't see it, you can't do it: Use good lighting and magnification.

9. Make an appropriately sized flap and treat the flap with respect.

10. Relax! Give yourself time and be patient. More complications are caused by rushing than taking too long to do the procedure.

11. Suture: Suturing promotes primary intention healing that ensures quicker, more comfortable, and more healing. Suture fresh-cut epithelium to epithelium. Never suture under tension.

12. Use proper medications after the procedure: Use antibiotics if there is overwhelming infection or other conditions that compromise the patient. But do not use antibiotics automatically. Use proper pain medications.

CONCLUSION

Most exodontic procedures are surgical extractions. If permitted by law and practice policy, the technician should receive advanced, hands-on training of exodontic technique. Great harm can be done to patients when inexperienced or untrained staff members perform these procedures. Box 12-3 lists a summary of the instruments used in this chapter.

BOX 12.3   Exodontia Packs

#1 Small Animal
Luxators 2, 3 mm
Winged elevators 1, 2, 3, 4
301S, 301SS, 301S forked (Cislak EX-5HXS)
Cislak WA2/WA3 Double-Ended Root Tip Pick or Miltex 78 root tip pick
Cislak EX-7 Feline Periosteal elevator

#2 Medium Animal
Luxators 3, 4 mm
Winged elevators 2, 3, 4, 5
301 elevator
Cislak WA2/WA3 Double-Ended Root Tip Pick or Miltex 78 root tip pick
Cislak EX-7 Feline Periosteal elevator

#3 Large Animal
Luxators 3, 4, 5 mm
Winged levators 3, 4, 6, 8
Cislak WA2/WA3 Double-Ended Root Tip Pick or Miltex 78 root tip pick
Kit #3: Molt #9 Periosteal elevator (Cislak EX-1)
Suture Packs:
Needle holder
Scalpel handle
Thumb forceps
Suture cutting scissors (1)
Each pack should have gauze so that sterilized gauze is available

CHAPTER 12 WORKSHEET

1. Exodontics may be indicated if the tooth is judged nonsalvageable or if the client is unable or unwilling to perform _____.
2. The client should be consulted for _____ before any teeth are extracted.
3. With regard to extraction, _____ vary from state to state.
4. The law of some states permits _____ of teeth by registered veterinary technicians.
5. The law of some states forbids registered veterinary technicians from performing _____.
6. _____ _____ are instruments that are used to engage teeth and raise them from the root socket.
7. _____ are used to grasp the tooth and remove it from the socket.
8. The _____, _____, and _____ are fine elevators that are good for extracting very small teeth.
9. The _____ root tip pick and HB10/11 root tip picks are useful in extracting retained root tips.
10. Use of _____ _____ forceps is recommended.
11. Because extraction is a surgical procedure and the instrument often enters tissue, _____ _____ should be used.
12. The _____ technique breaks bone (and tooth root) and causes more trauma than necessary.
13. The use of elevators to fracture bone by excessive force is _____.
14. A _____ motion rather than a "seesaw" motion should be used.
15. _____-rooted teeth are the incisors, the canines, the first premolars, and mandibular third molar in the dog, and the incisors, canines, and maxillary second premolar in the cat.
16. In _____ rotation, the elevator parallel to the root is used.
17. Splitting _____ teeth before extracting them is almost always the easiest method.
18. A _____ -shaped cut can be made on the maxillary first molar.
19. _____ _____ may be helpful in making sure that all the root tissue has been removed.
20. Occasionally, stubborn roots or root tips remain. The preferred treatment in this situation is to create a _____ and elevate the tooth buccally.

Advanced Veterinary Dental Procedures: Periodontal Surgery, Endodontics, Restorations, and Orthodontics

OUTLINE

LEARNING OBJECTIVES

When you have completed this chapter, you will be able to:
- Describe indications for periodontal surgery and list instruments needed for these procedures.
- Discuss indications, contraindications, and general procedure for performing gingivoplasty.
- Discuss the indications and general procedure for performing open flap and root planing and mandibular frenoplasty.

- Define oronasal fistula and list three techniques used to repair this condition.
- Define endodontics and describe equipment and supplies needed to perform these procedures.
- List and describe commonly performed endodontic procedures.
- Describe the general procedure for performing conventional, nonsurgical root canal therapy.

- List and describe restorative materials used in veterinary dentistry.
- Describe the stages for performing orthodontic procedures.

KEY TERMS

Absorbent points	File	Normograde
Alginate	Frenectomy	Odontoblastic cells
Ankylosis	Frenula	Oronasal fistula
Apicoectomy	Full-coverage metal crowns	Orthodontics
Barbed broach	Gingivectomy	Osteomyelitis
Canine tooth	Gingivoplasty	Periosteal elevator
Carious erosion	Glass ionomers	Plugger
Carnassial tooth	Gutta-percha	Porcelain-fused-to-metal crowns
Closed periodontal debridement	Halitosis	Pulp
Composites	Iatrogenic	Pulpectomy
Dental models	Iatrogenic pulpal exposure	Reamer
Dentinal tubules	Impression tray	Restorative dentistry
Direct pulp-capping	Indirect pulp-capping	Root canal sealant
Double palatal/pedicle flap	Inflammatory resorption	Simple buccal sliding flap
Double palatal/sliding flap	LaGrange scissors	Sodium hypochlorite
Endodontic therapy	Locking cotton	Spreader
Endo-ring	Mucogingival junction	Vital pulpotomy

At one time, veterinary dentistry meant either scraping calculus from the teeth or extracting them if they could not be saved by conservative techniques. Fortunately for the patient, veterinary dentistry has made significant advances. Although not all practices have the resources to perform advanced procedures, the veterinary staff should have an idea of the range of procedures that can be performed to save teeth, what each procedure entails, and the type of equipment necessary. Some practices may perform many advanced dental procedures, and this chapter briefly addresses the most common ones. Prior to using any of these techniques, training by a board-certified veterinary dentist is recommended.

PERIODONTAL SURGICAL TECHNIQUES

Periodontal surgical techniques are employed after more conservative measures, such as closed periodontal debridement, have been attempted without success or have been ruled out as impossible. In periodontal surgery, flaps are created to expose the tooth root and associated bone. The bone may be reshaped or augmented, and the gingiva may be sutured back to the initial position. Alternatively, the gingival height may be changed apically by gingival or bone surgery to decrease the pocket or coronally with guided tissue regeneration to increase the height of attachment.

Evaluation for Procedure

A periodontal probe and dental radiographs are used diagnostically before the procedure to determine the location of the pocket and to aid in the selection of an appropriate form of therapy.

Goal of Periodontal Surgery

The goal of periodontal surgery is to eliminate pockets harboring subgingival plaque and calculus. The ultimate aim is to prevent subgingival plaque and calculus from returning.

Instruments and Materials

Periodontal surgery requires various instruments and materials (Box 13.1). The No. 3 handle is the standard type for scalpels. A variety of different blades may be used, including special periodontal knives. The No.

BOX 13.1   Instruments and Materials for Periodontal Surgery

No. 3 (or similar) scalpel handle
15c scalpel blades
Small tissue scissors (LaGrange)
Periosteal elevator: Molt (No. 2, No. 4, or No. 9), ST-No. 7
Scaling curette
Sterile saline solution
Chlorhexidine (0.1% to 0.2%): diacetate or gluconate (gluconate preferred)
Tissue forceps
Needle holders, spring locking (Castroviejo)
4-0 or 5-0 absorbable or nonabsorbable suture material with reverse FS-2 cutting needle
High-speed handpiece
#2 or #4 round burs, appropriate for handpiece used
Bone files

15c blade is extremely fine and therefore useful in periodontal surgical procedures. In addition, small tissue scissors, such as LaGrange scissors, are helpful in trimming periodontal tissue. Periosteal elevators are used to lift the gingiva away from the bone. Several types are available. The Molt elevator is one type; the Molt No. 9 is particularly popular. Many practitioners also like the ST-No. 7 instrument. Having a variety of periodontal surgical instruments available makes treating various anatomic and pathologic conditions less difficult.

Solutions for irrigating the tissue are also important in periodontal surgery. Sterile saline solution and chlorhexidine are most common. Chlorhexidine is used in a 0.1% to 0.2% solution and is available in two forms: diacetate and gluconate. Gluconate is preferred.

Tissue forceps and needle holders are necessary for suturing. Although expensive, the best is the spring-locking Castroviejo-type needle holder. For the sutures themselves, 4-0 or 5-0 absorbable material with a reverse cutting FS-2 needle is used. The high-speed handpiece is used in the removal of bone, and burs may be added for the removal of granulation tissue. Round burs (#2 or #4), crosscut fissure burs (#701L), or pear-shaped burs (#330) may be used in the appropriate handpiece. Bone files may be used to contour bone.

Treatment Techniques

Hyperplastic Gingiva

Because gingivoplasty (gingivectomy) is performed only when hyperplastic gingiva is present, patients must be selected carefully. Gingivoplasty should not be used for treatment of deep periodontal pockets or as part of the routine prophy. This procedure is contraindicated when attached gingiva is minimal or absent or horizontal or vertical bone loss is present below the mucogingival junction, which is the line of demarcation where the attached gingiva and alveolar mucosa meet. These characteristics are prevalent in certain breeds and breed lines, particularly boxers and collies.

Gingivoplasty technique. The pocket depth and contour are determined by inserting a probe to the depth of the pocket at several areas around the tooth. The corresponding depth is measured on the outside of the gingiva, also with the probe. A bleeding point is made by placing the tip of the probe perpendicular to the gingiva and applying slight pressure to make a small hole or by using a small-gauge needle. Bleeding points are made around the contour of the pocket and are used as a guide for the gingivectomy. The gingivectomy is made at an angle apical to the bleeding point to create a beveled margin. At least 2 mm of healthy, attached gingiva must be present apical to the base of the incision. A multifluted bur, laser, scalpel blade, or electrosurgery blade is used to excise the gingiva by cutting below the bleeding points, with the blade held at approximately a 45-degree angle and the tip of the blade toward the crown. The ends of the excision should be tapered into the surrounding gingiva to create the normal scalloped contour, particularly if several adjacent teeth are treated. Gingival tags can be removed with the blade or a sharp curette. The exposed tooth and root surface can now be scaled and planed smooth. Hemorrhage is controlled by applying pressure with wet gauze pads or hemostatic agents. If electrosurgery is being performed, caution must be exercised because the collateral damage may extend past the desired surgical line. In Fig. 13.1, a periodontal probe is used to measure and mark the pocket depth. Once marked, a scalpel blade is used to perform the gingivoplasty.

Deep Periodontal Pocket

Treatment of deep periodontal pockets beyond the range of closed periodontal debridement requires either extraction of the tooth or creation of a periodontal flap

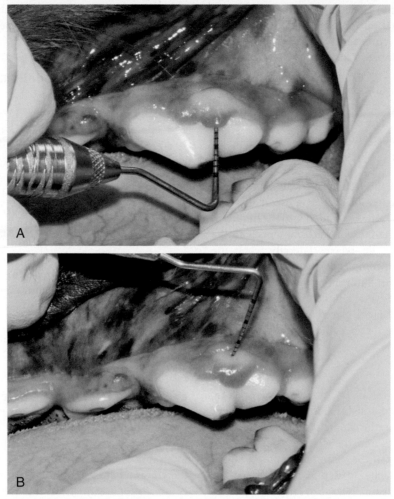

Fig. 13.1 A, Periodontal probe gingivoplasty measurement. B, Periodontal gingivoplasty probe marking the pocket depth.

and then treatment. The flap allows visualization of subgingival tissues. By creating a flap and reflecting the periodontal tissues off the tooth surface, the practitioner can see the tooth surface where periodontal debridement or root planing is being performed.

Indications for open flap and root planing. Generally, it is best to attempt the more conservative treatment of closed periodontal debridement before performing open surgery, if the pocket is greater than 5 mm in depth. After the flap is created, periodontal debridement or root planing is performed.

Open flap and root planing technique. The gingiva is disinfected. An incision should be made that follows the contour of the tooth running in the sulcus. Releasing incisions are created, starting at the line angle of the teeth mesial and distal to the surgery site. The gingiva is elevated with the periosteal elevator lingually/palatally and labially/buccally without exposing the marginal alveolar bone. The exposed root surfaces are planed until they are smooth and hard. Before closure, the area is flushed with chlorhexidine solution. The flap is repositioned and sutured with interrupted sutures placed interdentally.

Excessive Attachment of Frenula

Dogs have two mandibular frenula, located distal to the mandibular canine teeth. Although these frenula help hold the lower lip close to the gums, they may be too tight in some patients. Excessive tightness allows an accumulation of debris on the distal side of the canine teeth. The frenoplasty procedure is designed to relieve the tightness in the lip from the gingiva.

A mandibular frenoplasty (frenectomy) is indicated in patients with gingival recession or pocket formation on the distal side of the canine teeth caused by the presence of the frenulum. The objective of the procedure is to minimize the accumulation of food in the anterior portion of the mouth and improve self-cleansing of this area.

The attachment of the frenulum to the mandibular gingiva near the first premolar is cut horizontally with scissors or a blade. The cut is extended into the frenulum to release the pull of the muscular attachments with the blade or scissors. The lip relaxes laterally when the attachments have been completely cut. The cut surfaces create a diamond shape. Suturing brings the mesial and distal edges together. Several simple interrupted sutures of an absorbable material are placed to prevent reattachment. The root surfaces of the canines should be planed smooth and polished.

Oronasal Fistula

An oronasal fistula (ONF) is an abnormal opening between the oral and nasal cavities. Three techniques are used in ONF repair: the simple sliding flap, the double palatal/sliding flap, and the double palatal/pedicle flap. All are variations of the same procedure.

The simple buccal sliding flap is usually used for smaller fistulas. If the fistula is large or chronic, a double palatal/sliding flap is recommended. The margins of the fistula are debrided of necrotic and epithelialized tissue around the entire circumference of the lesion so you are suturing fresh, bleeding connective tissue to fresh, bleeding connective tissue.

The alveolar bone may require recontouring to allow better positioning of the flap. Recontouring is accomplished with a small rongeur, chisel, or curette. The flap is elevated and undermined such that the wound edges can be brought together and sutured in a tension-free manner. The flap is sutured with 3-0 or 4-0 sutures. If the simple flap fails, a variety of advanced flaps can be placed.

Postoperative care of ONF is very important. Home-care instructions should include soft food for 2 weeks and not handling the mouth for 2 weeks. If at all possible, medications should be administered voluntarily

(Pill Pockets, Greenies). If there is any chance of pawing, an Elizabethan Collar should be placed to prevent pawing and rubbing.

Follow-Up Recommendations for All Periodontal Surgery

After surgery the patient should be given a soft diet for 1 to 7 days. Oral antibiotics are administered, as appropriate. The oral cavity is flushed once or twice daily with chlorhexidine solution for 2 weeks. After the patient's wounds have healed, oral hygiene should be performed in the home to minimize future plaque accumulations.

After the surgical site has healed, home care must be continued. The product selected for use depends on the patient's particular situation. Postsurgical checkups are important to monitor the patient's progress. A minimum of two follow-up appointments should be scheduled for 10 days and 1 month after the procedure. Additional appointments may be scheduled if necessary. Because patients that have had periodontal surgery sometimes experience a relapse, monthly or quarterly follow-up visits may be necessary.

ENDODONTICS AND RESTORATIONS

At one time, veterinarians did not treat fractured teeth. Consequently, many patients suffered silently as the tooth first died and then became abscessed. Endodontic therapy is a better option. Endodontic therapy is a general term for treatment of the dental pulp that may be used to save vital pulp, remove live or dead pulp, and prevent or treat infection (Fig. 13.2).

Pulp tissue consists of blood vessels, nerves, and connective tissues that support the odontoblastic cells lining the pulp chamber and root canal. Throughout life the odontoblasts produce dentin that fills in the canal. As a result, the dentin layer thickens with age.

Bacteria usually gain entry to the pulp chamber via a fractured tooth. The pulpal tissue becomes inflamed and edematous and dies. Then bacteria move into the apical region of the tooth. From this area, they spread through the canals in the apical delta of the tooth, which formerly served as tunnels for the nerves and blood vessels. Once the bacteria enter the apical bone, an abscess starts. The periapical abscess may eventually (i.e., years later) become walled off, cause inflammatory resorption of the root, spread along the periodontal ligament, and

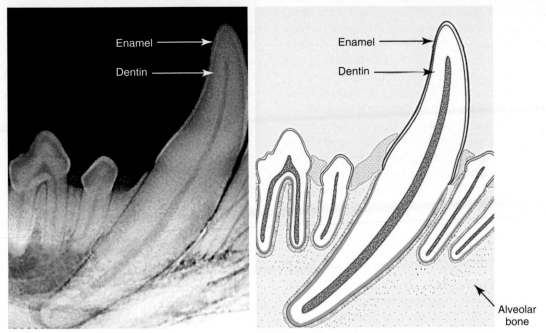

Enamel

Dentin

Enamel

Dentin

Alveolar bone

Fig. 13.2 The endodontic system.

cause ankylosis (fusion) of the tooth root with the surrounding bone.

Discolored teeth, especially those that are pink or purple, indicate pulpal hemorrhage. Pulp tissue responds to such physical trauma like any other bodily tissue—inflammation, pain, and swelling. If the apex of tooth is completely developed, the swelling of the pulp is restricted by the confines of the hard dental tissue. The blood flowing into and out of the pulp through the apical delta of the tooth is limited. As a result, inflammatory swelling within the pulp results in compressive strangulation of the blood vessels in the pulp and tissue ischemia results. Red blood cells begin to break apart, and hemosiderin and other blood-breakdown products leach into the dentin of the tooth to cause discoloration. Dentin is composed of very small dentinal tubules that generally run perpendicular to the pulp cavity. When the ENTIRE crown is discolored, it is likely (>90% of the time) that the pulp tissue is completely devitalized. This does NOT mean that the pulp tissue is septically contaminated (which would typically occur if the pulp was exposed to oral bacteria). The right bacteria at the wrong time could enter the tooth through a process called anachoresis and the pulp chamber would become infected.

Treatment considerations are dependent on the age of the patient and when the discoloration occurred. If the patient is between approximately 6 and 15 months of age, the pulp cavity is relatively large, the dentinal walls are relatively thin, and the apex is large, the vessels going in and out of the pulp tissue are relatively wide in diameter compared with that of an older dog. Therefore, it is possible that the tooth MIGHT recover from this traumatic event and that the death of pulp tissue might only be restricted to the most coronal portion of the pulp. If the event that caused the pulpal hemorrhage is witnessed or the client is very astute and recognizes the injury right away, nonsteroidal antiinflammatories might be beneficial. Intraoral radiographs should be taken as a baseline; they will show that the pulp cavity diameters are all about the same in the four canine teeth. At the very least, all of the other canine teeth should be radiographed, although it is recommended that all teeth be studied when an opportunity such as this arises. A larger pulp chamber and thinner walls of the discolored tooth compared with that of the other teeth is a poor sign and indicates that the trauma occurred earlier than first recognized. If the teeth look fairly identical, the radiographs should be followed up in 4 to 6 months. If the discolored tooth remains vital, continued maturation will be seen. If the discolored tooth is nonvital, further maturation will not occur and the tooth will have a wider pulp cavity, thinner dentinal walls, and immature apex compared with the other teeth. An immature dead tooth has a poor prognosis, and depending on wall thickness, exodontics may be the only alternative. If the tooth has developed further and the wall is developed, treatment for a nonvital permanent tooth should be endodontic therapy. It is much less traumatic for the patient, the tooth and its occlusal partner stay functional and it could have the same fee or less than extracting such a tooth in a larger patient.

An older patient may present with a discolored tooth for a different reason—the odontoblasts throughout the life of the tooth have created dentin. Eventually this dentin may occlude the apex of the tooth, walling it off from the rest of the body. The tooth may be dead, but without the inflammatory process previously discussed. Radiographs of these teeth in patients more than 10 years of age may show a wisp of a pulp chamber and normal bone around the apex of the tooth.

Indications for Endodontic Therapy

The most common indication for root canal therapy is fractured teeth. If the tip of the crown appears black, the patient is a candidate for a work-up and evaluation of the tooth. Cats are particularly susceptible to canine tooth abscess. The pulp chamber extends close to the tip, and any exposure of dentine allows bacteria into the pulp chamber. Chronic abscess of the canine teeth is extremely common in cats; all fractured teeth necessitate root canal therapy, extraction, or close monitoring.

A worn tooth with a brown covering in the area where the pulp chamber used to be indicates that the wear has occurred slowly enough that secondary dentin was deposited by the odontoblasts lining the root canal and pulp chamber. In this case, the tooth should be evaluated radiographically. Occasionally, teeth that are completely normal in appearance may have apical disease that can be diagnosed only radiographically.

The rationale for endodontic treatment is to maintain optimal health. A tooth with endodontic disease produces various signs, including pain and irritability. Many patients with endodontic disease exhibit fluctuations in appetite. Clients frequently report halitosis, or bad breath, in pets with undiagnosed endodontic disease.

Once pulpal death occurs, most dogs and cats do not show pain. However, if the tooth is alive and recently traumatized, many patients flinch when the tooth is percussed with a probe or other instrument. Some animals chew food only on the side of the mouth opposite the traumatized tooth, or they drool and produce increased calculus on the injured side. Hunting dogs may refuse their training dummies, utility dogs may refuse their dumbbells, and attack dogs may either hesitate or bite and release repetitively because of the pain (this is referred to as *typewriting*). Dogs that are used for tracking scents may be less effective than usual because of the odor from the oral infection, which overwhelms the scent.

When pulp exposure is secondary to a coronal fracture or a carious erosion, pathogenic bacteria soon descend into the pulp canal and cause an abscess either within the canal itself or periapically by extension of the infection. Infection that has penetrated the apical end of the root canal can cause osteomyelitis and the subsequent loss of surrounding bone. Periapical infection can spread, contributing to pathologic fractures of the lower jaw, or the infection can extend through weakened necrotic bone and develop into an ONF from any of the maxillary teeth.

Advantage of Endodontic Therapy

Endodontic therapy is much less invasive than surgical extraction of a large canine tooth, which is a large, single-rooted tooth designed for puncturing, tearing, and grasping, or a carnassial tooth, which is a shearing tooth that is the upper fourth premolar and lower first molar in the dog and cat. This therapy can therefore be performed more easily and quickly than a surgical procedure. Standard root canal therapy is less traumatic for the patient and more aesthetically pleasing to the owner than surgical extraction. Moreover, the cost of root canal therapy is equivalent to that of surgical extraction. Another advantage of small animal endodontics is that a well-done procedure is less likely to fail in the pet's lifetime because the patient has a relatively short life span.

Endodontic Procedures
Vital Pulpotomy

Vital pulpotomy is indicated for recent fractures to preserve healthy dental pulp in the dog. This procedure should be performed within 48 hours of the fracture of a mature tooth. In an incompletely developed adult tooth, this time can be extended to 2 or 3 weeks after the fracture. In such a case, the young tooth will ideally develop a thicker and stronger dentinal wall during the extended time period, even if persistent infection later necessitates standard root canal therapy. The procedure is not recommended in the cat.

A vital pulpotomy is performed by removing the exposed, contaminated pulp and gently disinfecting the remaining pulp and access site. Calcium hydroxide is applied to stimulate the formation of a dentinal bridge, and a strong base interface is installed to support the surface restoration material of metal or a composite.

Direct Pulp-Capping

Direct pulp-capping resembles vital pulpotomy but is performed after purposeful or accidental iatrogenic pulpal exposure. The pulp may be intentionally exposed during a disarming procedure in which all four canines are coronally reduced to the level of the adjacent incisors. This procedure may also be performed on one or two maloccluded mandibular canines to relieve traumatic penetration of the upper gingiva or palate. This procedure is performed aseptically. The materials installed are the same as those used in a vital pulpotomy. The pulp does not require disinfecting, however, because the teeth are invaded in a sterile manner.

Indirect Pulp-Capping

Indirect pulp-capping is a restorative procedure performed when the preparation of a carious lesion does not penetrate the pulp but is perilously close (0.5 mm) to it. For such incidences, a therapeutic and insulating base layer of quick-setting calcium hydroxide paste is installed to protect the pulp. It is followed by the preparation for and the installation of an appropriate surface restoration.

Standard Root Canal Therapy

Standard root canal therapy (formerly called *conventional root canal therapy*) is also known as *pulpectomy*. In this procedure the pulp canal is approached in a normograde direction (from the crown to the apex). The entire pulp is removed through either the fracture site or one or more drilled access holes.

Standard root canal therapy is indicated for adult teeth that are discolored and endodontically dead or contaminated with long-standing infection. In a mature

tooth, a long-standing infection is one in which the pulp has been contaminated for more than 48 hours. In an immature tooth, long-standing infection means that the pulp has been contaminated for more than 2 weeks.

The radiograph in Fig. 13.3A, taken at the time of root canal therapy, shows a lytic area of bone around the apex of the tooth. The radiograph taken 3 years later (Fig. 13.3B) shows resolution of the lytic area. The endodontic procedure was successful.

Endodontic Equipment

Endodontic therapy requires various instruments and materials (Box 13.2). The equipment required includes barbed broaches, reamers, files, irrigating needles, mixing slab (or paper pad), spatula, pluggers, and spreaders (Fig. 13.4). Materials are discussed in more detail later in this chapter.

Barbed Broaches

A barbed broach (Fig. 13.5) is manufactured by making deep incisions in a soft iron wire, creating flared barbs. This instrument is not strong, but it is useful in removing intact pulp. The broach can also be used to remove from the root canal absorbent points, cotton pellets, separated file tips, and other foreign material such as dirt, gravel, and grass.

Files and Reamers

Files and reamers are used to clean the canal and remove dead or infected tissues (Fig. 13.6). Reamers are an earlier style of file but are still preferred by some practitioners. They are twisted, square metal rods with fewer flutes (or twists) per millimeter than on a file. Reamers are used in a twisting, auger-like motion that delivers filings from the depth of the canal to the access site.

The K-files and K-reamers are stiffer and stronger, size for size, than the Hedström files because of the way they are manufactured. To create K-files, a square, rhomboid, or triangular rod is twisted, creating cutting flutes. The K-file is similar in design to a reamer but has a tighter twist and is operated either by making a push-and-pull motion or by rotating clockwise 90 degrees and pulling coronally. It will break easily if is lodged tightly in the canal and then twisted counterclockwise in an effort to dislodge it. K-files produce a clean, smooth canal wall and, because of their design, are best used to cleanse and shape the apical portion of the canal.

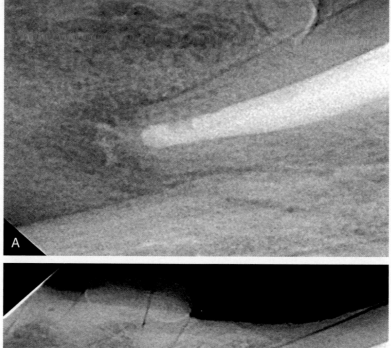

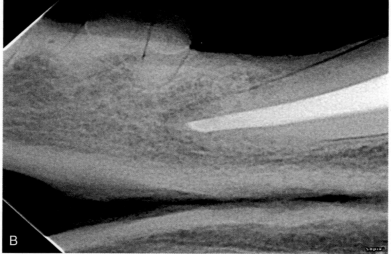

Fig. 13.3 A, Postoperative radiograph. B, Three-year follow-up radiograph.

BOX 13.2 **Endodontic Equipment, Instruments, and Materials**

Cutting bur: Tapered crosscut fissure burs #170L, round burs #2, #4, pear-shaped burs #330
Barbed broaches
K-files and Hedström files: Numbers 06, 08, 10, 15, 20, 25, 30, 35, 40, 45, 50, 55, 60, 70, 80, 90, 100 in 31 and 45 mm (minimum—longer files may be necessary)
Endodontic stops
Endodontic rings
Irrigation needles
Mixing slab and spatula

RC-Prep: Premier, PA, USA.
Canal irrigant: Sodium hypochlorite, chlorhexidine
Paper absorbent points: Similar size to files
Root canal sealer: Zinc oxide–eugenol (ZOE) or advanced sealers
Gutta-percha
Endodontic point forceps: Cotton or college pliers
Pluggers and spreaders: Short and long length
Restorative materials
Finishing disks, points, or stones

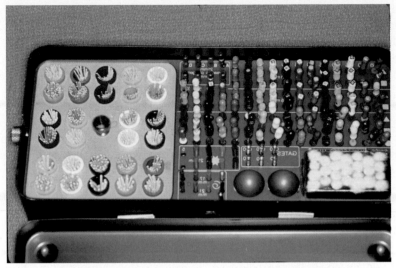

Fig. 13.4 This tray provides compact storage for materials.

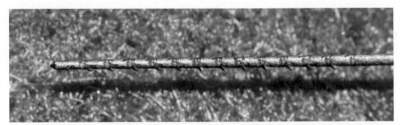

Fig. 13.5 Close-up of a barbed broach.

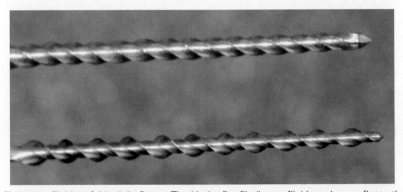

Fig. 13.6 K-file (upper file) has fairly tight flutes. The Hedström file (lower file) has sharper flutes than the K-file. These styles are manufactured for different distributors and can be purchased in premium or economy grades.

A Hedström file is created when a spiral groove is machined into the rod. It is weaker than a K-file because its core has been reduced in diameter by the machine. The shape of a Hedström file is that of inner-stacked cones. Its carrier effect is produced by a straight pull of the file. Hedström files produce a clean but not cylindrical or smooth wall. They are used to cleanse and shape the coronal or incisal portion of the canal.

Files and reamers have two dimensions: length and diameter. A millimeter notation indicates the length. Usually, two lengths are needed: 25 mm and 31 mm for incisors, premolars, and molars and 45 mm and 55 or 60 mm for canines (Fig. 13.7). The diameter is indicated by a number only, which represents the diameter of the file at the working end. A No. 10 file is 0.1 mm at the working end, and a No. 100 file is 1.0 mm at the working end. Files are stored in endodontic organizers. As they are pulled out and used, they may be stored (and cleaned) intraoperatively with an Endo-ring, which has an attached sponge and ruler. Before they are placed in the organizer, the files are cleaned and disinfected or sterilized.

Files and reamers are color coded to identify them by size. The numbers are repeated, however, so caution is necessary to prevent files of similar color but different size from being confused. The color-coding system is as follows:

Grey: 08
Purple: 10
White: 15, 45, 90, 150
Yellow: 20, 50, 100
Red: 25, 55, 110
Blue: 30, 60, 120
Green: 35, 70, 130
Black: 40, 80, 140

Newer types of files are available that increase by a percentage rather than by 0.05 mm or 0.1 mm. These files have their own color-coding system, which must be identified by the manufacturer.

Because an endodontic file is a cutting instrument, it operates most efficiently when sharp. The smaller sizes are delicate and prone to bending. They may also unravel, manifested by a shiny area between two cutting flutes, with repeated or improper use. Breakage occurs soon after a file has begun to unravel or after a file has been bent and subsequently straightened by the clinician (Fig. 13.8).

Endodontic Stops

Endodontic stops are pieces of rubber material placed on the file or reamer to aid in marking the length of the instrument. To find the apical working depth, smaller files are placed in the canal, the stop is moved to the

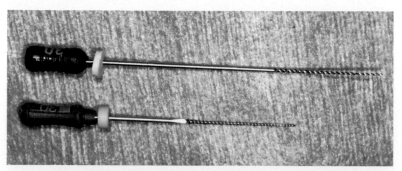

Fig. 13.7 File lengths: 31-mm and 55-mm files are compared.

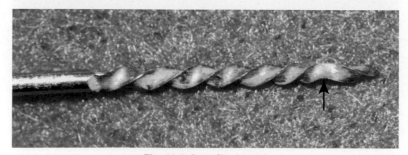

Fig. 13.8 Bent file *(arrow)*.

point where the file has entered the tooth, and a radiograph is taken. Once evaluated, the placement of the stop is adjusted so that the tip of the file reaches the apex when the stop just touches the access point. This distance is also measured.

Endo-Ring

An Endo-ring is a metal or plastic instrument that fits around the finger (Fig. 13.9). An attached disposable sponge, in which the files can be placed in ascending order of size, helps organize the files during the procedure. In addition, the sponge helps clean the files during the endodontic procedure.

Irrigation Materials

Irrigating solutions are introduced into the canal by means of a 27-gauge, blunt-tipped endodontic needle. Sodium hypochlorite helps break down and remove the organic material. When a file is being exchanged for a larger file (or whenever the canal is thought dry), the canal is flushed with a 1.5% sodium hypochlorite solution. This solution is made by mixing 1 part sodium hypochlorite to 3 parts water. RC Prep is an ethylenediaminetetraacetic acid (EDTA) chelating agent. This helps break down the inorganic material. A final flush is made with sodium hypochlorite.

Cotton or College Pliers

Locking cotton, also known as *college pliers,* are used to pick up paper points or gutta-percha without contaminating the container or points (Fig. 13.10).

Endodontic Materials

Absorbent points are used for drying the pulp canal after it has been prepared (debrided) and irrigated. Absorbent points are tightly rolled, tapered paper available in sizes 15 to 80, which correspond to file sizes. They are available in lengths of 25 mm, 31 mm, and 55 mm (Fig. 13.11). Absorbent points are disposable. Each size can be purchased in lots of 200 or fewer points, or they can be ordered in assorted sizes in conveniently organized packages. It is best to keep both lengths in every size on hand.

The root canal is sealed to prevent bacteria from entering the canal. Cements or pastes are used to seal the apical one-third of the root, dentinal tubules that radiate from the walls of the canal, and apical delta. There are several categories of root canal sealants, but two types are used most often in veterinary medicine. The first is a sealant made of zinc oxide–eugenol (ZOE). Used commonly in standard root canal procedures, it is best known for providing a long working time and being a good, nonirritating antimicrobial agent. Some dentists criticize it as being a temporary sealant because ZOE cements disintegrate after 5 to 8 years in the oral cavity. For most purposes, however, it is quite adequate for veterinary use because the life span of a dog or cat is much shorter than that of a person. The sealer is mixed by a figure-8 mixing motion.

Mixing should be performed on a glass slab or paper mixing pad. Noneugenol sealers, such as Nogenol, Sealapex, AH Plus, Tubliseal, and MTA, are used in place of ZOE. These sealers come in two-part systems (Fig. 13.12A). Usually, the parts are mixed equally on

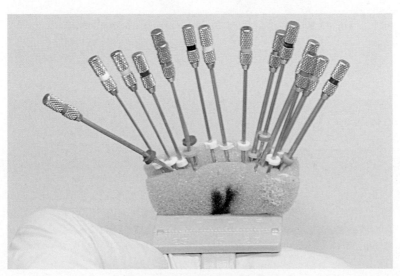

Fig. 13.9 An Endo-ring with files.

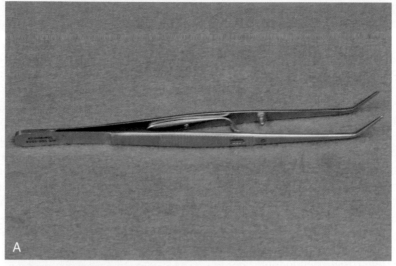

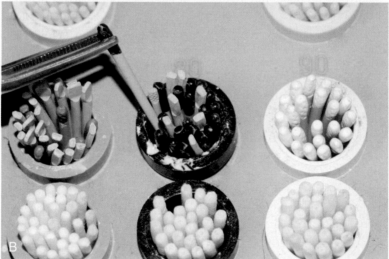

Fig. 13.10 A, Cotton pliers. B, Cotton pliers picking gutta-percha.

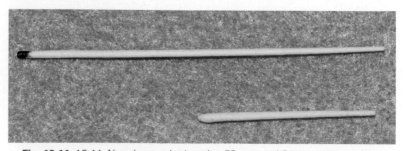

Fig. 13.11 13.11 Absorbent point lengths: 55-mm and 31-mm paper points.

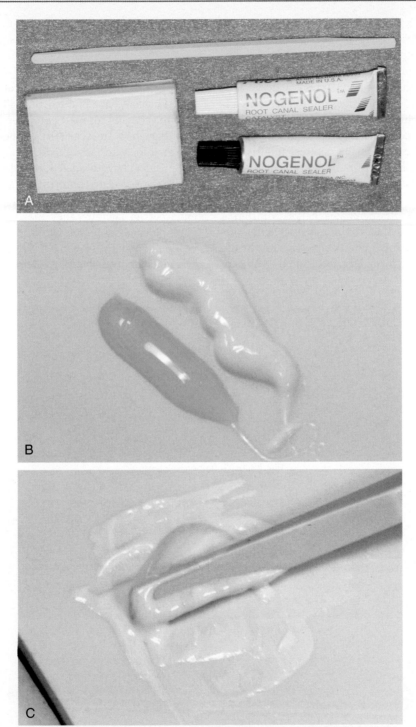

Fig. 13.12 A, Nogenol. B, Measuring Nogenol. C, Mixing Nogenol.

a paper pad (Fig. 13.12B). A figure-8 motion is used to mix the material (Fig. 13.12C). The mixture may be placed on the gutta-percha point and then carried into the canal with the gutta-percha.

Gutta-percha is the most popular core material used by veterinary practitioners. It does not irritate the periapical tissues and is highly condensable. It is used to help remove voids in the canal sealer and provide a better seal of the apex and openings to the dentinal tubules that radiate from the walls of the canal. Gutta-percha points, like absorbent points, are supplied in sizes 15 to 100 and in lengths of 30 mm and 55 mm to correspond with file sizes (Fig. 13.13). Gutta-percha is harvested from a rubber-type tree and is more commonly used in the softened beta form, which is more flexible and less brittle than the natural alpha form. Distributed to the clinician in the beta form, the material transforms to the less flexible and more brittle alpha form as its shelf-life expires.

Pluggers

A plugger is used to obtain vertical (apical) condensation. Pluggers have blunted tips (Fig. 13.14). They are used to vertically compact gutta-percha. Various lengths and diameters are available, including those specially designed for veterinary medicine.

Spreaders have a tapered, round shaft with a pointed tip. They are used to compress gutta-percha laterally and force sealant into dentinal tubules. By spreading the gutta-percha laterally, they make room for additional gutta-percha. Compared with the plugger, the spreader has a pointed tip (Fig. 13.15). Combination plugger-spreaders are available (Fig. 13.16).

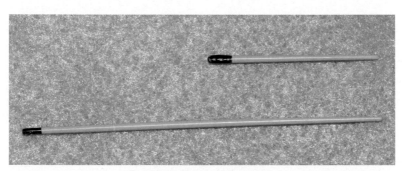

Fig. 13.13 Gutta-percha points.

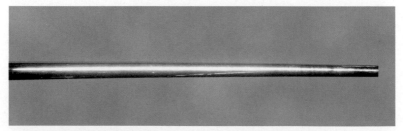

Fig. 13.14 Close-up of a plugger (note the blunt tip).

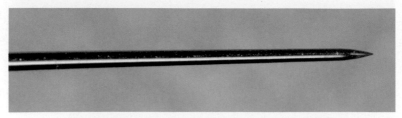

Fig. 13.15 Close-up of a spreader (note the pointed tip).

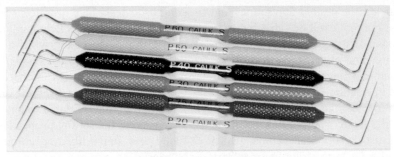

Fig. 13.16 Plugger-spreader set.

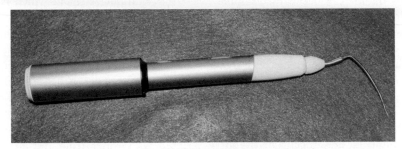

Fig. 13.17 Heated plugger.

Heated pluggers are used for cutting and softening gutta-percha to better conform it to the pulp chamber (Fig. 13.17).

Endodontic Technique

The following steps are performed in conventional, nonsurgical root canal therapy:
1. Evaluate the need for the procedure.
2. Expose the pulp chamber/root canal.
3. File and clean the canal.
4. Fill the canal with gutta-percha.
5. Prepare and fill the access site and any exposed fracture site.

Radiographs

Radiographs must be taken throughout the entire endodontic procedure. They are taken initially for diagnostic purposes. In the initial filing, a small rubber marker is placed on the file before insertion into the canal. The tooth is radiographed, which allows the practitioner to evaluate the length of the canal. When final filing of the canal is nearly complete, radiographs help the practitioner determine the depth and width of the filing procedure. After the canal has been filled (obturated), radiographs help the practitioner evaluate the seal and fill of the canal. If an apical seal is not obtained, the gutta-percha should be either condensed to seal or remove and the filling started over again.

Apicoectomy

Apicoectomy (retrograde or surgical) root canal therapy is indicated for peracute pulpal infections and as a treatment after standard root canal therapy has failed. It is also indicated when standard treatment presents anatomic or mechanical problems that prevent the completion of an adequate seal of the apical one-third of the root canal.

After standard root canal therapy, apicoectomy is performed on adult teeth in dogs and cats by approaching the apex of the root surgically through the alveolus. Once the necrotic debris is removed, the apex is sealed with a cement called MTA. This procedure is rarely required in small animals, but it is highly successful in treating difficult cases in which greater access and visibility are required.

RESTORATIVE DENTISTRY

Three types of dental restoratives are available to protect a tooth after endodontic treatment. The best material for the procedure depends on the desired appearance and the amount of trauma the tooth will be subjected to in the future. The purpose of restorative dentistry is to restore the form and function of damaged teeth.

Surface defects, whether iatrogenic (e.g., from drilling into a tooth) or caused by fracture, should be filled with a restorative material to protect the deeper filling materials used in treating the tooth. The cause of fractured and nonvital teeth is usually occlusal trauma, which occurs when the mandibular teeth strike the maxillary teeth or when an object is caught between the upper and lower teeth. This trauma can occur, for example, when a dog plays Frisbee or chews on objects harder than the teeth or when external forces are directed against the teeth. In most cases the patient will subject its teeth to further trauma after the tooth has been treated. A restoration protects the integrity of the crown and returns the tooth to its previous form and function. The restoration must be confluent with the margin of the defect and have the smoothest surface possible; this delays the formation of plaque and calculus on the surface of the restoration and prevents moisture leakage at its margins.

Two types of restoratives that are commonly used in veterinary dentistry are:
- Composites (plastics)
- Full-coverage metal or porcelain-fused-to-metal crowns

Composite Restoration

Composites are second only to metal restorations in hardness and are more aesthetically pleasing. Composites are installed on the rostral teeth and premolars. They must be applied in a dry environment. Composites are the most commonly used class of restorative material in veterinary dentistry. The use of light-cured composite restorations is recommended. Composites used in veterinary dentistry, like other dental restoratives, are manufactured for use in humans. However, dogs have a bite that is three times as powerful as that of humans. Dogs also abuse their teeth more than humans do.

The restoration site is prepared using a bur of the appropriate size and shape. As little of the tooth structure is removed as possible to prevent weakening but still allow for a macromechanical bond (mechanical retention) with the restorative material.

The site is cleaned with flour pumice to remove any surface oils that would interfere with adhesion to the composite resin. The pumice, which is commercially available, is a highly silicious material of volcanic origin. It should be mixed with oil-free (filtered) water until it reaches the consistency of a thick paste. Composites do not cure in a moist environment such as blood, saliva, or water. Even the oil from the operator's fingertips or contaminated water or air sprays will negatively affect the setting properties of composite resin. Blood also stains uncured composite. The site must be rinsed to remove the pumice residue and then air-dried.

A conditioner/etchant, which is an acid, is applied with a disposable brush to remove the powdered tooth debris (smear layer), 1 to 5 microns thick, created by the cutting bur (Fig. 13.18A). The conditioner makes tiny etches in the tooth's surface. Etching permits bonding agents to later penetrate into the etch-induced micro-irregularities and thereby form interlocking tags (Fig. 13.18B).

After application, the acid-etch is thoroughly rinsed with water from the air-water syringe. After rinsing, the tooth is gently air-dried with air from a three-way syringe or a hair dryer set on low. Caution should be used not to burn the gingiva if a hair dryer is used. Once dry, the enamel will appear chalky white (Fig. 13.18C).

Next, a bonding agent is applied to the tooth (Fig. 13.19A and B). The bonding agent often contains unfilled resin and a hydrophilic agent, an agent that will attract water and aid in the evaporation of water from the restoration surface.

After applying the bonding agent the area is gently blown dry with air from a three-way syringe and light-cured according to the manufacturer's recommendations, usually 10 to 20 seconds (Fig. 13.19C).

Finally, the defect is filled with composite, leaving no voids. First, a layer of composite no more than 2 to 3 mm thick is applied (Fig. 13.19D). This layer is light-cured for 40 to 60 seconds, according to the manufacturer's instructions. Layering continues in this manner until the defect is slightly overfilled and the composite overlaps the margins of the defect. A plastic working instrument is used to smooth out the composite in preparation for the final finishing (Fig. 13.19E).

Once contoured, the final layer of composite is light-cured. It is important not to look at the light-cure gun or tooth without special glasses or filters covering the light-curing process (Fig. 13.20).

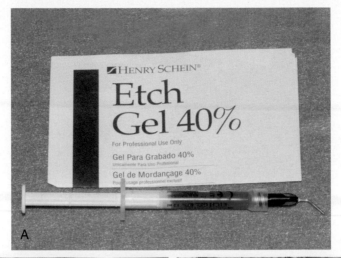

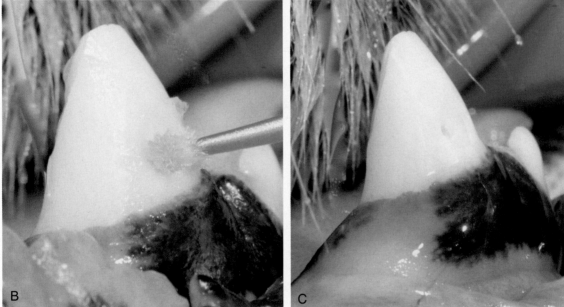

Fig. 13.18 A, Acid-etch gel. B, The acid-etch gel is placed on the tooth before placement of the restoration. C, The dry enamel appears chalky white.

The restored tooth is finished, or smoothed, until its surface is shiny and flawless. Finishing methods vary and include the use of the following instruments:

1. A fine, followed by an extra-fine, garnet sandpaper abrasive disk on a low-speed contra angle (Fig. 13.21A).
2. A composite finishing green stone followed by a white Arkansas stone bur (Fig. 13.21B) on a low- or high-speed handpiece

3. 12-, 16-, and then 30-fluted finishing burs. Finishing disks work best for fairly flat, broad surfaces. Rotating stones are useful when working close to the gingival margin or when recreating a developmental groove in the tooth's surface.

One alternative to a full composite restoration is to apply a base layer of glass ionomer prior to placing the composite restoration. This technique must be used when the older ZOE endodontic sealers are placed.

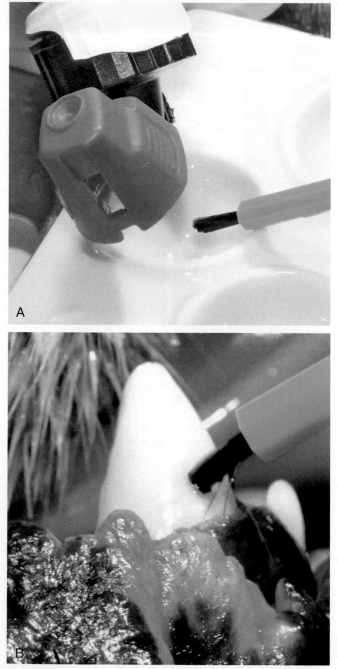

Fig. 13.19 A, Placing bonding agent into dappen dish. B, The bonding agent primer is placed on the tooth surface with a disposable brush.

Continued

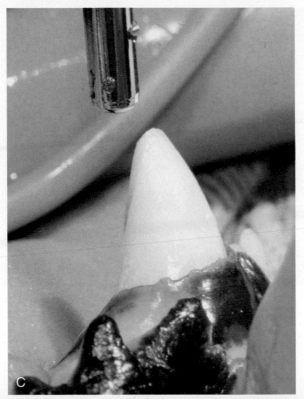

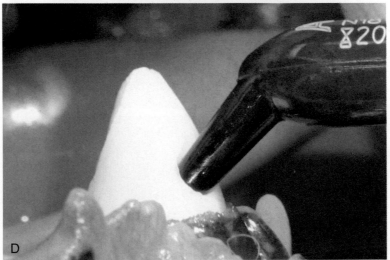

Fig. 13.19, cont'd C, Air-drying the bonding agent. D, Applying composite.

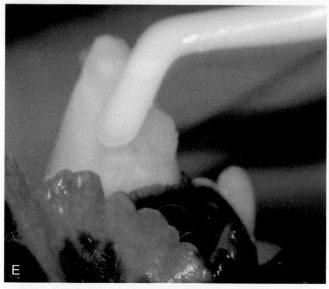

Fig. 13.19, cont'd E, A plastic working instrument is used to place the composite material.

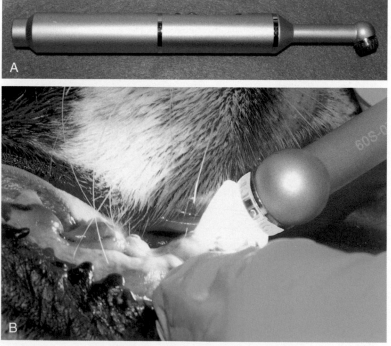

Fig. 13.20 A, Light-cure gun. B, Light curing.

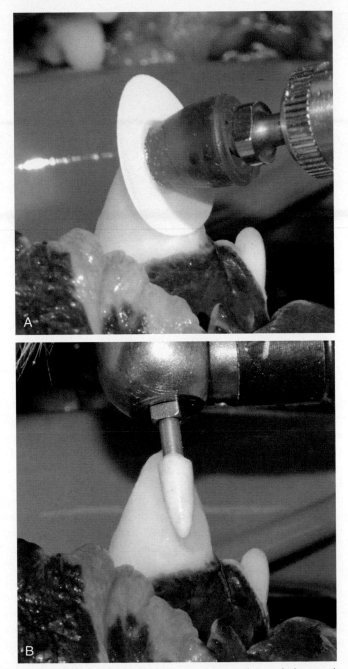

Fig. 13.21 A, Sanding disk. B, A white stone is used to shape and smooth the cured composite resin.

Crown Restorations

Full-coverage metal crowns are used to protect the surface of the endodontically treated tooth from further injury and to provide renewed height, shape, and function of severely deformed, fractured teeth. However, preparing the tooth to receive the crown can weaken the tooth. Porcelain-fused-to-metal (PFM) crowns are more cosmetically pleasing than metal crowns. With any type of full-coverage crown, careful evaluation of tooth size, stage of tooth development, and oral habits

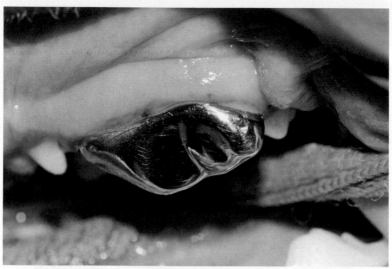

Fig. 13.22 Crown 208. The patient has had crown therapy to protect the left maxillary fourth premolar tooth.

of the patient is imperative to achieve successful results. In many patients, installing full-coverage crowns, whether metal or PFM, is unwise. Crown therapy is the best choice of restoration of the caudal, chewing teeth. Creation of a metal shield around the tooth protects it from chip fractures but does not prevent "catastrophic" fracture. Crowns require a great deal of effort in terms of design and preparation; installing a crown is therefore an advanced procedure.

Although metal crowns may provide renewed shape and function to the tooth, the clinician must be careful to avoid building the crown too high or torque forces will accumulate. Metal crowns are custom made and require preparation of the tooth and construction of a model (Fig. 13.22).

ORTHODONTICS

The term *orthodontics* refers to the correction of dental malocclusions. Before accepting the patient for orthodontic correction, the practitioner must advise the client of potential legal and ethical implications of these procedures. Orthodontic procedures should not be performed on animals intended for breeding or show, and whenever possible, animals should be neutered prior to the procedure.

Bite Evaluation

Orthodontic diagnosis and management require a three-dimensional evaluation of the relationships between the bone, teeth, and soft tissue structures within and between the dental arches. Although the incisor relationship is important, bite evaluation entails more than just observing the incisor relationship. Some commonly used lay terms such as "overbite" or "underbite" are not universally defined and can be interpreted differently. It is best to use scientific nomenclature that has been carefully worded and defined by the AVDC. The classes of occlusion are normal, class 1, class 2, class 3, and class 4. Normal occlusion is a scissor bite in which the lower incisors occlude on the cingulum on the palatal surface of the upper incisors. The upper and lower premolars are in an interdigitated relationship with the maxillary teeth buccal to the mandibular teeth. The upper and lower arches are symmetric. The reader is referred to Chapter 2 for the classes of malocclusion.

Good-quality photographs, taken with the macro setting that shows the arrangement of the rostral teeth and side view of the caudal maxillary and mandibular teeth with the mouth held closed and the lips retracted, are often helpful for evaluation and consultation.

Interceptive Orthodontics

It is recommended that deciduous teeth be selectively extracted as treatment of malocclusions for several reasons:

1. The patient currently is feeling pain as the sharp crown cusp of the deciduous mandibular canine tooth penetrates the palatal tissue whenever the

mouth is closed. Patients with malocclusion tend to be more "mouthy" than other animals because they would rather have a shoe or piece of furniture in their mouth than having that misaligned tooth or teeth penetrate their soft tissues and cause them pain.

2. An abnormally displaced deciduous tooth can interfere with jaw development by interlocking and preventing forward and side-to-side jaw growth. The four arches grow independently from the growth centers located in the caudal regions of the mandible and maxilla. The time the deciduous teeth are present corresponds to the most active period of growth. Although the arches are not physically joined together, they grow in a coordinated fashion owing to the interdigitation of the teeth. With soft tissue penetration on one side or even both sides, free forward and side-to-side growth can be inhibited, leading to a more serious malocclusion as the permanent teeth erupt.

3. The pointed crown cusp of a deciduous mandibular canine tooth will penetrate the palatal tissue in the location of the nonerupted and developing crown of the permanent, maxillary canine tooth and can lead to developmental damage.

Interceptive orthodontics does not cause the jaws to grow more, but it can allow the full genetic potential of the jaws to develop.

Dental Models

Dental models are made for orthodontic evaluation and treatment and the manufacture of restorative crowns. Many instruments and materials are used (Box 13.3). The following section includes a fundamental technique that provides basic information on the creation of a model. All techniques require instruction and practice.

Orthodontic correction usually requires a three-stage process (Box 13.4). In the first stage, an impression and dental model are made. An appliance is created from the

---

BOX 13.3 **Instruments and Materials for Making Models**

Impression trays
Alginate
Mixing bowls
Spatula
Dental stone
Vibrator

BOX 13.4 **Orthodontic Correction: Three-Stage Process**

Stage I (Impression)
Radiograph materials
Impression trays
Impression material: Alginate
Laboratory stone
Bite-register material
Mailing supplies for laboratory

Stage II (Placement)
Orthodontic cement kit
Appliance
Orthodontic buttons
Appliance adjustment instruments
Hand scaler
Ultrasonic scaler
Flour pumice
Low-speed handpiece with new prophy cup
Power cord
Elastics

Stage III (Removal)
Ultrasonic scaler
Band-removing forceps
Prophy angle, cups, and paste

---

model. In the second stage, the appliance is placed in the patient's mouth using orthodontic cement. Once the appliance is in place, the patient is carefully monitored at home and is returned to the practice for periodic rechecks. The third stage is the removal of the appliance after treatment is complete.

Materials for Making Models

Impression trays may be purchased from commercial sources (Fig. 13.23). Trays designed specifically for dogs and cats should be used, although impression trays used in human dentistry will work for some veterinary impressions. Custom trays may be made out of plastic materials.

When mixed with water, alginate forms an agar suspension that hardens to a gel in minutes. The actual rate of this process depends on the chemical formulation. Fast-setting and normal-setting varieties of alginate are available. Fast-setting alginate hardens in 1 to 2 minutes and is also known as *type I alginate*. Normal-setting alginate sets in 2 to 4.5 minutes and is

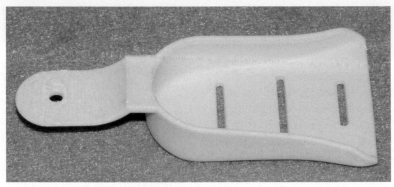

Fig. 13.23 Impression tray.

known as *type II alginate*. The setting rate of alginate also varies according to water and environmental temperatures. Heat speeds up the setting rate, whereas coldness slows it down. The trays should be tested in the mouth to make sure they fit before the alginate is mixed.

Alginate is mixed in flexible rubber mixing bowls. Either metal or plastic spatulas are used for stirring. Dental stone is hardened gypsum stone. The material is mixed, allowed to set, crushed, mixed, allowed to set once more, and then crushed again several times. Its hardness and resistance to shrinkage distinguishes dental stone from plaster of Paris, which is also frequently used. A dental vibrator is used to agitate the mixed dental stone material so that bubbles emerge and escape before hardening. Also, this vibration causes the material to flow more readily.

Technique for Making Models

Before alginate is mixed, the trays should be tested in the mouth. Specific product directions should always be consulted beforehand. The alginate jar should first be lightly shaken to "fluff up" the material and give it a uniform volume. Alginate is measured by volume with the measuring spoon provided (Fig. 13.24A). The alginate is then placed in a mixing bowl (Fig. 13.24B). A measuring cup for the water is provided with the alginate (Fig. 13.24C).

Next, the water is added to the bowl. Measuring systems are available in various sizes. The correct ratio of alginate to water is important, so the vessels should be marked if alginate from different manufacturers is being used. The alginate is mixed in a figure-8 mixing motion with a metal or plastic spatula. The bowl is rotated during mixing to ensure uniformity (Fig. 13.24D). The mixed alginate is transferred by spatula to a tray of appropriate size. The alginate must be mixed, poured, and quickly placed because it will harden in only a few minutes. Once the alginate reaches a smooth consistency, it is transferred to the tray (Fig. 13.24E). Spreading the material evenly in the tray with a spatula before inserting it into the mouth helps prevent the formation of air pockets and bubbles in the impression (Fig. 13.24F). The tray is placed in the posterior portion of the mouth first, and the anterior portion of the tray is rotated forward and held in position until it sets (Fig. 13.24G and H).

The last step is having the patient take a bite registration. Two types of materials are used: bite wax and two-part bite-registration compounds. The two models (maxillary and mandibular) can be matched up with a bite registration. Bite-registration material assists the laboratory in lining up the occlusion before laboratory work (Fig. 13.25).

The next step is pouring the stone model: measurement of the powder and liquid is important in the mixing process. Most dental stones are measured by weight as opposed to volume (Fig. 13.26). The measured water is placed in the bowl, and the dental stone is mixed. A vibrator is used to assist in the flow of the dental stone and to remove bubbles (Fig. 13.27). A base may be poured. This adds thickness to the model and may allow for easier removal of the model from the impression.

The model should be removed from the impression as soon as it has hardened. It is important that the alginate remains moist; if the models are not removed immediately, the model, alginate, and tray should be kept wrapped with damp towels in a plastic bag. Removing the tray before the alginate is removed from the model may be helpful. Care should be taken not to break the teeth as the alginate is being removed.

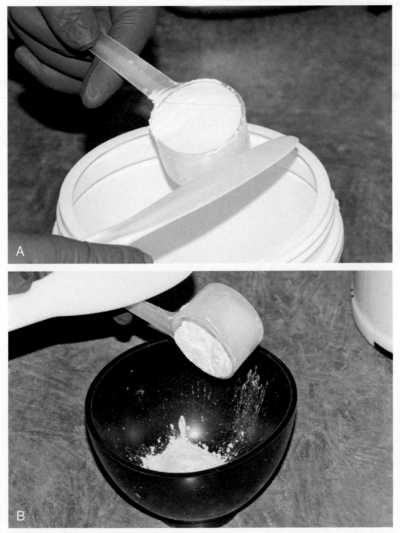

Fig. 13.24 A, A dry spatula is used to level the amount of alginate in the measuring spoon. B, The alginate is placed in the rubber mixing bowl.

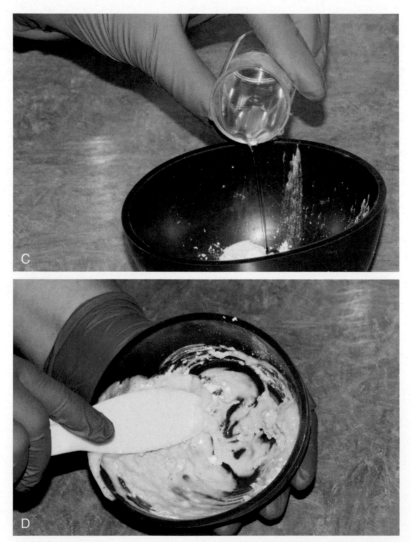

Fig. 13.24, cont'd C, The directions on the alginate bottle should always be followed; usually, one scoop of algi-nate requires one measure of water. D, A spatula is used to transfer the alginate into the tray.

Continued

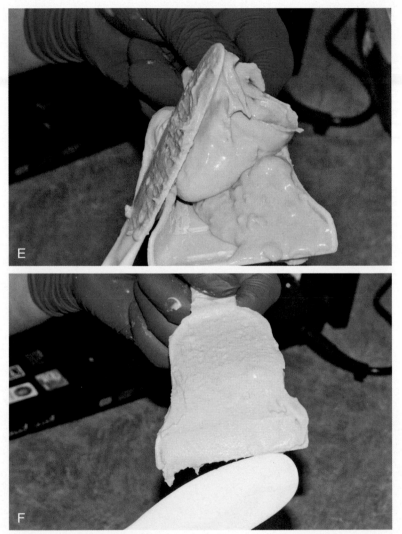

Fig. 13.24, cont'd E, Transferring to tray. F, A spatula is used to smooth the alginate before placing it in the mouth.

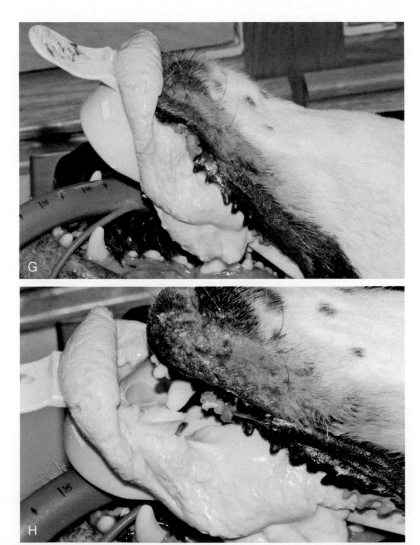

Fig. 13.24, cont'd G, An alginate tray is placed in the mouth and held steady until the alginate hardens. H, Removing alginate from mouth.

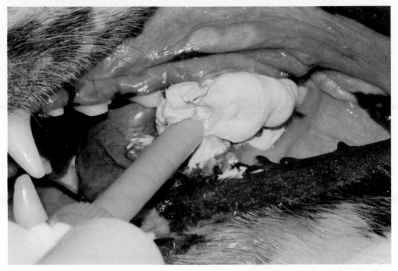

Fig. 13.25 Bite-registration material is placed in the mouth and allowed to harden.

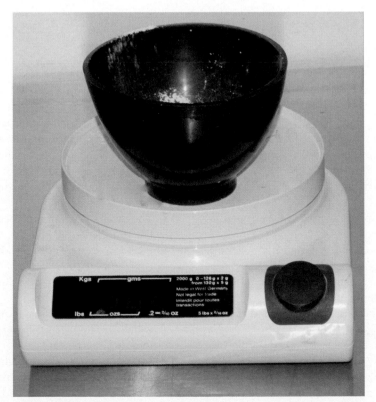

Fig. 13.26 A gram scale is used to measure the powder portion of the dental stone.

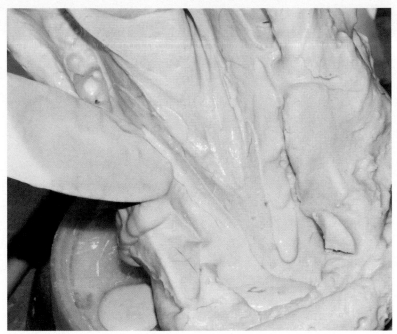

Fig. 13.27 A dental vibrator is used to help the dental stone to flow into the impression more readily.

CHAPTER 13 WORKSHEET

1. Periodontal flaps are created to expose _____ and associated _____.
2. A _____, _____ and _____ _____ are used diagnostically before the procedure to determine the location of the pocket and to aid in the selection of an appropriate form of therapy.
3. The No. _____ handle is the standard scalpel handle.
4. _____ is only performed in cases where hyperplastic gingiva is present.
5. The frenoplasty procedure is designed to relieve the _____ from the gingiva.
6. _____ _____ is a general statement indicating treatment of the dental pulp.
7. Most commonly, bacteria gain entry into the pulp chamber via a _____ _____.
8. A discolored tooth, especially if pink or purple, indicates _____ _____.
9. If the tip of the crown appears _____, the patient is a candidate for a work-up and evaluation of the tooth.
10. Compared with most extractions, standard root canal therapy is _____ traumatic for the patient.
11. Vital pulpotomy is indicated within _____ hours of the fracture of a mature tooth.
12. _____ _____ _____ therapy is indicated for adult teeth that are discolored and endodontically dead or that have been contaminated with long-standing infection.
13. The two most common types of files are the _____ file and the _____ file.
14. Files and reamers have two dimensions: _____ and _____.
15. _____ have blunted tips. They are used to vertically compact gutta-percha.
16. A _____ _____ is an abnormal occlusal pattern in which the upper and lower incisors occlude cusp to cusp.
17. In _____ _____ or in lingually displaced canine teeth the tips of the mandibular canine teeth are displaced lingually and occlude on the hard palate.

18. A _____ _____ is an abnormal occlusion caused by a difference in length of the two maxillas and mandibles.

19. _____ _____ are made for orthodontic evaluation and treatment and the manufacture of restorative crowns.

20. _____ _____ _____ are used to mix alginate. The mixing bowl is flexible, allowing better mixing.

14

Lagomorph, Rodent, and Ferret Dentistry

Alexander M. Reiter and Ana C. Castejon-Gonzalez

OUTLINE

LEARNING OBJECTIVES

When you have completed this chapter, you will be able to:

- Define the term *heterodont dentition* and explain how it applies to lagomorphs, rodents, and ferrets.
- Define the terms *aradicular hypsodont, brachyodont, elodont,* and *peg teeth* and explain how they apply to lagomorphs, rodents, and ferrets.
- Describe the unique structure of the peg teeth in lagomorphs and aradicular hypsodont cheek teeth of lagomorphs and rodents.

- List the dental formulas of the adult rabbit, guinea pig, chinchilla, hamster, rat, gerbil, and ferret.
- List the equipment needed for dental care of lagomorphs, rodents, and ferrets.
- List and describe common oral problems and diseases and treatments in lagomorphs and rodents.
- List and describe common oral problems and diseases and treatments in ferrets.

KEY TERMS

Abrasion
Acepromazine
Anisognathic jaw relationship
Aradicular hypsodont
Atraumatic malocclusion
Attrition
Blind intubation
Bone substitute
Brachyodont
Buccotomy
Calcium hydroxide
Caries
Carnivore
Cheek pouch impaction
Cheek retractors
Chinchilla
Diastema
Enamel hypomineralization
Endoscopic intubation
Endotracheal intubation

Ferret
Files
Floating
Gingivitis
Guinea pig
Herbivore
Heterodont dentition
Intermediate plexus
Intubation
Isoflurane
Ketamine
Lagomorph
Laryngoscope
Manipulation
Mouth gag
Occlusal equilibration
Odontoplasty
Omnivore
Otoscope
Palpation

Patency
Periodontal abscess
Periodontal disease
Periodontal-endodontic abscess
Periodontitis
Rabbit
Rasps
Retrograde intubation
Rodent
Scurvy
Sevoflurane
Slobbers
Stethoscope-aided intubation
Stomatitis
Tongue entrapment
Tongue retractors
Tooth elongation
Tracheotomy intubation
Traumatic malocclusion
Vital pulp therapy

This chapter discusses the basics of lagomorph, rodent, and ferret dentistry, including equipment, supplies, and techniques for oral examination, diagnosis, and treatment. Relevant anatomy is reviewed.

GENERAL INFORMATION

Lagomorphs

The order Lagomorpha includes the domestic rabbit, hare, and cottontail. Lagomorphs were once grouped with rodents; a separate order was later created owing to distinct differences in the number of incisor teeth. The rabbit is the only member of this order commonly kept as a family pet. Adult rabbits have between 26 and 28 teeth.

Rodents

The term "rodent" comes from the Latin word *rodere,* meaning "to gnaw." The order Rodentia is the largest order of the class Mammalia and contains a great diversity of species. Smaller animals within this order that are kept as pets are the rat, mouse, guinea pig, hamster, gerbil, chinchilla, gopher, squirrel, and prairie dog. Most adult pet rodents have between 12 and 22 teeth.

Ferrets

Ferrets belong to the order Carnivora and the family Mustelidae. Ferrets have deciduous and permanent dentitions. Adult ferrets have 34 teeth.

DENTAL ANATOMY

Dentition in the Lagomorph, Rodent, and Ferret

All lagomorphs and most rodents are herbivores, eating leaves, grass, and other lush green plants; however, some rodents are omnivores, eating plants and other animals. Lagomorphs and rodents have a dental formula that features variation in tooth size and shape among the incisors, premolars, and molars, known as a *heterodont dentition.* Lagomorphs and rodents do not have canine teeth but instead have a long diastema (toothless area) between the incisors and cheek teeth. Ferrets are carnivores with a heterodont dentition consisting of incisors, canines, premolars and molars. Lagomorphs differ from rodents in that they have two pairs of maxillary incisor teeth. The rostral row of incisors consists of two larger functional teeth; a second row of two rudimentary incisors (sometimes referred to as "peg" teeth) sits immediately behind the first row.

Type of Teeth in the Lagomorph

Both the incisors and cheek teeth of lagomorphs are of the aradicular hypsodont type (continuously growing and erupting throughout life, also referred to as elodont) (Fig. 14.1). These teeth have clinical crowns visible intraorally and reserve crowns submerged below the gingival margin. They continue to grow and erupt as the teeth undergo normal wear. These teeth never form roots.

Type of Teeth in the Rodent

Two basic types of teeth are found in the rodent: the aradicular hypsodont (continuously growing and erupting) and, in some species, aradicular hypsodont incisors and brachyodont cheek teeth. The brachyodont tooth is the same type of tooth found in humans, cats, and dogs (i.e., a tooth with true distinction between crown and root structure that does no longer grow once fully erupted). Guinea pigs (Fig. 14.2) and chinchillas (Fig. 14.3) have aradicular hypsodont teeth for both the incisors and cheek teeth, whereas mice and rats have aradicular hypsodont incisors and brachyodont cheek teeth.

Type of Teeth in the Ferret

Ferrets have long, thin canine teeth, with the mandibular canine teeth occluding into the space between the maxillary third incisors and canines, thus forming a tight dental interlock when the mouth is closed. Incisor teeth are small, with three incisors in each quadrant. The maxillary fourth premolar and mandibular first molar teeth are sectorial, closing in a scissor-like fashion. Hourglass-shaped maxillary first molar teeth are a common dental finding of the family Mustelidae (Fig. 14.4). The relatively small size of the teeth and oral cavity, coupled with the animal's active nature, makes it difficult to thoroughly assess oral health in conscious ferrets, and therefore oral pathology can easily be overlooked without sedation or anesthesia. Ferrets, being carnivores, have a highly specialized brachyodont dentition.

Incisor Teeth of Lagomorphs and Rodents

The maxillary and mandibular incisor teeth of lagomorphs and rodents, with the exception of the peg teeth of lagomorphs, come to a chisel-like point. These teeth have enamel on the front and lateral sides, but typically just cementum and dentin on the palatal/lingual surface. Cementum and dentin wear much faster than enamel, resulting in a chisel edge that is longer labially. The enamel of incisors in most rodents takes on a yellow-orange color—an exception is seen in the

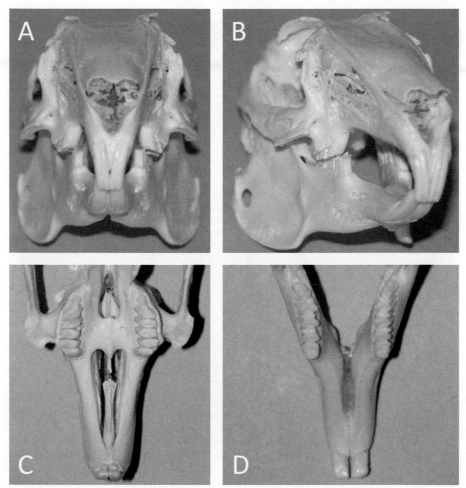

Fig. 14.1 Rabbit skull. A, Frontal view. B, Frontolateral view. C, Upper jaw occlusal view. D, Lower jaw occlusal view. (Copyright 2017, Alexander M. Reiter.)

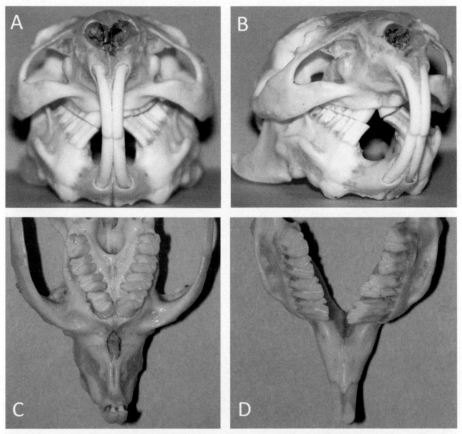

Fig. 14.2 Guinea pig skull. A, Frontal view. B, Frontolateral view. C, Upper jaw occlusal view. D, Lower jaw occlusal view. There is elongation of the clinical crowns (intraorally) and reserve crowns (periapically; note the bony bumps at the ventrolateral aspect of both mandibles and medial aspect of the left orbit) of the cheek teeth. (Copyright 2017, Alexander M. Reiter.)

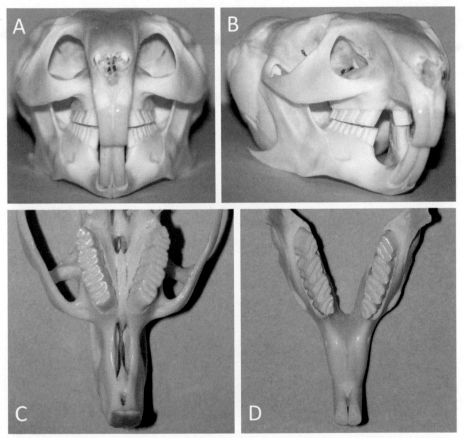

Fig. 14.3 Chinchilla skull. A, Frontal view. B, Frontolateral view. C, Upper jaw occlusal view. D, Lower jaw occlusal view. (Copyright 2017, Alexander M. Reiter.)

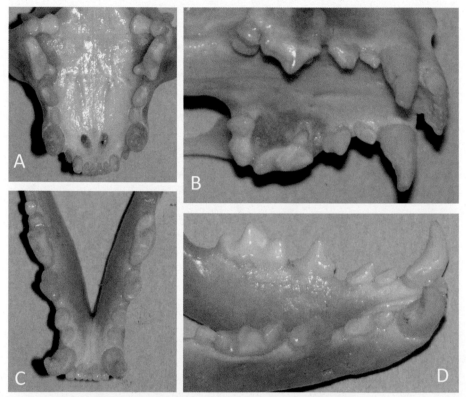

Fig. 14.4 Ferret skull. A, Upper jaw occlusal view. B, Upper jaw lateral oblique view. C, Lower jaw occlusal view. D, Lower jaw lateral oblique view. (Copyright 2017, Alexander M. Reiter.)

guinea pig. Incisor teeth are very long and curved. The location of the apex of these teeth varies with the species of animal. In most species the apex of the maxillary incisor teeth lies in the area of the diastema. However, in rats and mice, the mandibular incisor apices are distal to the roots of the last cheek tooth, whereas rabbits and chinchillas usually have their mandibular incisor apices near the mesial surfaces of the first cheek teeth.

Hypsodont Cheek Teeth of Lagomorphs and Rodents

Because of their unique function, hypsodont cheek teeth often have an angled rather than a flat occlusal table surface. The highest point of the chisel tip of the maxillary cheek teeth is on the labial side, angling dorsally toward the soft tissue of the hard palate. The bevel of the mandibular cheek teeth goes in the opposite direction. The chisel point of the mandibular cheek teeth is on the lingual side, and the tooth's occlusal table angles toward the soft tissue of the cheek. These wear patterns are owing to the fact that the maxillary cheek teeth are spread wider apart from the midline than are the mandibular teeth. This is known as an anisognathic, or naturally unequal, jaw relationship, in which the upper dental arch is slightly wider than the lower dental arch. Healthy rabbits have only a very slight angulation to the occlusal plane of the cheek teeth (~10-degree angle from dorsolingual to ventrobuccal), healthy guinea pigs have a relatively steep angulation (~30-degree angle from dorsobuccal to ventrolingual), and healthy chinchillas have a level occlusal plane.

Periodontal Ligament

The periodontal ligament (PDL) of permanent aradicular hypsodont teeth may differ from that of permanent brachyodont teeth owing to the presence of an intermediate plexus between its tooth and bone attachments. This plexus may allow continuously growing teeth to move coronally as they grow. This adaptation of hypsodont teeth is thought to explain how the PDL allows for continued eruption, although the presence of the intermediate plexus has been debated.

Adult Lagomorph Dental Formulas

Rabbit: 2 × (I 2/1, C 0/0, P 3/2, M 2-3/3) = 26 to 28 total teeth
Hare: 2 × (I 2/1, C 0/0, P 3/2, M 3/3) = 28 total teeth

Adult Rodent Dental Formulas

Guinea pig and chinchilla: 2 × (I 1/1, C 0/0, P 1/1, M 3/3) = 20 total teeth
Degu: 2 × (I 1/1, C 0/0, P 1/1, M 3/3) = 20 total teeth
Rat: 2 × (I 1/1, C 0/0, P 0/0, M 2-3/2-3) = 12 to 16 total teeth
Hamster: 2 × (I 1/1, C 0/0, P 0/0, M 2-3/2-3) = 12 to 16 total teeth
Gerbil: 2 × (I 1/1, C 0/0, P 0/0, M 3/3) = 16 total teeth
Squirrel: 2 × (I 1/1, C 0/0, P 1-2/1, M 3/3) = 20 to 22 total teeth

Adult Ferret Dental Formula

Ferret: 2 × (I 3/3; C 1/1; P 3/3; M 1/2) = 34 total teeth

INSTRUMENTS AND EQUIPMENT USED TO TREAT LAGOMORPHS, RODENTS, AND FERRETS

The following instruments and equipment are used in the treatment of oral disorders in lagomorphs, rodents, and ferrets:

Towels are helpful for restraint and for maintaining normothermia during procedures.

Anesthesia is available in two forms: injectable and inhalant. Injectable medications such as ketamine and acepromazine usually result in a longer recovery time than inhalants. Some injectables are reversible. Inhalants such as isoflurane and sevoflurane are preferred for maintenance of anesthesia for most procedures. Anesthesia masks can be used for induction of anesthesia prior to intubation or for the maintenance of anesthesia using an off-and-on mask approach during the actual dental procedure. Induction may also be administered in an anesthesia chamber, although small mammals may hold their breath because of the odor of the inhalant. Anesthesia and oxygen may also be delivered through an endotracheal tube. A laryngoscope with a small pediatric straight blade is used for endotracheal intubation to maintain the airway and administer anesthesia. Endotracheal tubes in sizes 1.5, 2.0, 2.5, or 3.0 Cole or a standard endotracheal tube may be used, depending on the patient's size. A wire stylet placed in the tubes makes passage much easier (Fig. 14.5).

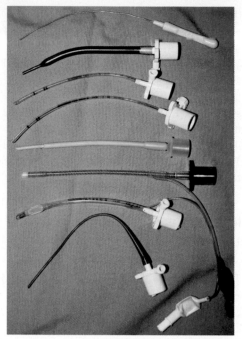

Fig. 14.5 Standard, Cole type, and hand-made endotracheal tubes and a stylet for use during tube placement. (Copyright 2017, Alexander M. Reiter.)

An **otoscope** with ear cones or a nasal speculum may be used to visualize the teeth and oral cavity of small mammals. In addition, these can be used as an aid in passing endotracheal tubes.

Intravenous (IV) catheters (12 to 14 gauge) can be used as an endotracheal tube for smaller rodents if the stylet is removed. These catheters can often be passed with the use of an otoscope as a laryngoscope.

Umbilical tape is used to anchor the endotracheal tube by snugly tying it to the tube and then behind the pet's head.

Cotton-tipped applicators are used during dental procedures to clear the oral cavity of food, saliva, and debris.

Explorers/probes are used to examine teeth and their attachment structures.

Handpieces, both high-speed and low-speed, can be used with burs to shape, trim, prepare, or extract teeth.

Mouth gags aid in keeping the mouth open during inspection and treatment. Most are spring activated, or they may expand with a screw device (Fig. 14.6).

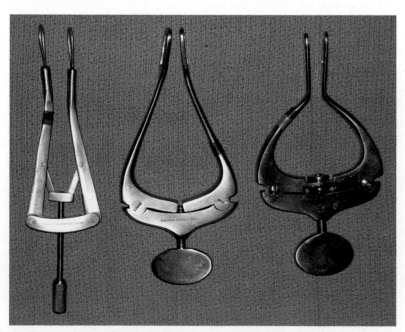

Fig. 14.6 Mechanical mouth gags. Care should be taken to avoid excessive force by opening the mouth only as wide as needed for visualization of the oral cavity. (Copyright 2017, Alexander M. Reiter.)

Cheek retractors are single-bladed instruments that retract the cheek on a single side or double-bladed instruments with a spring wire that can spread apart both cheeks at the same time (Fig. 14.7).

Tongue retractors are generally instruments with a single, flat blade used to move the tongue away from the area to be inspected or treated (Fig. 14.8).

Burs are used for removal of hard tissue. The most common types are diamond burs, carbide round burs, carbide tapered fissure burs, and white stone points (Fig. 14.9). A cylindrical diamond bur works well for incisors and cheek teeth. Carbide burs are more aggressive than diamond burs and white stones. Of the carbide burs, the 701L tapered fissure and #1 and #2 round ball burs are helpful. Of the white stone abrasive points, the flame-shaped point works well. Friction grip (FG) burs are used on high-speed handpieces when working in the rostral oral cavity, but straight handpiece (HP) burs are necessary for use on the cheek teeth of most lagomorphs and rodents owing to poor accessibility with the high-speed handpiece. A safety guard can be used to effectively protect soft tissues from being traumatized by the bur. The use of a diamond disk without safety guard is strongly discouraged.

Files/rasps (sometimes referred to as "floats") are instruments used to level an abnormally uneven occlusal table of the teeth or remove excess dental hard tissue causing trauma to adjacent soft tissue (Fig. 14.10). The hand floats used in the small mouths of lagomorphs and rodents are typically either modified bone files or rasps. The rasps cut both on the push and pull stroke, whereas the files typically cut only on the pull stroke. The rabbit molar file is a float specifically developed for use in rabbits. Most have a large handle for better control and a working end that is similar to a bone rasp. A smaller diamond-coated rasp works well for final smoothing of jagged tooth surfaces after use of a bur or larger file to reduce an overgrown tooth (Fig. 14.11).

Tooth cutters may be modified hard-tissue nippers, pin and wire cutting pliers, or side-cutting rongeurs (Fig. 14.12). However, some have been developed specifically for use in rabbits.

Luxators and elevators are used to work circumferentially around a tooth in the PDL space to aid in the tooth's removal (Fig. 14.13). Hypodermic needles, sizes 18- to 22-gauge (or smaller), can often be used for this function in lagomorphs and rodents (Fig. 14.14). However, standard elevators can also be used, such as No. 1 and 2 winged elevators, 301 apical elevators, and specific rabbit luxators.

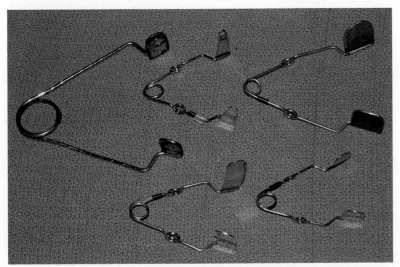

Fig. 14.7 Spring-loaded cheek retractors used to move the cheeks laterally for improved visualization of and access to the cheek teeth. (Copyright 2017, Alexander M. Reiter.)

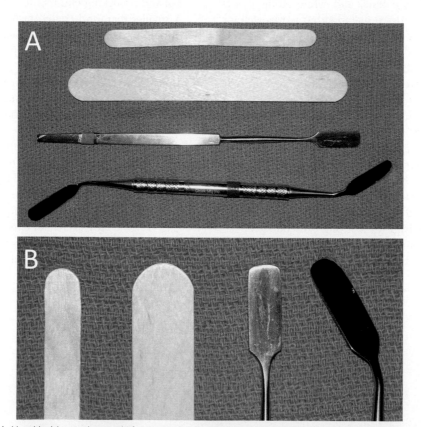

Fig. 14.8 A, Hand-held spatulas made from wood and metal for tongue and cheek retraction. B, Close-up view of their working ends. (Copyright 2017, Alexander M. Reiter.)

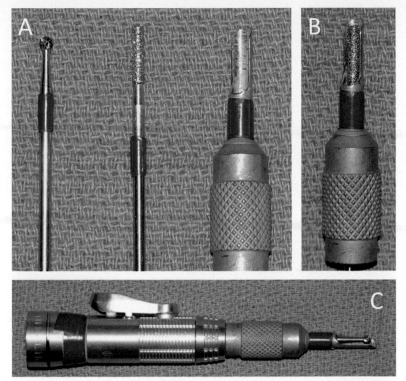

Fig. 14.9 Power tools for trimming overgrown teeth. A, Round carbide bur, cylindrical diamond bur, and safety guard. B, Cylindrical diamond bur within safety guard (note the opening on one side which will face the area of the tooth to be worked on). C, Round carbide bur, safety guard, and low-speed handpiece. (Copyright 2017, Alexander M. Reiter.)

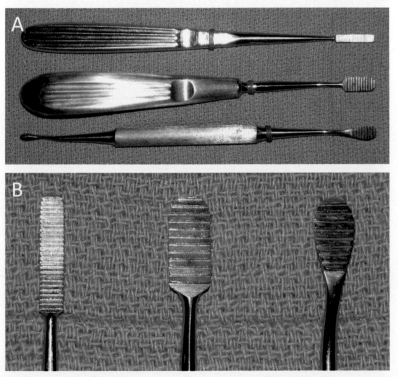

Fig. 14.10 A, Files used for floating of teeth in lagomorphs and rodents. B, Close-up view of their working ends. (Copyright 2017, Alexander M. Reiter.)

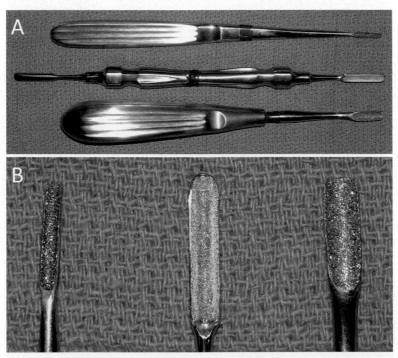

Fig. 14.11 A, Diamond-coated rasps used for fine-contouring of teeth in lagomorphs and rodents. B, Close-up view of their working ends. (Copyright 2017, Alexander M. Reiter.)

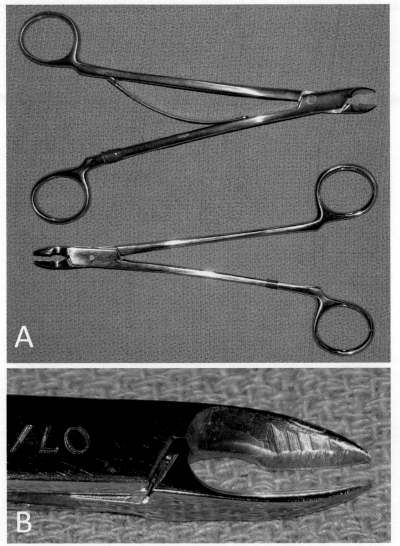

Fig. 14.12 A, Tooth cutters used for removal of small spurs on the clinical crowns of lagomorph and rodent teeth. B, Close-up view of the working end. (Copyright 2017, Alexander M. Reiter.)

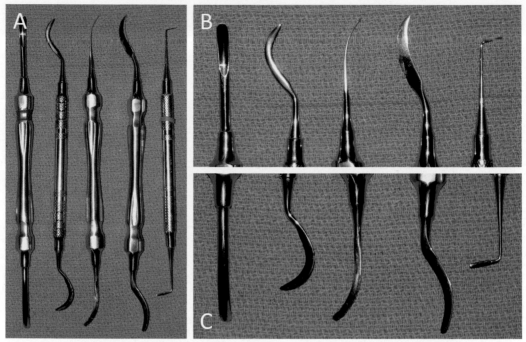

Fig. 14.13 A, Luxators and elevators for use on lagomorph and rodent teeth. B and C, Close-up views of their working ends. Note that the instrument on the right of each image is for luxation and elevation of cheek teeth, while all the others are for luxation and elevation of incisor teeth. (Copyright 2017, Alexander M. Reiter.)

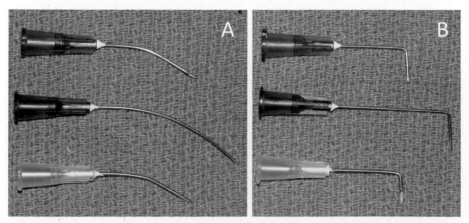

Fig. 14.14 Hypodermic needles used for luxation and elevation of lagomorph and rodent teeth. A, Curved needles for incisor teeth. B, Needles bent at a 90-degree angle for cheek teeth. (Copyright 2017, Alexander M. Reiter.)

Extraction forceps are used to grasp teeth loosened by elevation or severe disease. Most incisors can be handled with small animal extraction forceps. For the cheek teeth, a small 90-degree angled Halstead mosquito forceps or an angled root tip forceps can be useful. Some extraction forceps are specifically designed for use in rabbits and rodents (Fig. 14.15).

Bone substitutes are placed into areas in which periodontal or endodontic disease has resulted in bone loss. These grafts may be combined with an antibiotic or other medicament when placed in a bony void.

Antibiotic-impregnated beads may be placed for treatment of refractory infections. They may be nonabsorbable, such as polymethylmethacrylate beads. Polymethylmethacrylate releases heat during polymerization. Thus, a thermostable antibiotic (e.g., gentamicin) must be used. Calcium phosphate antibiotic-impregnated beads are typically absorbed within weeks after placement.

Paper points are commonly used to apply medicaments to exposed pulps.

Calcium hydroxide is commonly used in either a powder or paste form. It is placed over the exposed pulp of a tooth in an attempt to maintain its vitality. Its use has also been described as a packing material in infected draining abscesses, although this use can cause severe soft tissue necrosis owing to its high pH.

Restoratives used in small mammal and exotic pets are ordinarily temporary filling materials, such as reinforced zinc oxide-eugenol (ZOE) cements, or glass ionomer restorative materials.

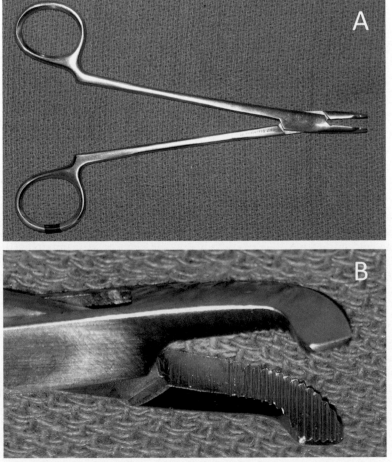

Fig. 14.15 A, Extraction forceps for cheek teeth of lagomorphs and rodents. B, Close-up view of the working end. (Copyright 2017, Alexander M. Reiter.)

COMMON ORAL PROBLEMS AND DISEASES IN LAGOMORPHS AND RODENTS

Common problems in lagomorphs and rodents are gingivitis, periodontitis, enamel hypomineralization/hypoplasia, caries, tooth fracture, malocclusion, tongue entrapment, tooth overgrowth (elongation), jaw abscess, cheek pouch impaction, stomatitis, oral tumors, and slobbers.

Gingivitis

Gingivitis in the rostral mouth of lagomorphs and rodents is often owing to trauma caused by rough edges on watering devices and food bowls. Treatment includes removal, repair, or replacement of the defective device causing the trauma. Once the source of irritation is removed, most patients respond positively without further treatment. However, if the situation warrants, the lesion can be treated with multiple coats of tincture of myrrh and benzoin or topical antibiotic ointments.

Periodontitis

Periodontitis is generally found in the cheek teeth of animals with brachyodont teeth, such as mice and rats. Treatment consists of professional dental cleaning and, if warranted, tooth extractions. Chinchillas also frequently suffer from periodontitis. Periodontitis may develop secondary to tooth elongation and/or tooth resorption in aradicular hypsodont cheek teeth of rabbits, chinchillas, and guinea pigs.

Enamel Hypomineralization/Hypoplasia

Hypomineralized/hypoplastic areas of enamel may be seen occasionally on incisor teeth. This may appear as a chalky white or brown discoloration on the labial surface of the tooth. Enamel abnormalities generally result from either a nutritional imbalance, infection, or inflammation that temporarily decreases enamel production. Generally, the only treatment required is correction of the initiating cause. Trauma to and subsequent death of ameloblasts may result in long-term enamel defects. The teeth seldom require any direct treatment, unless the weakened area of the tooth results in tooth fracture.

Caries

True caries lesions are generally found in only the cheek teeth of rodents with brachyodont teeth. Caries is considered to be uncommon, but detection of this problem is challenging because cheek teeth are difficult to examine. Caries may be on the occlusal surface of the crown, but many lesions are found on the root surfaces, making them even more difficult to detect. The most common treatment is extraction, although removal of the diseased dental structure with a bur and glass ionomer restorations have been used in some cases in an attempt to maintain the teeth as vital and functional.

Malocclusion

Malocclusion can be classified into two basic categories: traumatic and atraumatic.

Traumatic Malocclusion

Traumatic injuries to the teeth can result in broken crowns, which may cause overgrowth (elongation) of the opposing tooth because of the lack of normal attrition (tooth-to-tooth wear). Overgrowth of teeth opposite to previously lost or extracted teeth may also fall into this category.

1. Treatment of the overgrown opposing tooth can generally be controlled by periodic odontoplasty (occlusal equilibration) (Fig. 14.16).
2. Treatment of the fractured tooth includes initial inspection to determine if the tooth's pulp has been exposed. If the pulp is exposed and the tooth shows no clinical or radiographic evidence of not being vital, a vital pulp therapy should be performed to improve the chances of maintaining the tooth's vitality and return of normal occlusal interaction with the opposing tooth. If the tooth is nonvital, it and its opposing tooth may eventually require extraction.

Atraumatic Malocclusion

Atraumatic malocclusions are caused by hereditary factors or by nutritional or other atraumatic changes of the teeth, temporomandibular joints, mandibular symphysis, or bone that result in improper tooth alignment. Atraumatic malocclusion is found in three basic forms:

1. Short maxillary diastema results in the maxillary incisor teeth failing to meet properly with the mandibular incisors. This results in the overgrowth of one or more of the incisor teeth. This condition typically manifests

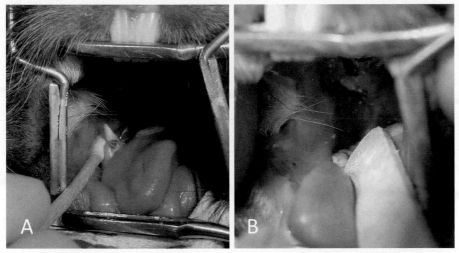

Fig. 14.16 Treatment of an overgrown (elongated) right mandibular cheek tooth in a rabbit. A, Before treatment. B, After occlusal equilibration and odontoplasty. (Copyright 2017, Alexander M. Reiter.)

within the first year of the animal's life and is generally considered to be of autosomal recessive inheritance in rabbits resulting in a shortened maxillary diastema. Treatment involves control of the overgrowth by routine odontoplasty of the incisor teeth.

2. Genetics, nutrition, or abnormal mandibular excursion may also result in malocclusion of the incisors or the cheek teeth. This condition usually manifests after 2 years of age. It has a poor long-term prognosis, and clients should be made aware of this fact. Treatment includes occlusal equilibration of the affected teeth, nutritional changes, and symptomatic treatment of secondary conditions that may arise. This may include the use of anti-inflammatory medications and fluid therapy.

3. Improper wear is usually also a result of insufficient chewing from feeding the wrong diet. Treatment consists of dietary correction, if required, and the periodic odontoplasty of overgrown teeth.

Tongue Entrapment

Tongue entrapment occurs when the clinical crowns of the mandibular cheek teeth elongate intraorally to meet at the midline, pinning the tongue in the intermandibular space (which is common in the guinea pig) (Fig. 14.17). Treatment involves trimming of the overgrown teeth to release the tongue and routine odontoplasty of these teeth in the future to prevent recurrence. Anti-inflammatory medication, fluids, hand feeding, and other supportive therapies may be required. Long-term prognosis may be poor.

Incisor Tooth Overgrowth

When not complicated by cheek tooth involvement, incisor tooth overgrowth (elongation) (Fig. 14.18) can usually be treated and controlled by one of the following methods:

1. Odontoplasty, which reestablishes a functional occlusion.

2. Extraction, which removes the occlusal interference and trauma while establishing a functional occlusion.

Cheek Tooth Overgrowth

Once cheek tooth overgrowth (elongation) (Fig. 14.19) and periapical disease begins, a serious, life-threatening process ensues. Cheek tooth overgrowth results in a chronic inflammatory disease that causes gradual weight loss and many secondary health problems. The condition can be controlled by odontoplasty, antibiotics, anti-inflammatory medications, and supportive care.

Jaw Abscess

Teeth may develop abscesses as a result of periodontal or endodontic/periapical disease. Treatment may involve endodontic procedures, but extraction of the diseased tooth is generally necessary. The actual abscess may require excision, extraction of involved teeth, wound debridement, lavage, closure or marsupialization.

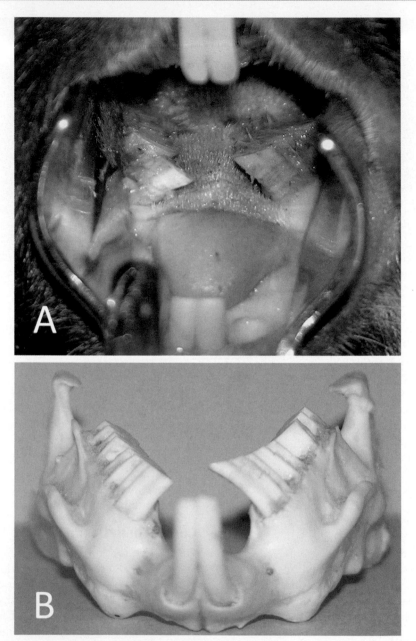

Fig. 14.17 Tongue entrapment in guinea pigs. A, Clinical patient. B, Dry specimen showing elongation of the clinical crowns of the mandibular cheek teeth. (Copyright 2017, Alexander M. Reiter.)

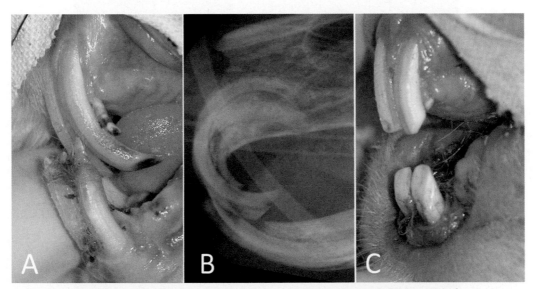

Fig. 14.18 Overgrowth (elongation) of incisors in a rabbit. A, Before treatment. B, Radiograph before treatment. C, After treatment. (Copyright 2017, Alexander M. Reiter.)

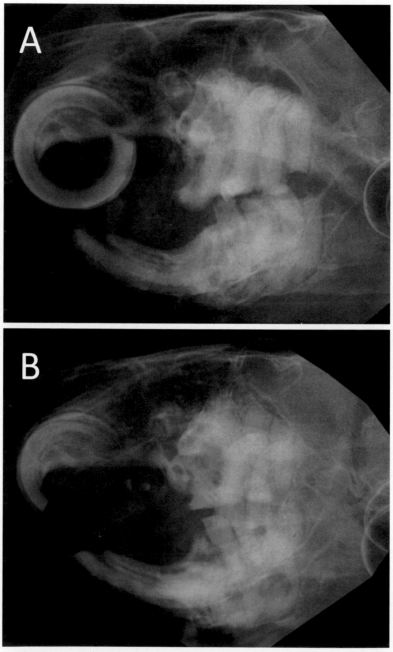

Fig. 14.19 Overgrowth (elongation) of incisors and cheek teeth in a chinchilla. A, Radiograph before treatment. B, Radiograph after treatment. (Copyright 2017, Alexander M. Reiter.)

Cheek Pouch Impaction

Occasionally, food becomes impacted in the cheek pouches, causing mild buccal irritation or stomatitis. Treatment consists of removal of the impacted material. In severe cases, antibiotic therapy may be warranted.

Stomatitis

Most cases of stomatitis are secondary to a non-oral cause, such as hypovitaminosis C, which results in scurvy. Scurvy leads to gingivitis, periodontitis, oral hemorrhage, mobile or lost teeth, anorexia, and loss of body weight. Treatment should be immediately initiated with vitamin C supplements and supportive care, which may include fluid therapy and tube feeding. The diet should be enhanced with fruits and vegetables rich in vitamin C. If a commercial diet is being used, its expiration date should be closely inspected because vitamin C in commercial diets gradually depletes with time. These diets are usually dated for safety.

Oral Tumors

Many oral tumor types can be seen in small mammals and exotic pets. Odontogenic tumors (odontoma, pseudo-odontoma, elodontoma) have been reported in lagomorphs and rodents. A diagnosis is made by means of incisional or excisional biopsy, and the choice of treatment greatly depends on histopathologic findings. In cases of odontoma, pseudo-odontoma, and elodontoma, radiographs are usually very suggestive of the disease. However, the prognosis is often poor to guarded because the tumors tend to grow and invade adjacent structures.

Slobbers

Slobbers, or wet dewlap, is a condition in which excess drooling saliva results in a moist dermatitis and hair loss around the mouth, neck, and front limbs. Many of the previously described oral diseases may result in slobbers. Treatment includes control of the initiating disease. Dermatitis is treated by clipping the hair, cleansing, and topical treatment with antibiotics if secondary infection is present.

COMMON ORAL PROBLEMS AND DISEASES IN FERRETS

Common oral problems and diseases in ferrets include tooth extrusion, tooth abrasion, tooth fracture, endodontic and periapical disease, crowding of mandibular incisor teeth, and periodontal disease.

Tooth Extrusion

Tooth extrusion can be seen when the root surface is exposed in the absence of gingival recession. As is commonly seen in domestic cats, extrusion of the canine teeth results in a longer than normal clinical crown. Based on a study of 63 rescued ferrets, extrusion was seen in one or more of the canine teeth in 93.7% of ferrets. Although extrusion itself does not require treatment, it may predispose the extruded tooth to fracture or luxation.

Tooth Abrasion

Abrasion (wear owing to contact of a tooth with a non-dental material) was seen in 76.2% of rescued ferrets and 63.2% of client-owned ferrets. Abrasion can be seen in nearly every tooth, although the prevalence differs depending on the population investigated. Abrasion is most commonly seen on the mandibular and maxillary third premolar teeth in rescued ferrets, whereas the rostral teeth were more affected in client-owned ferrets. The progression of abrasion may be slowed by minimizing exposure to hard toys, although ferrets will often still chew on housing and cage bars. Abrasion can result in pulp exposure if the rate of wear occurs more rapidly than the odontoblasts on the inside of the tooth can produce tertiary dentin. If pulp exposure is not present and the tooth is not sensitive, treatment may not be required.

Tooth Fracture

Tooth fractures were seen in 31.7% of rescued ferrets and 73.7% of client-owned ferrets, with 60% of fractured teeth having evidence of pulp exposure, also referred to as a *complicated tooth fracture*. The most commonly affected tooth is the canine tooth. No treatment may be needed for uncomplicated fractures (without pulp exposure) other than monitoring. Treatment of complicated tooth fractures involves either extraction or endodontic therapy. Endodontic therapy is recommended over extraction for a fractured maxillary canine tooth to avoid upper lip ulceration owing to contact with the ipsilateral mandibular canine tooth.

Malocclusion

Malocclusion is rare in ferrets, with the exception of mild crowding of the mandibular incisors, which results in a more lingual position of the mandibular second incisors in 95.2% of rescued ferrets. This malocclusion does not require specific treatment, but any crowding of teeth may be associated with an increased risk of developing periodontal disease.

Periodontal Disease

Clinical evidence of periodontal disease was seen in 65.3% of rescued ferrets and 100% of client-owned ferrets. Periodontal pockets in ferrets are present if the probing depth of the gingival sulcus is > 0.5 mm. Occasionally, facial swelling may be seen; this is caused by endodontic infection secondary to severe periodontal disease.

PREPARATION FOR PROCEDURES

Preanesthesia Examination

The preanesthesia examination has two parts. The first is a thorough general physical examination in preparation for anesthesia. The second is examination of the oral cavity and associated structures to assess the type of problems that may be encountered so that appropriate equipment, instruments, and supplies can be prepared for further diagnostics and treatment. However, the conscious oral examination may not be particularly informative because of the small size of the oral cavity in small mammal and exotic pets. The use of an otoscope with an ear cone inserted into the mouth sometimes allows a degree of visualization of the teeth and surrounding tissues in tolerant lagomorph and rodent pets.

Preanesthesia Preparation

Preanesthesia preparation is an integral part of the procedure. The planned procedure and its risks are discussed with the client. An estimate of cost and procedure time should be provided so that clients do not become unnecessarily anxious during the procedure. If the client will not be present during the procedure, a contingency plan should be arranged in case any additional problems arise or are discovered during the procedure. If the client has failed to provide direction or cannot be contacted during a procedure, only the agreed-upon procedures and those necessary to maintain the patient should be performed. Antibiotics, if indicated, may be given before or during anesthesia. Preanesthesia restriction of food and water is often not required in lagomorphs or rodents because their digestive system does not ordinarily allow for regurgitation of stomach contents. In compromised patients, even short-term nutritional restriction may be contraindicated.

Inhalant Anesthesia

Ether has been used in the past as an inhalant anesthetic, but because of its flammability and safety concerns its use in general practice is not recommended. Isoflurane and sevoflurane are currently the inhalant anesthetics of choice for general usage in lagomorphs, rodents, and ferrets.

Anesthesia Induction

Induction of anesthesia is done in one of three ways: (1) restraint and use of injectable anesthetics, (2) restraint and masking with inhalant anesthetics, or (3) placement of the pet in an anesthesia chamber and use of inhalant anesthetics.

Anesthesia Maintenance

Maintenance of anesthesia is also typically accomplished in one of three ways: injectable anesthetics, alternating off/on masking of inhalants, or intubation for delivery of inhalants. Possible disadvantages of injectable anesthesia include administration site hair loss and abscess, prolonged recovery time, and sensitivity in chronically ill animals. The advantage of injectable anesthesia is the ability to administer it to almost any animal fairly easily. Disadvantages of strict inhalant anesthesia are potential for severe hypotension and airway irritation owing to higher concentrations of inhaled anesthetics. Once an animal is induced, the technique of alternating off/on masking, or keeping the nares covered with a small mask while working in the mouth, allows time for treatment of minor oral conditions and easily accessed incisors and other more rostrally located teeth. This technique can also be used for more complicated treatments in the mouth, but it is not necessarily recommended since it can greatly prolong procedure time because of waiting to reestablish the desired plane of anesthesia. Treatment in the oral cavity, especially the cheek teeth, is easier to perform and recovery is usually rapid and uneventful when intubation can be accomplished.

Intubation

Intubation of lagomorphs and rodents can be difficult. Intubation of ferrets can be accomplished relatively easily with a cuffed endotracheal tube (inner diameter 2.5 mm). With practice, intubation can be accomplished in many of the small mammal and exotic pets. To avoid accidental extubation, one can also suture the endotracheal tube to the skin of the lip in addition to having it tied with umbilical tape behind the ears.

Blind Intubation

Used primarily in rabbits, chinchillas, and larger rodents, blind intubation is often the most simple and effective way of intubating these animals. The patient is usually placed in sternal recumbency. An endotracheal tube (inner diameter 2.0, 2.5, or 3.0 mm) is cut to the appropriate length depending on the animal to be intubated. A wire stylet is made with a loop on one end for easy removal from the connector end of the tube. The wire is cut so that it is approximately 1 to 2 mm short of the end of the tube. This reduces the chance of trauma to the soft tissues caused by the wire extending beyond the end of the tube. The wire is bent 1 cm from the beveled end of the endotracheal tube at a 45-degree angle. A section of umbilical tape is tied around the tube for its eventual anchorage. The tube is then inserted into the oral cavity with the bent tip contacting the roof of the mouth, causing the tip of the tube to enter the trachea. Typically, a light gagging reflex will be induced; with transparent tubes, condensation is visible with each breath. The umbilical tape should be tied behind the ears to anchor and stabilize the tube. Should the first attempt fail, another attempt should be made before attempting the next intubation technique.

Pediatric Laryngoscope

Pediatric laryngoscope blades may be used primarily in rabbits, chinchillas, larger rodents, and ferrets. The straight blade seems to more accurately provide the needed visualization for intubation than the angled blade. The lighted blade is first inserted into the mouth. The endotracheal tube with a wire stylet is introduced parallel to and outside of the blade track to maximize visualization of intubation. An alternative procedure, which is sometimes easier, is to first pass a No. 5 French urinary catheter into the trachea. The endotracheal tube is slid down over the urinary catheter, and finally the urinary catheter is removed. The endotracheal tube should be secured by tying umbilical tape around the tube and behind the ears.

Otoscope or Endoscopic Intubation

Intubation using an otoscope with an endotracheal tube or intravenous (IV) catheter is primarily used with rats,

hamsters, gerbils, chinchillas, and smaller lagomorphs and rodents. This form of intubation calls for the use of an ear cone in a size appropriate for the size and depth of the animal's oral cavity. The otoscope is advanced until the laryngeal area can be identified. An endotracheal tube can be advanced beside the otoscope and then into the trachea by visual placement. The plastic sheath of an IV catheter with the stylet removed may be advanced down the actual inside of the otoscope into the trachea. The otoscope and cone must then be removed without disturbing the positioning of the catheter. The use of IV catheters for intubation allows for a patent airway, but regulation of inhalant anesthesia through such small devices is suboptimal because they can quickly become blocked with mucus or debris. Therefore, their patency should be closely observed and maintained.

Stethoscope-Aided Intubation

An endotracheal tube is attached to a standard clinical stethoscope using an appropriate adapter. An elliptic hole is made in the stethoscope tubing near the attachment to the endotracheal tube. The animal is placed in sternal recumbency, and the neck is extended. The endotracheal tube is advanced into the mouth over the base of the tongue. Using the stethoscope, it is possible to identify the inspiratory and expiratory phases of respiration to accurately place the end of the tube over the epiglottis. The endotracheal tube is advanced into the trachea during inspiration. Proper placement results in a cough reflex, which is vented through the hole in the stethoscope tubing. The endotracheal tube is removed from the stethoscope and is attached to the anesthesia tubing.

Retrograde Intubation

Retrograde intubation can be used in all sizes of lagomorphs and rodents. However, this method can be traumatic and irritating to the trachea and should be used only when the two previously described techniques have failed. In this technique, a needle is inserted through the midventral neck region between two of the tracheal rings and directed toward the head. The needle should be stopped as soon as it penetrates the trachea. A monofilament suture is then passed through the needle into the trachea and gently pushed until it exits into the mouth. The end of the suture is then grasped and passed through the endotracheal tube. The tube is then slid down over the suture into the trachea. Both ends of the suture should be held firmly to provide a smooth, taut guideline for the tube. Once the tube is in the trachea, the suture and needle are removed from the neck and the endotracheal tube is adjusted to the appropriate depth.

Tracheotomy Intubation

Tracheotomy intubation may be performed in all sizes of lagomorphs and rodents. However, this method should be reserved only for special or critical cases in which intubation is absolutely required and more conservative techniques have failed. Proper clipping of the hair and disinfection of the site with surgical scrub solutions should be performed. A tracheotomy is performed by making a longitudinal skin incision over the trachea midway between the larynx and thoracic inlet. A stab incision is made between two of the tracheal rings, and the endotracheal tube is passed into the trachea and then anchored with umbilical tape, which is tied to the tube and then around the animal's neck to prevent accidental extubation.

Stabilization and Monitors

Starting at the time of premedication, the patient should be monitored closely. A spare endotracheal tube should be available for emergencies. Oxygen flow should be at a minimum of 500 mL/min, and isoflurane is set at approximately 1% to 2.5% for maintenance. Once every 2 minutes, the tube patency should be checked by light positive pressure ventilation. If moisture or mucus blocks the tube, the tube should be disconnected and an open-end tom cat catheter inserted down the tube. A syringe can be attached and light negative pressure used to remove the debris. Should patency not be immediately reestablished, the tube should be removed and the patient masked, until the spare tube can be placed or the patient awakened. Pulse oximeters have been shown to be useful in lagomorphs and rodents. Knowledge of basic physiologic parameters is needed for proper monitoring (Table 14.1).

Complete Oral Examination

Once the patient has been anesthetized and monitors show the patient is stable, a detailed examination of the oral cavity is performed. This will confirm a diagnosis for an appropriate treatment plan. External palpation, jaw manipulation, and visual and radiographic examination all play a part in an accurate diagnosis of the problem.

TABLE 14.1 Patient Physiologic Monitoring Data			
Species	Respiration (breaths/ min)	Heart Rate (beats/ min)	Body Temperature (° C)
Rabbit	32–60	130–325	38.0–39.6
Guinea pig	42–104	230–380	37.2–39.5
Chinchilla	40–65	40–100	36.1–37.8
Rat	70–115	250–450	35.9–37.5
Hamster	35–135	250–500	37.0–38.4
Gerbil	70–120	260–600	38.1–38.4

Palpation and Manipulation

Palpation of the head, face, jaws, neck and throat area should be carefully performed to locate sites of swelling, discharge, or fluctuancy, which might indicate a pathologic condition. Subtle lumps under the ventrolateral aspect of the mandible can be a normal anatomic finding in some species, but prominent bony swellings may suggest periapical disease of the cheek teeth.

The jaws should be gently manipulated to examine for resistance to normal occlusal movements. Is there reasonable vertical movement, and do the edges of the maxillary and mandibular incisors meet in an appropriate scissors bite? When the lower jaw is moved from side to side in a horizontal movement, is the occlusion forced open on one side or can crepitus be felt? If so, this suggests there is an overgrowth (elongation) of teeth on the side opposite the open bite.

Visual Examination and Aids

The use of a mouth gag, cheek retractor, tongue retractor, good lighting, and appropriate magnification can greatly enhance the visual examination (Fig. 14.20). When proper soft tissue retraction cannot be attained, visual inspection typically reveals little. While inspecting the teeth, the practitioner should look for hooks, vertical blades of enamel, uneven occlusal planes, general tooth elongation, increased interdental spaces between cheek teeth, gingival enlargement, and dental defects. It is common for cheek tooth elongation to be on the opposite side of the face to that of incisor tooth elongation.

Diagnostic Imaging Examination

Radiographs are highly useful diagnostic and monitoring tools for small mammals and exotic pets. The use

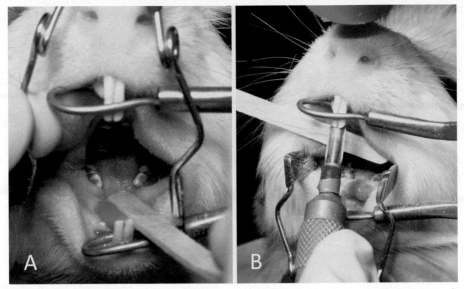

Fig. 14.20 Oral examination and occlusal equilibration in a guinea pig. A. Mouth gag, cheek retractor, and tongue depressor allow for proper visualization of the oral cavity (odontoplasty had already been performed on the cheek teeth). B, Low-speed handpiece, safety guard, and cylindrical diamond bur used to trim the maxillary incisors. (Copyright 2017, Alexander M. Reiter.)

of dental films, phosphor plates, or sensor pads is more convenient and can give greater distinction of detail (even when used extraorally), but standard x-ray films can also be used. Helpful for small mammals and exotic pets are sizes 0, 1, 2, and 4. An intraoral technique can be used, depending on the size of the patient. A modification of the size 3 of the phosphor plates (slim plate) is useful for obtaining intraoral radiographs of the cheek teeth. The use of intraoral radiographs allows for isolation of incisor teeth and cheek teeth. The size 4 dental films or phosphor plates are used extraorally and can be used for dorsoventral or ventrodorsal, lateral, lateral oblique, and rostrocaudal views of the entire head, including dentition and temporomandibular joints. The lateral and lateral oblique views are commonly most diagnostic, revealing hooks, elongation, uneven occlusal planes, and periapical pathology.

Computed tomography (CT), cone beam CT (CBCT), and micro-CT are other diagnostic imaging options for evaluation of diseases of the oral cavity and associated structures, allowing for assessment of lesions without superimposition of other structures. However, in very small patients CT might not have enough resolution to identify abnormalities. When CBCT was compared to conventional CT, CBCT was superior for evaluation of dental structures. Micro-CT has been used for evaluation of small exotic pets without the use of anesthesia. All of these diagnostic imaging modalities also allow for 3D reconstruction that can make it easier to visualize lesions and explain them to the client.

CHARTING

All detected pathologic conditions should be recorded in an appropriate chart as thoroughly as possible. The use of charts customized to small mammal and exotic pet species can be helpful.

TREATMENT

Professional Dental Cleaning

Lagomorph, rodent, and ferret teeth can be cleaned in a fashion similar to that of most other species (see Chapter 7). Because of the small oral aperture and risks of fluids entering the respiratory tract, care should be taken when considering use of water spray, particularly if the patient has not been intubated. Therefore, hand instruments or mechanical scalers that produce little heat are helpful; certain sonic scalers may meet this requirement. The teeth can be polished with a prophy cup on a low-speed handpiece except in very small patients where access is limited. Excess polish and debris should be cleaned from the mouth with cotton-tipped applicators.

Floating or Odontoplasty of Teeth

The term *floating* refers to creating a level occlusal surface; *occlusal equilibration* is the equivalent medical term. *Odontoplasty* refers to the process of recontouring a tooth surface, which is not limited to leveling an occlusal surface. Both terms are used almost interchangeably when referring to adjustment of aradicular hypsodont teeth. Instruments used for adjustment of the teeth include tooth cutters, rasps, files, and various burs and abrasive points.

Tooth Cutters

Tooth cutters are available in two types: incisor cutters and molar cutters. They are typically either burs or edge-cutting hand instruments. The edge-cutting hand instruments should generally be used only for cutting tooth spurs and hooks and not for attempting to actually reduce an elongated clinical crown. When used to cut teeth and reduce occlusal height, they are likely to break, crack, or shatter teeth. Dog toenail clippers should be avoided when reducing tooth height.

Burs

When cutting incisors, burs on a low or high speed handpiece provide a smooth, even cut, reestablishing the chisel-shaped edges, which slope caudally and toward the palatal and lingual gingiva. White stone flame-shaped points, fluted burs, carbide burs, and diamond burs all work well, although stones and diamond burs are inherently less aggressive and thus safer. Edge-cutting hand instruments should be used with caution because shattering and crushing of the teeth are common. These should be used on incisors only to remove spurs or hooks and not to reduce actual tooth height.

When dealing with cheek teeth, high-speed handpieces are difficult to use efficiently and safely because of the right angle and short shank of the bur. A low-speed handpiece with a straight handpiece (HP) carbide or diamond bur is useful with careful attention to avoid damage to the tongue, gingiva, or alveolar, sublingual, and buccal mucosa.

Rasps and files. Rasps and files can be used to gradually reduce the clinical crowns of cheek teeth while also recontouring them into a reasonable reestablishment of the proper occlusal table angulation (Fig. 14.21). Files cut primarily on the pull stroke. Rasps usually cut on both the push and pull strokes, which may result in a more rapid reduction of the tooth surface. Diamond-coated rasps are particularly helpful, although they do

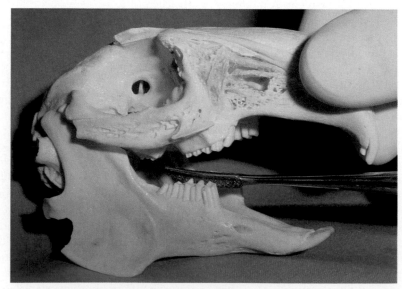

Fig. 14.21 Demonstration of a diamond-coated rasp being used on the right mandibular cheek teeth of a rabbit skull. (Copyright 2017, Alexander M. Reiter.)

not cut as aggressively compared to other instruments. Care should be taken in the push stroke on mandibular cheek teeth, particularly in rabbits, where trauma to a branch of the inferior alveolar vessels can occur beneath the caudal oral mucosa, resulting in rapid and unexpected bleeding.

Abscess Treatment

Diseased teeth may develop jaw abscesses (periodontal, periapical, or a combination of periodontal-periapical abscesses). Medical therapy alone is extremely unlikely to result in a favorable long-term outcome. Most dental-related abscesses are detected by the clients usually on the face or lower jaw.

Periodontal Abscesses

Abscesses of this nature are typically caused by food or other debris being forced into the PDL space of a tooth. This results in an abscess along the gingival or alveolar mucosal surface adjacent to the tooth. The abscess is lanced and debrided, systemic antibiotics may be initiated, and the causative substances should be removed from the diet. Stemmy hays and roughage are often found within these lesions.

Periapical Abscesses

Periapical abscesses frequently result from some form of trauma that has exposed the pulp and resulted in devitalization of the tooth. Root canal therapy can be performed on these teeth, but long-term success in aradicular hypsodont teeth is rare. Extraction is usually the most prudent approach to treatment. The tooth should be extracted and the fistulous tract debrided. In addition to treatment of the tooth/teeth of origin, treatment of the abscess includes removal of the abscess capsule, debridement and lavage of the wound, suturing of the intraoral tissues, and possibly leaving a portion of the surgical site open externally (marsupialization) to allow for postoperative lavage and second intention healing. In some cases, the abscess may have caused considerable bone loss, and fracture of the jaw is possible during extraction. Placement of antibiotic-impregnated beads may be considered in some cases where the surgical site is closed primarily (Fig. 14.22). If the wound is left open externally, a paste or slurry form of an antibiotic, such as ampicillin, clindamycin, tetracycline, doxycycline or minocycline, can be placed into the surgical site and replaced every 2 weeks until the defect heals

from the inside out by second intention. The patient may be placed on postoperative antibiotics, especially if the surgical site is left open for drainage and flushing and if remaining bone is significantly diseased.

Periodontal-Periapical Abscesses

Periodontal-periapical abscesses occur owing to extension of periodontal disease apically to enter the pulp of a fractured or worn tooth with pulp exposure. Treatment is similar to that described for periapical abscesses.

Extractions

Extractions can be broken down into two categories, depending on whether the tooth is an incisor or cheek tooth. Each type of extraction requires different techniques and equipment.

Incisor Teeth

Incisor teeth in ferrets usually are removed in a closed fashion (i.e., without creating a flap). Because of the highly curved reserve crown structure and the fragile nature of incisor teeth in lagomorphs and rodents, use of appropriate technique and equipment is required (Fig. 14.23). Most of the strength of the PDL holding the tooth in place is found in the gingival third of the reserve crown and on the mesial surface. This means the primary area to be elevated is the reserve crown near the gingival surface. Curved hypodermic needles sometimes can be quite useful for this purpose. The 18- to 22-gauge 1½ inch needle has been used for many years in rabbits. However, the No. 1 and No. 2 winged elevators and specific ("Crossley") rabbit luxators are well designed for this function. Elevation of the tooth is achieved by pressing the elevator into the PDL space between the tooth and alveolar bone and gently rotating it. These incisor teeth are fragile, especially in the apical portion of their reserve crowns. Once the teeth are loosened, extraction forceps can be used to grasp the tooth and remove it. The operator should recall that the tooth curves in an arch and the extraction pull must be made in that same circular plane. Once the tooth has been extracted, the alveolus is debrided and rinsed and the gingiva sutured with absorbable material.

Teeth broken during extraction must be evaluated carefully. They are generally categorized as non-diseased and diseased. Nondiseased teeth with no preexisting infection, such as teeth being extracted because of an

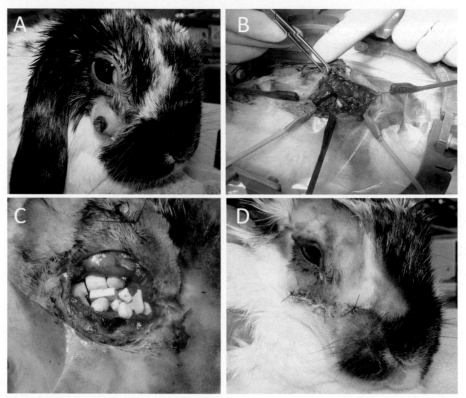

Fig. 14.22 Abscess in a rabbit. A, Right-sided facial swelling. B, Incision, removal of abscess capsule, and debridement and lavage of the wound. C, Placement of antibiotic-impregnated beads. D, Wound closure. (Copyright 2017, Alexander M. Reiter.)

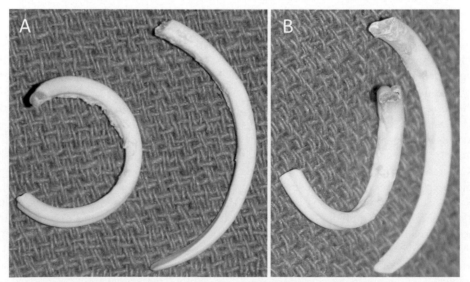

Fig. 14.23 Extracted rabbit first incisors. A, Lateral view. B, Apicolateral view. Note the difference in curvature of the maxillary incisor (on the left of each image) versus the mandibular incisor (on the right of each image). (Copyright 2017, Alexander M. Reiter.)

atraumatic malocclusion, may have a growth center at the apex that is intact and active. If this is the case, the tooth will typically regrow in 1 to 4 months, and a second attempt at extraction can be made at that time if still needed. Diseased teeth are characterized by preexisting infection, pulp exposure, abscess, or traumatic malocclusion. Most are associated with some form of trauma to the tooth or gums. Should an infected tooth fracture during extraction, every reasonable attempt should be made to retrieve the entire tooth because the remaining portion usually continues to cause problems. If the segment cannot be removed, local or systemic antibiotics may be warranted. If the retained piece of reserve crown continues to cause problems, a surgical approach will be necessary to remove it and debride the wound.

Canine Teeth in Ferrets

Canine teeth in ferrets are found on oral examination to exhibit fractures with pulp exposure owing to their long, thin crown shape. Fractured teeth with pulp exposure can be treated by performing root canal therapy or extraction. Root canal therapy is performed through the fracture site and is preferred to extraction in ferrets, particularly for fractured maxillary canine teeth. Similar to cats, extraction of the maxillary canine tooth in a ferret allows the upper lip to fall into a more medial position, resulting in upper lip trauma from the sharp cusp of the ipsilateral mandibular canine tooth (Fig. 14.24). If extraction of a ferret canine tooth is necessary, care is taken to raise a mucoperiosteal flap, and a stay suture is placed in the extremely thin flap to retract it and avoid trauma with forceps. Bone is removed over the labial aspect of the canine tooth with a No. 1 or 2 round carbide bur attached to a water-cooled high-speed handpiece. After elevation of the tooth, the alveolus is debrided, and the site is closed with 5-0 absorbable suture in a simple interrupted pattern. In the case of maxillary canine tooth extraction, careful odontoplasty of the cusp of the ipsilateral mandibular canine tooth may help to decrease trauma to the upper lip, but only approximately 1 mm may be removed before risking iatrogenic pulp exposure.

Cheek Teeth

Brachyodont cheek teeth of rats, mice, and ferrets are usually easier to extract than the aradicular hypsodont cheek teeth of lagomorphs, guinea pigs, and chinchillas.

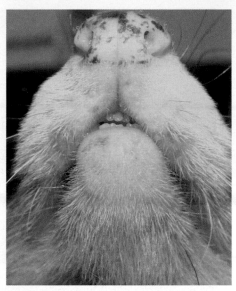

Fig. 14.24 Bilateral upper lip irritation caused by trauma from the opposing mandibular canine teeth noticed 24 hours after extraction of the maxillary canine teeth in a ferret. (Copyright 2017, Alexander M. Reiter.)

In ferrets, closed and open extraction techniques can be employed similar to what is done in cats (Fig. 14.25). In rats and mice, the No. 2 Molt surgical elevator and an 18- to 22-gauge 1½ inch needle bent at a 90-degree angle work reasonably well as elevators for intraoral extraction of brachyodont cheek teeth. Aradicular hypsodont cheek teeth have a more complex and deeper reserve crown structure compared with the roots of brachyodont teeth. Therefore, extractions are usually more difficult. However, the same basic techniques as previously described for brachyodont teeth can be used, but tooth repelling or even buccotomy may also be required. In many smaller rodents, suturing the extraction site may not be possible because of lack of access.

Tooth repelling is the procedure of making an access hole below the tooth and pressing a small, blunt metal rod against the bottom of the tooth to push it into the oral cavity. Often with diseased teeth, only light hand pressure is required to accomplish the repelling of the tooth into the mouth. Alternatively, the cheek tooth can sometimes be retrieved through the extraoral incision. Buccotomy is a full-thickness incision through the skin, mucosa, and subcutaneous tissue to allow for direct visualization and ability to treat cheek teeth.

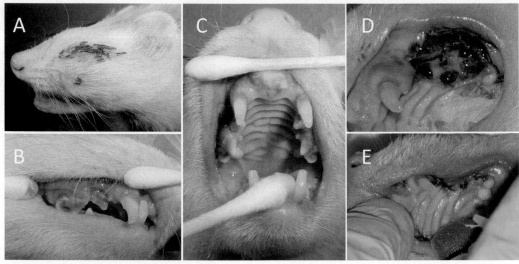

Fig. 14.25 Tooth extraction in a ferret. A, Periorbital swelling/bleeding at the left eye and sinus tract formation at the left upper lip skin. B and C, Note the use of cotton-tipped applicators to retract lips/cheeks and open the mouth for conscious oral examination. D. Maxillary cheek teeth removed using an open extraction technique. E, Wound closure. (Copyright 2017, Alexander M. Reiter.)

This procedure can leave permanent scars, which some clients may find objectionable. Because many of these species actively use the cheek pouch during eating and may store food in the pouch, complication of infection and dehiscence of the suture line may occur.

Vital Pulp Therapy

Vital pulp therapy, performed to maintain tooth vitality, may be required when injury or iatrogenic action causes exposure of the pulp. Any instrument or material coming in contact with exposed pulp tissue must be sterile. The site of exposure should be cleaned with lactated Ringer's solution. The coronal portion of the pulp is removed with a small round carbide bur or a small round diamond bur on a high-speed handpiece (partial pulpectomy). A paper point is dipped into a dappen dish of lactated Ringer's solution. The moistened end is then dipped into a dappen dish of calcium hydroxide powder. The powder adheres to the paper point, which is then placed into the pulp chamber of the injured tooth until it contacts the pulp. The paper point is then gently tapped against the pulp to place a small coating of the calcium hydroxide on the pulp (direct pulp capping). The walls of the access site are cleaned, and a restorative, such as a glass ionomer or reinforced ZOE cement, is placed over the exposure to seal the tooth (restoration).

Tooth Fillings

Because of the small size of the teeth generally involved, restoratives that easily bond to enamel and dentin are preferred for fillings. Among these are materials, such as the glass ionomers, reinforced ZOE cements, and composites.

Glass ionomers are used for restoration in lagomorphs and rodents. The dental lesions should be prepared and the glass ionomer applied according to the manufacturer's recommendations. Composites, when used with bonding agents, are also well suited for use in lagomorphs, rodents, and ferrets, although they are more technique-sensitive than glass ionomers. Composites that flow easily are often less difficult to apply in the restricted space of these small oral cavities. Reinforced or macro-fill composites should be avoided in lagomorphs and rodents because their wear pattern might be slower than that of the associated tooth structure.

Drug Treatment

Various antibiotics and other drugs are used in treatment whose dosages must be calculated not only by weight but also by species. CAUTION: Some lagomorphs and rodents are sensitive to certain antibiotics; some drugs may even cause death. In rabbits, hamsters, and guinea pigs the potential of fatal colitis caused by the use of antibiotics, especially oral antibiotics, is always present. Therefore, antibiotics should be carefully selected and dosages checked before administering.

Home-Care Instructions

Clients should closely observe food and water intake during the first 4 hours after recovery from surgery in lagomorphs and rodents. Seriously ill patients may be reluctant to eat and drink after dental and oral surgical procedures. If the patient fails to ingest food and water within the first 4 hours after treatment, hand feeding with liquid concentrates and water should be instituted until normal intake resumes. Prolonged inappetence is generally an indication of a more severe secondary problem, which may require administration of fluids, antibiotics, anti-inflammatory medications, and other supportive care and treatments.

▌CHAPTER 14 WORKSHEET

1. Lagomorphs have _____ teeth that continually grow and erupt throughout the animal's life, whereas rodents may have _____ and _____ teeth.

2. Lagomorphs and rodents have a heterodont dentition and have _____, _____, and _____, but no _____ teeth.

3. Continual growth and eruption of aradicular hypsodont teeth may be possible by a special feature of the periodontal ligament known as the _____ _____.

4. Malocclusions are generally grouped into two categories: _____ or _____.

5. Extraction of a maxillary canine tooth in a ferret may result in long-term trauma to the ipsilateral _____ _____.

6. If a lagomorph or rodent fails to ingest food and water within the first _____ hours after an anesthetic procedure, hand feeding with liquid concentrates and water should be instituted until normal intake resumes.

7. The condition in which excess drooling saliva results in a moist dermatitis is often referred to as _____.

8. _____ _____ _____ is a term describing the discrepancy of widths of the upper and lower dental arches.

9. The bright yellow/orange color on the labial surfaces of the incisor teeth is the _____.

10. Food and water should be restricted for how long before surgery on lagomorphs and rodents? _____.

FURTHER READING

Böhmer E, Crossley D. Objective interpretation of dental disease in rabbits, guinea pigs and chinchillas. Use of anatomical reference lines. *Tierarztl Praxis* 2009;37: 250-260.

Böhmer E. *Dentistry in Rabbits and Rodents*. Ames, Iowa, 2015, John Wiley & Sons, Ltd.

Capello V, Lennox A, Ghisleni G. Elodontoma in two guinea pigs. *J Vet Dent* 2015;32: 111-119.

Capello V, Lennox A. Advanced diagnostic imaging and surgical treatment of an odontogenic retromasseteric abscess in a guinea pig. *J Small Anim Pract* 2015;56: 134-137.

Capello V. Diagnostic imaging of dental disease in pet rabbits and rodents. *Vet Clin Exot Anim* 2016;19: 757-782.

Capello V. Surgical treatment of facial abscesses and facial surgery in pet rabbits. *Vet Clin Exot Anim* 2016;19: 799-823.

Capello V, Cauduro A. Comparison of diagnostic consistency and diagnostic accuracy between survey radiography and computed tomography of the skull in 30 rabbits with dental disease. *J Exot Pet Med* 2016;25: 115-127.

Capello V, Gracis M, Lennox AM. *Rabbit and Rodent Dentistry Handbook*, Lake Forth, FL, 2005, Zoological Education Network.

De Rycke LM, Boone MN, Van Caelenberg AI, et al. Micro-computed tomography of the head and dentition in cadavers of clinically normal rabbits. *Am J Vet Res* 2012;73: 227-232.

Donnelly TM, Vella D. Anatomy, physiology and non-dental disorders of the mouth of pet rabbits. *Vet Clin Exot Anim* 2016;19: 737-756.

Eroshin V, Reiter AM, Rosenthal K, et al. Oral examination results in rescued ferrets: clinical findings. *J Vet Dent* 2011;28: 8-15.

Gardhouse S, Sanchez-Migallon Guzman D, Petritz OA, et al. Diagnosis and treatment of sialectasis in domestic rabbit (Oryctolagus cuniculus). J Exot Pet Med 2016;25: 72-79.

He T, Friedel H, Kiliaridis S. Macroscopic and roentgenographic anatomy of the skull of the ferret (Mustela putorius furo). Lab Anim 2002;36: 86-96.

Gracis M. Clinical technique: Normal dental radiography of rabbits, guinea pigs, and chinchillas. J Exot Pet Med 2008;17: 78-86.

Jekl V, Hauptman K, Knotek Z. Quantitative and qualitative assessments of intraoral lesions in 180 small herbivorous mammals. Vet Rec 2008;62: 442-449.

Jekl V, Hauptman K, Jeklova E, et al. Dental eruption chronology in degus (Octodon degus). J Vet Dent 2011;28: 16-20.

Jekl V, Krejcirova L, Buchtova M, et al. Effect of high phosphorus diet on tooth microstructure of rodent incisors. Bone 2011;49: 479-484.

Jekl V, Redrobe S. Rabbit dental disease and calcium metabolism. The science behind divided opinions. J Small Anim Pract 2013;54: 481-490.

Johnson-Delaney CA. Anatomy and disorders of the oral cavity of ferrets and other exotic companion carnivores. Vet Clin North Am Exot Anim Pract 2016;19: 901-928.

Legendre L. Oral examination and occlusal equilibration in rodents and lagomorphs. J Vet Dent 2011;28: 52-57.

Legendre L. Treatment of oral abscesses in rodents and lagomorphs. J Vet Dent 2011;28: 30-33.

Legendre L. Rodent and lagomorph tooth extractions. J Vet Dent 2012;29: 204-209.

Legendre L. Anatomy and disorders of the oral cavity of guinea pigs. Vet Clin Exot Anim 2016;16: 825-842.

Long CV. Common dental disorders of the degu (Octodon degus). J Vet Dent 2012;29: 158-165.

Mancinelli E, Capello V. Anatomy and disorders of the oral cavity of rat-like and squirrel-like rodents. Vet Clin Exot Anim 2016;19: 871-900.

Mans C, Jekl V. Anatomy and disorders of the oral cavity of chinchillas and degus. Vet Clin Exot Anim 2016;19: 843-869.

Meredith AL, Prebble JL, Shaw DJ. Impact of diet on incisor growth and attrition and the development of dental disease in pet rabbits. J Small Anim Pract 2015;56: 377-382.

Minarikova A, Hauptman K, Jeklova E, et al. Diseases in pet guinea pigs: a retrospective study in 1000 animals. Vet Rec 2015;177(8): 200. https://doi.org/10.1136/vr.103053.

Minarikova A, Fictum P, Zikmund T, et al. Dental disease and periodontitis in a guinea pig (Cavia porcellus). J Exot Pet Med 2016;25: 150-156.

Müller J, Clauss M, Codron D, et al. Growth and wear of incisor and cheek teeth in domestic rabbits (Oryctolagus cuniculus) fed diets of different abrasiveness. J Exp Zool 2014;321A: 283-298.

Nemec A, Zadravec M, Račnik J. Oral and dental diseases in a population of domestic ferrets (Mustela putorius furo). J Small Anim Pract 2016;57: 553-560.

Norman R, Wills A. An Investigation into the relationship between owner knowledge, diet, and dental disease in guinea pig (Cavia porcellus). Animals 2016;6: 73. https://doi.org/10.3390/ani6110073.

Okuda A, Hori Y, Ichihara N, et al. Comparative observation of skeletal-dental abnormalities in wild, domestic, and laboratory rabbits. J Vet Dent 2007;24: 224-229.

Regalado A, Legendre L. Full-mouth intraoral radiographic survey in rabbits. J Vet Dent 2017;34: 190-200.

Reiter AM. Pathophysiology of dental disease in the rabbit, guinea pig and chinchilla. J Exotic Pet Med 2008;17: 70-7.

Riggs GG, Arzi B, Cissell, et al. Clinical application of cone-beam computed tomography of the rabbit head: Part 1—Normal dentition. Front Vet Sci 2016;3: 93. https://doi.org/10.3389/fvets.2016.00093.

Riggs GG, Cissell DD, Arzi B, et al. Clinical application of cone beam computed tomography of the rabbit head: Part 2—Dental disease. Front Vet Sci 2017;4: 5. https://doi.org/10.3389/fvets.2017.00005.

Sasai H, Iwai H, Fujita D, et al. The use of micro-computed tomography in the diagnosis of dental and oral disease in rabbits. BMC Vet Res 2014;10: 209. https://doi.org/10.1186/s12917-014-0209-4.

Schumacher M. Measurement of clinical crown length of incisor and premolar teeth in clinically healthy rabbits. J Vet Dent 2011;28: 90-95.

Schweda MC, Hassan J, Böhler A, et al. The role of computed tomography in the assessment of dental disease in 66 guinea pigs. Vet Rec 2014;175: 538-543.

Taylor M, Beaufrere H, Mans C, et al. Long-term outcome of treatment of dental abscesses with a wound-packing technique in pet rabbits: 13 cases. J Am Vet Med Assoc 2010;237: 1444-1449.

Tyrrell KL, Citron DM, Jenkins JR, et al. Periodontal bacteria in rabbit mandibular and maxillary abscesses. J Clin Microbiol 2002;40: 1044-1047.

Van Caelenberg A, De Rycke LM, Hermans K, et al. Comparison of radiography and CT to identify changes in the skulls of four rabbits. J Vet Dent 2011;28: 172-181.

Wyss F, Muller J, Clauss M, et al. Measuring rabbit (Oryctolagus cuniculus) tooth growth and eruption by fluorescence markers and bur marks. J Vet Dent 2016;33: 39-46.

Marketing Veterinary Dentistry

OUTLINE

LEARNING OBJECTIVES

When you have completed this chapter, you will be able to:

- Describe strategies for marketing veterinary dental services.
- Describe the "smile book" and explain how this is used in marketing veterinary dental services.
- List possible topics for the dentistry section of a practice newsletter.
- Explain how estimate and consent forms can be used as tools for marketing veterinary dental services.
- State examples of veterinary dental marketing materials.
- Discuss methods of internet marketing.
- Describe methods that can be used to market dental services during regular patient examinations and list suggested topics for client education in the examination room.

KEY TERMS

Clip art
Consent form
Dental models
Estimate

Handouts
Internet marketing
Marketing
Oral bacteria examination tool

Recall system
Smile book
Social media sites

Marketing is a system of activities designed to identify and satisfy consumer needs and desires. During the patient examination the veterinarian must determine the patient's medical needs and then inform the clients in such a manner that they want the services. The first step in effectively marketing a product or service is to determine the patient's needs. In veterinary medicine, practitioners must first educate themselves and become familiar with all aspects of the anticipated service. However, despite what many practitioners assume, marketing is more than merely presenting this information to the client. In reality, marketing begins with developing your product through education.

Another way to look at marketing is that it is really "doctoring." It entails examining the patient, advising the client on the needs of the patient and on the capability of the practice to deliver the recommended services. A variety of methods reinforce the importance of veterinary dentistry in maintaining overall health.

Between the writing of the first edition and this text, the internet revolution has widened the opportunities for marketing veterinary dentistry. Some things stay the same and a practice still must market its services when clients are in the facility, but there are many new opportunities for getting them into the facility and having them return.

MARKETING STRATEGIES

Gathering Client Information

Along with patient information, client information, such as e-mail addresses and permission to contact by e-mail, are essential to marketing.

Practice Brochures

The investment of time, effort, and money in the creation of a practice brochure can be extremely rewarding. The practice brochure should cover all aspects of service, including, of course, dental procedures. The brochure may provide information on practice policies, equipment, and commonly performed procedures; with the addition of illustrations, it can also be a pictorial guide to the practice. The brochure should be handed out in the practice as well as be available online.

Smile Book

A "smile book" is a pictorial description of procedures performed in the practice. One effective strategy is to include "before and after" photographs of dental procedures. This type of visual aid can be used to educate the client with regard to expected outcomes. It also can be used to describe the various steps of a recommended procedure or alternative procedure. Professional books can be made relatively easily through programs such as iphoto for Macintosh or online through websites such as www.Blurb.com, www.shutterfly.com, www.kodakgallery.com, and many others.

Posters and Transparencies

A variety of posters and transparencies are available that graphically illustrate dental disease. Some posters can be framed and hung in the reception area or examination room. Others can be backlit in the examination room on x-ray view boxes.

Newsletters

The practice newsletter should include a section on dentistry. Potential topics include the cause of periodontal disease, treatment techniques for the prevention and treatment of periodontal disease, fractured teeth, dietary considerations in dentistry, veterinary dental orthodontics, tooth resorption, and dental home-care products. Clip art, which is available from several commercial sources, can be used to enliven the textual content. With the advent of the internet, mailing lists can be collected and newsletters can be sent out through companies such as www.constantcontact.com.

Messages on Hold

Rather than listening to music (or, worse yet, silence) while they are on hold, clients can hear informative messages about veterinary medicine and veterinary dentistry. Subjects may include the need to take care of teeth, periodontal disease, fractured teeth, home care, and other important information.

Handouts

Handouts give the client additional information on the procedure or procedures that must be performed. Several pharmaceutical companies distribute helpful handouts and transparencies that may mention the company's products on the back page but focus primarily on delivering objective information. Handouts are also available for purchase through commercial companies. Fig. 15.1 is an example of a handout produced by Hills.

The practice can also customize, print, and make available on line original handouts. This allows customization of the handout to inform the client of the need for the procedure. Handouts can be general, covering all branches of veterinary dentistry, or specific, dealing only with the procedure recommended for the particular patient. Handouts on periodontal disease should cover the need for prevention through the complete prophy. Handouts on endodontic disease should discuss the reasons for performing root canals and the consequence of no treatment. The preoperative handout can be in the

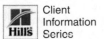

Client
Information
Series

**Reducing the Risks of
Canine Periodontal Disease**

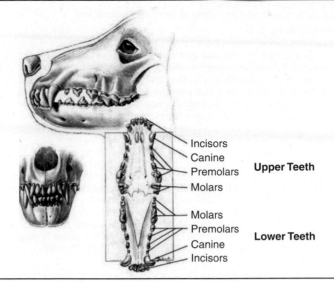

Incisors
Canine
Premolars — **Upper Teeth**
Molars

Molars
Premolars — **Lower Teeth**
Canine
Incisors

Reducing the Risks of Canine Periodontal Disease

Periodontal disease, or inflammation of the structures that support the teeth, is the primary cause of tooth loss in dogs. Dental care in young adults will prevent irreversible damage. This client education sheet will help you learn more about the risks of periodontal disease and will review your veterinarian's plan for keeping your dog healthy, as well as follow-up with the veterinary health care team.

Risk Factor Management for Canine Periodontal Disease

A risk factor is a condition or characteristic that predisposes an animal to disease. For example, high blood pressure in human beings increases the risk of stroke and heart and kidney failure. The importance of identifying risk factors is that sometimes the risk factor (high blood pressure, for example) can be eliminated or controlled to prevent or lessen the severity of the disease (stroke, for example). Veterinarians also recognize risk factors in pets. The extent to which such risk factors are managed will help determine the length and quality of your pet's life.

Risk Factors

Periodontal disease is very common. More than 80 percent of dogs three years old and older have some degree of periodontal disease. Although periodontal disease is found more frequently in older pets, its effects start in younger animals. Inflammation of the gums (gingivitis) often develops by the time a pet is one or two years old, and without proper care will progress causing irreversible damage and potentially infecting other organs such as the heart, liver and kidneys.

Risk factors for periodontal disease include:
- Lack of home dental care.
- Age.
- Overcrowding of teeth in small dogs, especially in those with short, wide skulls.
- Malocclusion (poor alignment) of teeth.
- Chewing on hard objects.
- Retained baby teeth.
- Other diseases, such as chronic kidney failure or diabetes.

Fig. 15.1 Example of a handout produced by Hill's Pet Nutrition. (Courtesy Hill's Pet Nutrition, Topeka, KS.)

Continued

Detecting Risk Factors

Frequent and complete veterinary checkups are especially important as your pet ages. These checkups can help detect underlying causes of periodontal disease as well as the disease itself. These checkups are warranted once a year, or more frequently according to your pet's oral health and your veterinarian's instructions.

Managing Risk Factors

Your veterinarian will prescribe a routine periodontal management program for your dog. This program will eliminate or minimize as many risk factors as possible. A thorough professional examination and dental cleaning that includes removal of plaque and calculus above and below the gum line will be provided by your veterinary health care team as the first step.

Home care is the most important part of therapy for preventing and managing periodontal disease. Frequent removal of plaque from your dog's teeth will help prevent periodontal disease and tooth loss. Plaque removal should begin in young animals because periodontal disease starts when pets are young.

Your veterinarian will show you how to care for your pet's teeth. The key to plaque removal is to make it a pleasant routine for your pet. Begin by handling your pet's muzzle. (You can hold a small dog in your lap while you do this.) When your pet is comfortable with this, you can try to brush a small number of teeth, such as the incisor (front) teeth. When your pet accepts this, you can gradually work the brush around the sides of your pet's mouth to reach the premolar and molar teeth. If your pet won't tolerate a brush, you should try a soft cloth. Your veterinarian has special toothpastes for your pet. Do not use human tooth paste on your pets.

Your veterinarian will probably schedule routine office visits to check your pet's teeth. These visits will allow him or her to help you combat periodontal disease through dental scalings and other necessary procedures designed to help your pet keep its teeth.

Nutritional Plan

If your pet has periodontal disease, your veterinarian may suggest a dietary change. Optimal nutrition provides for a pet's need based on age and activity level, and reduces the health risks associated with feeding excess sodium, calcium, phosphorus, protein, and calories. Foods that avoid these harmful excesses and also reduce the tartar and plaque that contribute to periodontal disease and bad breath include Hill's® Prescription Diet® t/d® Canine Dental Health.

Transitioning Food

Unless recommended otherwise by your veterinarian, gradually introduce any new food over a seven-day period. Mix the new food with your pet's former food, gradually increasing its proportion until only the new food is fed.

If your pet is one of the few that doesn't readily accept a new food, try warming the canned food to body temperature, hand feeding for the first few days, or mixing the dry food with warm water (wait ten minutes before serving). Feed only the recommended food. Be patient but firm with your pet. This is important because the success or failure of treatment depends to a large degree on strict adherence to the new food.

Presented as an educational service by

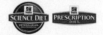

Home Care Instructions
Client's Name: _____
Patient's Name: _____
Medication(s): _____
Nutritional Recommendation: _____
Follow-Up Appointment: _____ (Hospital Stamp Area Above)
Regular visits will help our veterinary health care team provide for your pet's best interest.

Fig. 15.1, cont'd

form of a dental estimate that discusses fees, expected outcomes, and possible complications associated with the individual patient's disease process.

Computer systems can generate handouts on demand. For example, after a patient with stage 1 disease undergoes a prophy, a handout describing the stage of the disease, treatment, and home care can be linked to the computerized record. This handout would be different for the patient with stage 4 periodontal disease undergoing periodontal therapy.

Estimate and Consent Forms

Although designed primarily for legal reasons, estimate and consent forms are valuable marketing tools. An estimate is an effective way to present the treatment plan before the procedure is performed. Unfortunately, many veterinarians determine their fees after they have already performed the procedure; usually, they decide that they are charging too much and subtract charges where they can. To be fair to the practice and client, the best method is to document all necessary costs beforehand. Developing a treatment plan and estimate is an excellent way to promote discussion of the patient's needs and the client's wishes.

When discussing the treatment plan, the practitioner should focus on the services that are being presented and why they are necessary. Go through each item on the list and explain what it is and why it is being done. Once clients understand the procedure, they are more willing to give their permission to proceed.

Of course, during the course of one procedure, practitioners often discover a need for another. One method to handle this is to give the client three choices on the standard estimate/surgical release/drop-off form. These choices may be presented as follows:

1. Do anything the doctor feels is necessary.
2. Call first; if I cannot be reached, do what is necessary.
3. Do nothing if you cannot contact me.

These three choices eliminate the frustration of trying to contact a client who is difficult to reach while the patient is under anesthesia.

Recall System

Recall cards or e-mail is a valuable method of reminding the client to return for repeat visits. Recall reminders should be customized according to the patient's needs. Clients with generally healthy pets and pets with gingivitis should be reminded to come in for annual visits. Patients with established periodontal disease should be seen every 3 to 6 months, and patients with advanced periodontal disease should be seen every 3 months. Many practice management systems will automatically create a list of reminders when due. Some will send out e-mail messages to clients.

Dental Models

Plastic dental models are available for use in client education (Fig. 15.2). This education should focus on the patient's condition and recommended procedures for

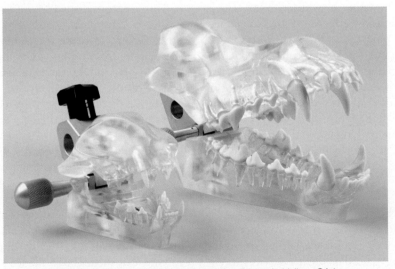

Fig. 15.2 Model. (Courtesy Dentalaire, Fountain Valley, CA.)

treatment. Three companies currently distribute plastic dental models of the canine and feline oral anatomy and disease conditions. Butler Company (800-344-2246) and Henry Schein Company (800-872-4346) market models with excellent representations of dental abnormalities and pathology. Dr. Shipp's Laboratories (800-442-0107) offer models with plastic teeth embedded in clear plastic. All three varieties are excellent for demonstrating root structure.

Special Events

Many practices sponsor special events to draw attention to dental health. These are an excellent way to increase awareness of this important aspect of veterinary medicine, and the entire staff can become involved. Participation in National Pet Dental Health Month (currently in February) allows the practice to use professional resources for advertising and other materials. In "Pet Dental Checks" veterinarians perform examinations (focusing on the oral cavity) on large numbers of patients. Clients receive report cards after participating. "The Great Brush Off" is a contest demonstrating toothbrushing techniques and dog obedience. A "Dog Walk" can be a community "fun run" or walk. These can be tied into "Pet Dental Checks." Veterinarians and staff can also host booths at health fairs intended for human health. These opportunities vary from area to area and practice to practice.

Internet Marketing

Unlike traditional marketing in which the message is put out by business and received by the consumer, internet marketing puts the computer in control of the marketing. Consumers control the medium by participating by having conversations, sharing resources, and forming their own community. Like a school of fish, no one individual controls the activity. Marketing is no longer passive, but requires participation by the company and consumer. This marketing is conducted by e-mail, creating a great website, and then participating in social forums such as Facebook, Twitter, and LinkedIn.

E-Mail Marketing

Collecting e-mail addresses, receiving permission to e-mail, and sending e-mail comprise a fairly inexpensive method of marketing veterinary dental services to clients. E-mails can be sent out for reminder of treatments due, such as dental recalls, and with newsletters from the practice.

Websites

Clients expect a practice to have a website. There are a number of computer programs that can help develop a website. Many companies, such as Go Daddy, Register.com, and Intuit, will provide hosting and fairly simple-to-use website design. Programs such as iweb for the Macintosh, Dreamweaver, and Web Image Studio can be used, or professional website designers can be hired.

However, designing the website is only a part of the process. The consumer must be drawn to the website and, once there, be enticed to stay there by the design, structure, and content. The design must make the reader think that it looks so good on the surface that the facility behind it must also do good work. The website should be structured so that it is easy for visitors to find what they are seeking. It should not have so many options that it is confusing; instead, the reader should be led through the website. They say "content is king." The purpose is to educate clients and potential clients and build expertise in their eyes. This content can include a virtual tour of the facility, photographs of the staff, photographs of patients (and clients with permission), hospital brochures, past newsletters, health tips, explanations of services provided, and many more items.

In addition to being snappy looking, the website should be optimized so that search engines can "see" it. This is accomplished by the search engine recognizing letters, numbers, words, phrases, image tags, and other factors. Because the number of webpages is in the billions (or who knows, trillions), it takes a lot of work to get your home page near the top of relevant search results. This usually will require professional assistance. Finally, the website needs to be maintained. Nothing looks worse than a website that contains old data.

Another feature of a good website would be a blog. A blog contains information from the practice; it is updated on a regular basis and is broken down into "posts." The blog may or may not have interaction whereby the readers can leave comments. Content can also be published in multiple places at the same time or syndicated via RSS (Really Simple Syndication) feed. Anyone can subscribe to the feed and use it by using a feed reader such as the Google Reader.

Social Media Sites

Facebook, Twitter, and LinkedIn are social media sites. There are currently more than twice the number of residents of the United States on Facebook worldwide, and before the next edition of this text, Facebook will have more users than China, the world's largest nation! People are not on Facebook to get information on veterinary dentistry, but rather to express themselves and connect with others. The goal of the marketer on Facebook is to build relationships with clients and potential clients and gain visibility, which drives the client to the veterinary dental practice and other services. The whole idea of social media is to make friends and get those friends to become clients. There are many good books on social media marketing; the reader is encouraged to read them.

MARKETING IN THE EXAMINATION ROOM

A dental examination should be conducted when the patient is 7 to 8 months of age to evaluate the occlusion and ensure that all primary teeth have exfoliated. At this time, further education may be provided to the client. Suggested topics include the recognition of dental disease, the importance of brushing and other home-care techniques, breed predilection for dental disease, and the need for regular professional teeth cleaning. If the patient is going under general anesthesia for spaying or neutering, the teeth can be scaled (or even just polished) at that time. Dental examinations should be included with the annual physical and may correspond with routine teeth-cleaning appointments. The key is to prevent disease, not let it start and then attempt to treat it. Dental examinations for older patients should be performed as appropriate; some require dental procedures every 3 months, and others need yearly checkups. Patients with periodontal disease should be rechecked every 1 to 2 weeks until the condition is under control. Then the patient should be recalled every 3 months to make sure that oral health is being maintained. Patients with tooth resorption should be checked 3 months after treatment to make sure the restoration is still in place. Patients that have had endodontic procedures (pulp-capping or root canal therapy) should be rechecked and radiographed under general anesthesia 6 months after the procedure.

Another tool that can be used in the examination room is disclosing solution, which is used to detect plaque that is not visible to the human eye. Disclosing solution, however, can be messy. A newer technology, the oral bacteria examination tool, uses a light-emitting diode (LED) to help identify evidence of bacteria in a pet's mouth. This technology is called *qualitative light-induced fluorescence* technology. A patient's mouth may appear to be healthy and free of bacteria; however, when using this dental examination tool, the veterinarian can show the client evidence of bacteria that may be early indications of further oral health problems. The bacterial by-products that fluoresce will be pink/orange.

OraStrip, discussed in Chapter 6, is an in-the-examination room test that can be performed on the cooperative awake patient. The test will instantly detect the presence of periodontal disease and can be a good marketing tool in convincing the client of the need for a Complete Oral Health Assessment and Prevention or Treatment (COAPT).

Every patient that comes through the practice door has a mouth, and these mouths have many problems that must be solved. Each problem may be viewed as a marketing opportunity and a way to provide better service to the patient.

Box 15.1 lists some common conditions that every practice should be diagnosing, know how to treat, and recognize when to refer for treatment.

BOX 15.1 Common Conditions/ Treatments Seen in the General Practice to Learn How to Treat or Refer for Treatment

1. Discolored teeth
2. Fractured teeth
3. Periodontal disease
4. Persistent deciduous teeth
5. Oral masses
6. Tooth resorption (both cat and dog!)
7. Worn teeth

CHAPTER 15 WORKSHEET

1. Traditionally, marketing is defined as a system of activities to _____ and _____ consumer _____ and _____.
2. Realistically, however, marketing is also _____.
3. A "_____ _____" is a pictorial description of procedures performed in the practice.
4. A variety of _____ are available that graphically illustrate dental disease.
5. _____ give the client more information on the procedure or procedures that need to be performed.
6. Computerized _____ may link the information presented to the individual patient's dental disease.
7. _____ _____ are a valuable method of reminding the client to return for repeat visits.
8. _____ (month) is National Pet Dental Health Month.
9. A dental examination should be conducted when the patient is 7 to 8 months of age to evaluate the _____.
10. Each problem that needs to be solved can be viewed as a marketing opportunity and a way to provide _____ _____ to the patient.
11. _____, _____, and _____ are social media sites.
12. The consumer must be drawn to the website and, once there, be enticed to stay there by the _____, _____, and _____.
13. Another feature of a good website would be a _____.
14. Collecting _____ addresses, receiving _____ to e-mail, and sending _____ comprise a fairly inexpensive method of marketing veterinary dental services to clients.
15. E-mails can be sent out for reminder of treatments due, such as _____, and with _____ from the practice.

Dental Equipment Inventory

HOSPITAL INVENTORY

The following table lists minimal equipment requirements that, in the author's opinion, are necessary to perform the treatments indicated. Many alternatives to the items mentioned here exist; this list is meant to be a starting point only!

BASIC

Hospital provides basic prophy services, exodontics, dental radiography, and the treatment of periodontal disease.

Item	Suggested	Number	Location
Safety glasses or face shield	One/technician		
Respirator mask	One/technician/day		
Examination gloves	*		
Ultrasonic scaler	One		
Supragingival insert	*		
Subgingival insert	*		
Sickle scaler (H6/7, N6/7, SH6/7, or Cislak P-12)	*		
Curette (Barnhardt 5/6 or Cislak P-10)	*		
Periodontal probe/explorer	*		
Compressed air system	One		
Slow-speed handpiece or electric motor handpiece	Two		
Prophy angle	Package		
Prophy cups	Package		
Prophy paste: Coarse	Package or jar		
Prophy paste: Fine	Package or jar		
Disclosing solution	One bottle		
Prophy angle lubricant	One bottle		
High-speed handpiece spray	One can		
Arkansas sharpening stone	One		
Arkansas conical sharpening stone	One		
High-speed handpiece	Two		
701L burs	One package		
301SS elevator	†		
301S elevator or Cislak EX-5	†		
301S elevator (modified) or Cislak EX-5H	Two		
301 elevator or Cislak EX-4	†		
303 elevator or Cislak EX-3	†		

Continued

Item	Suggested	Number	Location
Size 1 winged elevator or Cislak EX-W1			
Size 2 winged elevator or Cislak EX-W2			
Cislak Size 3 winged elevator or Cislak EX-W3			
Size 4 winged elevator or Cislak EX-W4			
Size 6 winged elevator or Cislak EX-W5			
Size 8 winged elevator or Cislak EX-W8			
Size 2 luxator straight and curved or Cislak LT-2S, LT2L, LT2R			
Size 3 luxator straight and curved or Cislak LT-3S, LT3L, LT3R LT3CA, LT3CB			
Size 4.5 luxator straight and curved Cislak LT-4.5S, LT4.5L, LT4.5R LT4.5CA, LT4.5CB			
Root tip picks: Heidbrink, 3HB10/11, Cislak 14, RT-1 for canines and WA-1 for felines or Miltex 76	†		
Feline extraction forceps	†		
Periosteal elevator: Molt #9 or Cislak EX-1/EX-1S	†		
Periosteal elevator Cislak EX-9			
Thumb forceps	†		
Mayo-Hegar needle holder	†		
3-0 Monocryl suture	Package		
4-0 Monocryl suture	Package		
5-0 Monocryl suture	Package		
Consil	Box		
Dental x-ray machine	One		
Digital x-ray system with computer, or if film system used, the following equipment is needed:			
Chairside darkroom	One		
X-ray developing solution	Bottle		
X-ray fixing solution	Bottle		
X-ray developing clips	Six		
Size 0, DF 57 x-ray film	Box		
Size 2, DF 58 x-ray film	Box		
Size 4, DF 50 x-ray film	Box		
X-ray film mounts	Box		
Doxirobe or Arestin	Box		
No. 3 (or similar) scalpel handle	†		
Small tissue scissors (LaGrange)	One		
Sterile saline solution	Bottle		
#15c blades	Box		

*Maximum number of prophy/periodontal therapy/day × 1 (this allows sterilization for each patient).
†Maximum number of procedures/day × 1 (this allows sterilization for each patient).

INTERMEDIATE AND ADVANCED

Hospital provides all veterinary dental services.

Items in the Basic list plus the following items:

Item	Suggested	Number	Location
Light-curing gun	One		
Assorted burs: Tapered crosscut fissure burs: 701L; round burs: #2, #4; pear-shaped burs: #330	Minimum five each type		
31-mm K-files: 06, 08, 10, 15, 20, 25, 30, 35, 40, 45, 50, 55, 60, 70, 80, 90, 100	Minimum six each type		
55-mm K-reamer files: 10, 15, 20, 25, 30, 35, 40, 45, 50, 55, 60, 70, 80, 90, 100	Minimum six each type		
60-mm Hedström files: 30, 35, 40, 45, 50, 55, 60, 70, 80	Minimum six each type		
Endodontic stops	One per file (placed on file before use)		
Endodontic irrigation needles, 27 gauge	Box		
Barbed broaches: Assorted sizes	Minimum two each		
Endodontic rings	One		
Endodontic sponges	Bag		
RC-Prep	Syringe		
Canal irrigant: Sodium hypochlorite, chlorhexidine	Stock bottle plus Luer-lock syringe		
Paper absorbent points: Similar size to files	Packages		
Root canal sealer: Zinc oxide–eugenol (ZOE) or advanced sealers	One box		
Mixing pad	One pad		
Mixing spatula	One		
Endodontic point forceps: Cotton or college pliers	One		
#30 Plugger and spreader: Canine size	One		
#50 Plugger and spreader: Canine size	One		
#65 Plugger and spreader: Canine size	One		
#90 Plugger and spreader: Canine size	One		
#25 Plugger and spreader: Human size	One		
#30 Plugger and spreader: Human size	One		
#35 Plugger and spreader: Human size	One		
#40 Plugger and spreader: Human size	One		
#50 Plugger and spreader: Human size	One		
#60 Plugger and spreader: Human size	One		
Light-cure restorative materials	One		
Finishing disks, points, or stones	Box		
Impression trays	One set		
Impression material: Alginate	Jar		
Laboratory stone	Box		
Dental laboratory vibrator	One		
Bite registration material	Box		
Orthodontic cement	Box		
Orthodontic buttons	Box		
Howe pliers	One		
Flour pumice	Jar		
Power cord: Assorted sizes	Reel		
Band-removing forceps	One		

AVDC Abbreviations for use in Case Logs Equine and Small Animal

This list of abbreviations has been recommended by the Nomenclature Committee and approved by the AVDC Board. The list is in alphabetical order.

Anatomic items are show in **black font.**

Conditions and diagnostic procedures appropriate for use in the Diagnosis column of a case log entry are shown in blue font.

Treatment procedure and related items suitable for inclusion in the Procedure column in the case log entry are shown in red font.

Note: Use of other abbreviations in AVDC case logs is not permitted—write out the whole word if it must be included in a case log entry.

For further information on the use of particular definitions, visit the Nomenclature page on the AVDC web site.

Abbreviation		Definition
A		**Alveolus**
AB		Abrasion
ABE		Alveolar bone expansion
ALV		Alveolectomy/alveoloplasty
ANO		Anodontia
AOS		Alveolar osteitis
AP		**Apex**
	AP/X	Apicoectomy
APN		Apexification
AT		Attrition
ATE		Abnormal tooth extrusion
B		Biopsy
	B/B	Bite biopsy
	B/CN	Core needle biopsy
	B/E	Excisional biopsy
	B/I	Incisional biopsy
	B/NA	Needle aspiration
	B/NB	Needle biopsy
	B/P	Punch biopsy
	B/S	Surface biopsy
BR		Bite registration
BRI		Bridge
BTH		Ball therapy
BUC		Buccotomy
BUP		Bullous pemphigoid

C		**Canine**
CA		Caries
	CA/INF	Infundibular caries (equines)
	CA/INF/D	Distal infundibular caries
	CA/INF/M	Mesial infundibular caries
	CA/PER	Peripheral caries (in equines)
CB		Crossbite
	CB/C	Caudal crossbite
	CB/R	Rostral crossbite
CC		Calcinosis circumscripta
CEJ		**Cementoenamel junction**
CFL		Cleft lip
	CFL/R	Cleft lip repair
CFP		Cleft palate
	CFP/R	Cleft palate repair
CFS		Cleft soft palate
	CFS/R	Cleft soft palate repair
CFSH		Soft palate hypoplasia
	CFSH/R	Soft palate hypoplasia repair
CFSU		Unilateral cleft soft palate
	CFSU/R	Unilateral cleft soft palate repair
CFT		Traumatic cleft palate
	CFT/R	Traumatic cleft palate repair
CHO		Calvarial hyperostosis
CL		Chewing lesion
	CL/B	Chewing lesion (buccal mucosa/cheek)
	CL/L	Chewing lesion (labial mucosa/lip)
	CL/P	Chewing lesion (palatal mucosa/palate)
	CL/T	Chewing lesion (lingual/sublingual mucosa/tongue)
CMO		Craniomandibular osteopathy
COM		Commissurotomy
CON		**Condylar process of the mandible**
	CON/X	Condylectomy
COO		Condensing osteitis
COR		**Coronoid process of the mandible**
	COR/X	Coronoidectomy
CPL		Cheiloplasty/commissuroplasty
CR		**Crown**
	CR/A	Crown amputation
	CR/AC	**Anatomic crown**
	CR/C	Ceramic crown (full)
	CR/C/P	Ceramic crown (partial)
	CR/CC	**Clinical crown**
	CR/L	Crown lengthening
	CR/M	Metal crown (full)
	CR/M/P	Metal crown (partial)
	CR/P	Crown preparation
	CR/R	Resin crown (full)
	CR/R/P	Resin crown (partial)
	CR/RC	**Reserve crown**

Continued

Abbreviation		Definition
	CR/PFM	Porcelain fused to metal crown (full)
	CR/PFM/P	Porcelain fused to metal crown (partial)
	CR/T	Temporary crown
	CR/XP	Crown reduction
CS		Culture/sensitivity
CT		Computed tomography
	CT/CB	Cone-beam CT
CTH		Chemotherapy
CU		Contact mucositis or contact mucosal ulceration
D		**Diastema**
	D/O	Open diastema
	D/ODY	Diastema odontoplasty (or widening)
	D/V	Valve diastema
DC		Diagnostic cast
	DC/D	Die
	DC/SM	Stone model
DI		Discharge
	DI/ND	Right nasal discharge
	DI/NS	Left nasal discharge
	DI/NU	Bilateral nasal discharge
	DI/OD	Right ocular discharge
	DI/OS	Left ocular discharge
	DI/OU	Bilateral ocular discharge
DMO		Decreased mouth opening
DP		Defect preparation (prior to filling a dental defect)
DT		**Deciduous tooth**
	DT/P	Persistent deciduous tooth
DTC		Dentigerous cyst
	DTC/R	Dentigerous cyst removal
E		**Enamel**
	E/D	Enamel defect
	E/H	Enamel hypoplasia
	E/HM	Enamel hypomineralization
	E/P	Enamel pearl
EM		Erythema multiforme
ENO		Enophthalmos
EOG		Eosinophilic granuloma
	EOG/L	Eosinophilic granuloma (lip)
	EOG/P	Eosinophilic granuloma (palate)
	EOG/T	Eosinophilic granuloma (tongue)
ER		Erosion
ESP		Elongated soft palate
	ESP/R	Elongated soft palate reduction
EXO		Exophthalmos
F		Flap
	F/AD	Advancement flap
	F/AP	Apically positioned flap
	F/CO	Coronally positioned flap
	F/EN	Envelope flap
	F/HI	Hinged (overlapping) flap
	F/IS	Island flap

	F/LA	Laterally positioned flap
	F/RO	Rotation flap
	F/TR	Transposition flap
FB		Foreign body
	FB/R	Foreign body removal
FOD		Fibrous osteodystrophy
FOL		Folliculitis
FRE		Frenuloplasty (frenulotomy, frenulectomy)
FT		Fiberotomy
FX		Fracture (tooth or jaw; see T/FX for tooth fracture abbreviations)
	FX/R	Repair of jaw fracture
	FX/R/EXF	External skeletal fixation
	FX/R/IAS	Interarch splinting (between upper and lower dental arches)
	FX/R/IDS	Interdental splinting (between teeth within a dental arch)
	FX/R/IQS	Interquadrant splinting (between left and right upper or lower jaw quadrants)
	FX/R/MMF	Maxillomandibular fixation (other than muzzling and interarch splinting)
	FX/R/MZ	Muzzling
	FX/R/PL	Bone plating
	FX/R/WIR/C	Wire cerclage
	FX/R/WIR/OS	Intraosseous wiring
GC		Gingival curettage
GE		Gingival enlargement (in the absence of a histologic diagnosis)
GF		Graft
	GF/B	Bone graft
	GF/C	Cartilage graft
	GF/CT	Connective tissue graft
	GF/F	Fat graft
	GF/G	Gingival graft
	GF/M	Mucosal graft
	GF/N	Nerve graft
	GF/S	Skin graft
	GF/V	Venous graft
GH		Gingival hyperplasia
GR		Gingival recession
GTR		Guided tissue regeneration
GV		Gingivectomy/gingivoplasty
HC		Hypercementosis
HS		Hemisection
HYP		Hypodontia
I1,2,3		**Incisor**
IM		Detailed imprint of hard and/or soft tissues (e.g., individual teeth or palate defect)
	IM/F	Full-mouth impression (i.e., imprints of teeth of upper and lower dental arches)
IMP		Implant
INF		**Infundibulum**
IOF		Intraoral fistula
	IOF/R	Intraoral fistula repair
IP		Inclined plane
	IP/AC	Acrylic inclined plane
	IP/C	Composite inclined plane
	IP/M	Metal (i.e., laboratory-produced) inclined plane
ITH		Immunotherapy

Continued

Abbreviation		Definition
LAC		Laceration
	LAC/B	Laceration (cheek skin/buccal mucosa)
	LAC/G	Laceration (gingiva/alveolar mucosa)
	LAC/L	Laceration (lip skin/labial mucosa)
	LAC/O	Laceration (palatine tonsil/oropharyngeal mucosa)
	LAC/P	Laceration (palatal mucosa)
	LAC/R	Laceration repair
	LAC/T	Laceration (lingual/sublingual mucosa)
LE		Lupus erythematosus
LIN		**Tongue**
	LIN/X	Tongue resection
LIP		**Lip/cheek**
	LIP/X	Lip/cheek resection
LN		**Lymph node** (regional, i.e., facial, mandibular, parotid, lateral and medial retropharyngeal)
	LN/E	Lymph node enlargement
	LN/X	Lymph node resection
M1,2,3		**Molar**
MAL		Malocclusion
	MAL1	Class 1 malocclusion (neutroclusion; dental malocclusion with normal upper/lower jaw length relationship)
	MAL1/BV	Buccoversion
	MAL1/DV	Distoversion
	MAL1/LABV	Labioversion
	MAL1/LV	Linguoversion
	MAL1/MV	Mesioversion
	MAL1/PV	Palatoversion
	MAL2	Class 2 malocclusion (mandibular distoclusion; symmetrical skeletal malocclusion with the lower jaw relatively shorter than the upper jaw)
	MAL3	Class 3 malocclusion (mandibular mesioclusion; symmetrical skeletal malocclusion with the upper jaw relatively shorter than the lower jaw)
	MAL4	Class 4 malocclusion (asymmetric skeletal malocclusion in a caudoventral, side-to-side or dorsoventral direction)
	MAL4/DV	Asymmetric skeletal malocclusion in a dorsoventral direction
	MAL4/RC	Asymmetric skeletal malocclusion in a rostrocaudal direction
	MAL4/STS	Asymmetric skeletal malocclusion in a side-to-side direction
MAR		Marsupialization
MET		Metastasis
	MET/D	Distant metastasis
	MET/R	Regional metastasis
MMM		Masticatory muscle myositis
MN		**Mandible/mandibular**
	MN/FX	Mandibular fracture
MRI		Magnetic resonance imaging
MX		**Maxilla/maxillary**
	MX/FX	Maxillary fracture
N		**Nose/nasal/nasopharyngeal**
	N/EN	Rhinoscopy
	N/LAV	Nasal lavage
	N/NS	Naris stenosis
	N/NS/R	Naroplasty

	N/NPS	Nasopharyngeal stenosis
	N/NPS/R	Nasopharyngeal stenosis repair
	N/POL	Nasopharyngeal polyp
	N/SCC	Nasal SCC (check abbreviations under OM for other tumors)
OA		Orthodontic appliance
	OA/A	Orthodontic appliance adjustment
	OA/AR	Arch bar
	OA/BKT	Bracket, button or hook
	OA/CMB	Custom-made OA/BKT
	OA/EC	Elastic chain, tube or thread
	OA/I	Orthodontic appliance installment
	OA/R	Orthodontic appliance removal
	OA/WIR	Orthodontic wire
OAF		Oroantral fistula
	OAF/R	Oroantral fistula repair
OC		Orthodontic counseling
ODY		Odontoplasty
OFF		Orofacial fistula
	OFF/R	Orofacial fistula repair
OLI		Oligodontia
OM		Oral/maxillofacial mass
	OM/AA	Acanthomatous ameloblastoma
	OM/AD	Adenoma
	OM/ADC	Adenocarcinoma
	OM/APN	Anaplastic neoplasm
	OM/APO	Amyloid-producing odontogenic tumor
	OM/CE	Cementoma
	OM/FIO	Feline inductive odontogenic tumor
	OM/FS	Fibrosarcoma
	OM/GCG	Giant cell granuloma
	OM/GCT	Granular cell tumor
	OM/HS	Hemangiosarcoma
	OM/LI	Lipoma
	OM/LS	Lymphosarcoma
	OM/MCT	Mast cell tumor
	OM/MM	Malignant melanoma
	OM/OO	Osteoma
	OM/OS	Osteosarcoma
	OM/MTB	Multilobular tumor of bone
	OM/PAP	Papilloma
	OM/PCT	Plasma cell tumor
	OM/PNT	Peripheral nerve sheath tumor
	OM/POF	Peripheral odontogenic fibroma
	OM/RBM	Rhabdomyosarcoma
	OM/SCC	Squamous cell carcinoma
	OM/UDN	Undifferentiated neoplasm
OMJL		Open-mouth jaw locking
	OMJL/R	Open-mouth jaw locking reduction
ONF		Oronasal fistula
	ONF/R	Oronasal fistula repair

Continued

Abbreviation		Definition
OP		Operculectomy
OR		Orthodontic recheck
OS		Orthognathic surgery
OSN		Osteonecrosis
OSS		Osteosclerosis
OST		Osteomyelitis
PA		**Periapical**
	PA/A	Periapical abscess
	PA/C	Periapical cyst
	PA/G	Periapical granuloma
	PA/P	Periapical pathology (if a distinction between granuloma, abscess or cyst cannot be made)
PCB		Post-and-core build-up
PCD		Direct pulp capping
PCI		Indirect pulp capping
PD		Periodontal disease
	PD0	Clinically normal
	PD1	Gingivitis only (without attachment loss)
	PD2	Early periodontitis (<25% attachment loss)
	PD3	Moderate periodontitis (25% to 50% attachment loss)
	PD4	Advanced periodontitis (>50% attachment loss)
PDE		Acquired palate defect
	PDE/R	Acquired palate defect repair
PEC		Pericoronitis
PEO		Periostitis ossificans
PH		**Pulp horn (in equines numbered by the du Toit system)**
	PH/D	Pulp horn defect
PHA		**Pharynx**
	PHA/IN	Pharyngitis
PM1-4		**Premolar**
POB		Palatal obturator
PRO		Professional dental cleaning (scaling, polishing, irrigation)
PTY		Ptyalism
PU		**Pulp**
	PU/M	Mineralization of pulp
	PU/S	Pulp stone
PV		Pemphigus vulgaris
PYO		Pyogenic granuloma
R		Restoration (filling of a dental defect)
	R/A	Filling made of amalgam
	R/C	Filling made of composite
	R/CP	Filling made of compomer
	R/I	Filling made of glass ionomer
RAD		Radiography
	RAD/SG	Sialography
RBA		Retrobulbar abscess
RCR		Retained crown-root or clinical crown-reserve crown or clinical crown-reserve crown and root
RCT		Standard root canal therapy
	RCT/S	Surgical root canal therapy

RO		**Root**
	RO/AC	**Anatomic root**
	RO/CR	**Clinical root**
	RO/X	Root resection/amputation
RP		Root planing
	RP/C	Closed root planing
	RP/O	Open root planing
RPA		Retropharyngeal abscess
RR		Internal resorption
RTH		Radiotherapy
RTR		Retained root or reserve crown
S		Surgery
	S/M	Partial mandibulectomy
	S/MB	Bilateral partial mandibulectomy (removal of parts of the left and right mandibles)
	S/MD	Dorsal marginal mandibulectomy (marginal mandibulectomy, mandibular rim excision)
	S/MS	Segmental mandibulectomy (removal of a full dorsoventral segment of a mandible)
	S/MT	Total mandibulectomy (removal of one entire mandible)
	S/P	Partial palatectomy
	S/X	Partial maxillectomy
	S/XB	Bilateral partial maxillectomy (removal of parts of the left and right maxillae and/or other facial bones)
SCI		Scintigraphy
SG		**Salivary gland**
	SG/ADC	Salivary gland adenocarcinoma (check abbreviations under OM for other tumors)
	SG/ADS	Sialadenosis
	SG/IN	Sialadenitis
	SG/MAR	Marsupialization
	SG/MUC/S	Sublingual sialocele
	SG/MUC/P	Pharyngeal sialocele
	SG/MUC/C	Cervical sialocele
	SG/NEC	Necrotizing sialometaplasia
	SG/RC	Mucous retention cyst
	SG/SI	Sialolith
	SG/X	Salivary gland resection
SHE		Shear mouth (increased occlusal angulation of equine cheek teeth)
SIN		**Sinus**
	SIN/CF	**Conchofrontal sinus**
	SIN/CF/F	Conchofrontal sinus flap
	SIN/CMX	**Caudal maxillary sinus**
	SIN/EN	Sinoscopy
	SIN/F	Sinus flap
	SIN/IN	Sinusitis (e.g., SIN/IN/RMX = rostral maxillary sinusitis)
	SIN/LAV	Sinus lavage
	SIN/MX/F	Maxillary sinus flap
	SIN/RMX	**Rostral maxillary sinus**
	SIN/SP	**Sphenopalatine sinus**
	SIN/TRP	Sinus trephination
	SIN/VC	**Ventral conchal sinus**
SR		Surgical repositioning
ST		Stomatitis

Continued

Abbreviation		Definition
	ST/CS	Caudal stomatitis
SYM		**Mandibular symphysis**
	SYM/R	Mandibular symphysis repair
	SYM/S	Mandibular symphysis separation
T		**Tooth**
	T/A	Avulsed tooth
	T/CCR	Concrescence
	T/DEN	Dens invaginatus
	T/DIL	Dilaceration
	T/E	Embedded tooth
	T/EL	Tooth elongation (abnormal intraoral and/or periapical extension of the coronal and/or apical portions of the tooth; e.g., T/EL/CC = elongation of the clinical crown)
	T/FDR	Fused roots
	T/FUS	Fusion
	T/FX	Fractured tooth (see next seven listings for fracture types)
	T/FX/EI	Enamel infraction
	T/FX/EF	Enamel fracture
	T/FX/UCF	Uncomplicated crown fracture
	T/FX/CCF	Complicated crown fracture
	T/FX/UCRF	Uncomplicated crown-root facture
	T/FX/CCRF	Complicated crown-root fracture
	T/FX/RF	Root fracture
	T/GEM	Gemination
	T/I	Impacted tooth
	T/LUX	Luxated tooth
	T/MAC	Macrodontia
	T/MIC	Microdontia
	T/NE	Near pulp exposure
	T/NV	Non-vital tooth
	T/PE	Pulp exposure
	T/RI	Tooth reimplantation (for an avulsed tooth)
	T/RP	Tooth repositioning (for a luxated tooth)
	T/SN	Supernumerary tooth
	T/SR	Supernumerary root
	T/TRA	Transposition
	T/U	Unerupted tooth
	T/V	Vital tooth
	T/XP	Partial tooth resection
TMA		Trauma
	TMA/B	Ballistic trauma
	TMA/E	Electric trauma
	TMA/BRN	Burn trauma
	TMA/R	Trauma repair
TMJ		**Temporomandibular joint**
	TMJ/A	Temporomandibular joint ankylosis (true or false)
	TMJ/A/R	Temporomandibular joint ankylosis repair
	TMJ/D	TMJ dysplasia
	TMJ/FX	Temporomandibular joint fracture
	TMJ/FX/R	Temporomandibular joint fracture repair
	TMJ/LUX	TMJ luxation
	TMJ/LUX/R	Temporomandibular joint luxation reduction

TON		**Palatine tonsil**
	TON/IN	Tonsillitis
	TON/X	Tonsillectomy
TP		Treatment plan
TR		Tooth resorption
TRP		Trephination
TS		Trisection
TT		Temporal teratoma
US		Ultrasonography
VPT		Vital pulp therapy
X		Closed extraction of a tooth (without sectioning)
XS		Closed extraction of a tooth (with sectioning)
	XS/ODY	Removal of interproximal crown tissue to facilitate transoral extraction of a tooth
XSS		Open extraction of a tooth
	XSS/APX/RPL	Extraction of a tooth after apicoectomy and repulsion
	XSS/BUC	Transbuccal extraction of a tooth after buccotomy
	XSS/BUC/ALV	Transbuccal extraction of a tooth after buccotomy and alveolectomy
	XSS/COM	Transbuccal extraction of a tooth after commissurotomy
	XSS/COM/ ALV	Transbuccal extraction of a tooth after commissurotomy and alveolectomy
	XSS/MIB	Extraction of a tooth via minimally invasive buccotomy (small incision made for introduction of straight instrumentation to elevate, section or drill into a cheek tooth for the purpose of facilitating its transoral extraction)
	XSS/RPL	Extraction of a tooth after repulsion
ZYG		**Zygoma (zygomatic arch)**
	ZYG/X	Zygomectomy

AVDC Nomenclature Introduction

NOMENCLATURE ADOPTED BY THE AVDC BOARD

Last updated March 2016

American Veterinary Dental College (AVDC) has adopted the following items as standard nomenclature for use in College documents. Residents making case log entries or submitting case reports or publications for AVDC credentials review are required to use these terms and these abbreviations.

Abbreviations: AVDC has approved a specific set of Abbreviations to match the definitions provided in this web page. Click Abbreviations List to download the full Abbreviations list file. The Abbreviations List is also available via a link in the Edit Case Log web page screen. Use of these abbreviations by residents in AVDC case logs is mandatory.

Abbreviations to be used in AVDC Case Logs are shown in **(blue brackets)**

DEFINITIONS OF VETERINARY DENTISTRY, EQUINE DENTISTRY AND BEAKOLOGY

Veterinary dentistry is a discipline within the scope of veterinary practice that involves the professional consultation, evaluation, diagnosis, prevention, treatment (nonsurgical, surgical, or related procedures) of conditions, diseases, and disorders of the oral cavity and maxillofacial area and their adjacent and associated structures; it is provided by a licensed veterinarian, within the scope of his/her education, training and experience, in accordance with the ethics of the profession and applicable law.

Equine dentistry is the practice of veterinary dentistry performed in equids (genus Equus: horses, asses, and zebras).

Beakology is the branch of science dealing with the anatomy, physiology, and pathology (including diagnosis and treatment of such pathology) of the beak and associated tissues of vertebrate animals that have beaks or beak-like structures.

DEFINITIONS OF ITEMS APPLYING TO MORE THAN ONE ORAL TISSUE OR DISEASE

Congenital: Of or relating to a disease, condition, or characteristic that is present at birth and may be inherited or result from an insult during pregnancy

Acquired: Of or relating to a disease, condition, or characteristic that develops after birth and is not inherited

Inherited: Of or relating to a disease, condition, or characteristic that results from the genetic make-up of the individual animal and may be present at birth or develop later in life

Culture/sensitivity (CS): Bacteria cultured in medium and analyzed for sensitivity to antibiotics

Laceration (LAC): A tear or cut in the gingiva/alveolar mucosa **(LAC/G)**, tongue/sublingual mucosa **(LAC/T)**, lip skin/labial mucosa **(LAC/L)**, cheek skin/buccal mucosa **(LAC/B)**, palatal mucosa **(LAC/P)**, or palatine tonsil/oropharyngeal mucosa **(LAC/O)**; debridement and suturing of such lacerations is abbreviated as **LAC/R**

Chewing lesion (CL): Mucosal lesion resulting from self-induced bite trauma on the cheek **(CL/B)**, lip **(CL/L)**, palate **(CL/P),** or tongue/sublingual region **(CL/T)**

Foreign body (FB): An object originating outside the body; removal of the foreign body is abbreviated with **FB/R**

Burn (TMA/BRN): Injury to skin, mucosa, or other body parts caused by fire, heat, radiation, electricity, or a caustic agent

Ballistic trauma (TMA/B): Physical trauma sustained from a projectile that was launched through space, most commonly by a weapon such as a gun or a bow

Electric injury (TMA/E): Physical trauma to skin, mucosa or other tissues when coming into direct contact with an electrical current

ANATOMY OF ORAL, DENTAL, AND RELATED STRUCTURES

Dental Anatomy

Pulp cavity: Space within the tooth

Pulp chamber: Space within the crown of a tooth

Root canal: Space within the root of a tooth

Apical foramen: Opening at the apex of a tooth, through which neurovascular structures pass to and from the dental pulp

Apical delta: Multiple apical foramina forming a branching pattern at the apex of a tooth reminiscent of a river delta when sectioned and viewed through a microscope; this occurs in some brachyodont teeth

Ameloblasts: Epithelial cells involved in the formation of enamel (amelogenesis)

Enamel (E): Mineralized tissue covering the crown of brachyodont teeth

Anatomic crown (CR/AC): That part of a tooth that is coronal to the cementoenamel junction (or anatomic root)

Clinical crown (CR/CC): That part of a tooth that is coronal to the gingival margin; also called erupted crown in equines

Anatomic root (RO/AR): That part of a tooth that is apical to the cementoenamel junction (or anatomic crown)

Clinical root (RO/CR): That part of a brachyodont tooth that is apical to the gingival margin

Cementoenamel junction: Area of a tooth where cementum and enamel meet

Reserve crown (CR/RC): That part of the crown of a hypsodont tooth that is apical to the gingival margin

Nomenclature and Numbering of Teeth

Incisor Teeth

The incisors will be referred to as (right or left) (maxillary or mandibular) first, second, or third incisors numbered from the midline.

Reference(s): Peyer B: *Comparative odontology*, ed 1, Chicago, 1968, University of Chicago Press, pp 1–347. Nickel R, Schummer A, Seiferle E, et al: Teeth, general and comparative. In *The viscera of domestic mammals*, ed 1, Berlin, 1973, Verlag Paul Parey, pp 75–99.

Premolar Teeth in the Cat:

In the cat, the tooth immediately distal to the maxillary **canine** is the second **premolar**, the tooth immediately distal to the mandibular canine is the third premolar.

Reference(s): Nickel R, Schummer A, Seiferle E, et al: Teeth, general and comparative. In *The viscera of domestic mammals*, ed 1, Berlin, 1973, Verlag Paul Parey, pp 75–99.

Tooth Numbering:

The existence of the conventional anatomic names of teeth as well as the various tooth numbering systems is recognized. The correct anatomic names of teeth are (right or left), (maxillary or mandibular), (first, second, third or fourth), (**incisor, canine, premolar, molar**), as applicable, written out in full or abbreviated. The **modified Triadan system** is presently considered to be the tooth numbering system of choice in veterinary dentistry; gaps are left in the numbering sequence where there are missing teeth (e.g., the first premolar encountered in the feline left maxilla is numbered 206, not 205. The two lower right premolars are 407 and 408, not 405 and 406).

Both the use of anatomic names and of the modified Triadan system are acceptable for recording and storing veterinary dental information. The use of anatomic names in publications is required by many leading journals and is recommended. It offers the advantage of veterinary dental publications being understandable to other health professionals and scientists with an interest in veterinary dentistry.

Reference(s): Floyd MR: The modified Triadan system: nomenclature for veterinary dentistry, *J Vet Dent* 8:18–19, 1991.

Comments:

In January 1972, the International Dental Federation adopted a new, two-digit, user-friendly nomenclature system for use in the human dental patient. This new system eliminated the plus and minus signs of the Haderup system and the brackets of the Winkel system. Following the acceptance of the new system for human dental nomenclature, Professor Dr. MedDent H.

Triadan, a dentist at the University of Bern, Switzerland, introduced a similar system for animals. Owing to the fact that many animals, including his canine model, have more than nine teeth in a quadrant, the Triadan system for animals utilizes three digits instead of two digits.

ABBREVIATIONS ASSOCIATED WITH TEETH:

Tooth (T): Hard structure embedded in the jaw; used for biting and chewing

Incisor (I): Incisor tooth

Canine (C): Canine tooth

Premolar (P): Premolar tooth

Molar (M): Molar tooth

Alveolus (A): Socket in the jaw for a tooth root or reserve crown (plural: alveoli)

Crown (C): Coronal portion of a tooth

Root (RO): Radicular portion of a tooth

Apex (AP): End of the root or reserve crown (plural: apices)

Generations of Teeth in Diphyodont Species

Deciduous and Permanent are the anatomically correct terms to denote the two generations of teeth in diphyodont species.

It is acceptable to use **"primary"** instead of **deciduous** in communicating with clients.

Reference(s): Anonymous. *Nomina anatomica veterinaria,* ed 4, Zurich and Ithaca, 1994, World Association of Veterinary Anatomists. Boucher CO, Zwemer TJ: *Boucher's clinical dental terminology—a glossary of accepted terms in all disciplines of dentistry,* ed 4, St. Louis, 1993, Mosby. Evans HE: *Miller's anatomy of the dog,* ed 3, Philadelphia, 1993, WB Saunders Co.

Comments: Deciduous is the scientific term used in biology, as well as in comparative anatomy and anthropology for both animal and plant structures that are regularly shed. As a substitute for temporary, the term primary appeared early in the literature and it is listed in both Anthony's and Otofy's dictionaries 1922–23. The style of the Journal of the ADA requires the term deciduous in all literature designed for the profession and allows primary only in discourse for non-professional persons.

Deciduous tooth (DT): Primary tooth replaced by a permanent (secondary) tooth.

The **deciduous dentition** period is that period during which only deciduous teeth are present.

The **mixed dentition** period is that period during which both deciduous and permanent teeth are present.

The **permanent dentition** period is that period during which only permanent teeth are present.

Reference(s): Anonymous: *Nomina anatomica veterinaria,* ed 4, Zurich and Ithaca, 1994, World Association of Veterinary Anatomists. Boucher CO, Zwemer TJ: *Boucher's clinical dental terminology—a glossary of accepted terms in all disciplines of dentistry,* ed 4, St. Louis, 1993, Mosby. Evans HE: *Miller's anatomy of the dog,* ed 3, Philadelphia, 1993, WB Saunders Co.

The term **"Persistent deciduous tooth"** is etymologically correct, although the term "retained deciduous tooth" is commonly used. The latter term, however, can be confused with an unerupted deciduous tooth.

Reference(s): Eisenmenger E, Zetner K: *Tierv§ rztliche Zahnheilkunde,* ed 1, Berlin, 1982, Verlag Paul Parey, pp 44–50.

SURFACES OF TEETH AND DIRECTIONS IN THE MOUTH

Vestibular/Buccal/Labial

Vestibular is the correct term referring to the surface of the tooth facing the vestibule or lips; **buccal** and **labial** are acceptable alternatives.

Reference(s): Anonymous. *Nomina anatomica veterinaria,* ed 4, Zurich and Ithaca, 1994, World Association of Veterinary Anatomists.

Comment(s): The term "facial" specifically refers to the surfaces of the rostral teeth visible from the front. According to Dr. A.J. Bezuidenhout, a veterinary anatomist at Cornell University, "facial" is a bit of a misnomer. Traditionally "facial" has been used in human dentistry for the aspect of teeth visible from the front (i.e., incisors and canines).

Lingual/Palatal

Lingual: The surface of a mandibular or maxillary tooth facing the tongue is the lingual surface. Palatal can also be used when referring to the lingual surface of maxillary teeth.

Mesial/Distal

Mesial and **distal** are terms applicable to tooth surfaces. The **mesial** surface of the first incisor is next to the median plane; on other teeth it is directed toward the first incisor. The **distal** surface is opposite from the mesial surface.

Rostral/Caudal

Rostral and **caudal** are the positional and directional anatomic terms applicable to the head in a sagittal plane in nonhuman vertebrates. **Rostral** refers to a structure closer to, or a direction toward the most forward structure of the head. **Caudal** refers to a structure closer to, or a direction toward the tail.

Anterior and *posterior* are the synonymous terms used in human dentistry.

TEETH ABNORMALITIES AND RELATED PROCEDURES

Enamel Abnormalities

Abrasion (AB): Tooth wear caused by contact of a tooth with a nondental object

Attrition (AT): Tooth wear caused by contact of a tooth with another tooth

Erosion (ER): Demineralization of tooth substance owing to external acids

Caries (CA): Degradation of dental hard tissue caused by demineralization owing to acids released during bacterial fermentation of carbohydrates

Enamel defect (ED): Lesion affecting the structural integrity of enamel

Enamel hypoplasia (E/H): refers to inadequate deposition of enamel matrix. This can affect one or several teeth and may be focal or multifocal. The crowns of affected teeth can have areas of normal enamel next to areas of hypoplastic or missing enamel.

Enamel hypomineralization (E/HM): refers to inadequate mineralization of enamel matrix. This often affects several or all teeth. The crowns of affected teeth are covered by soft enamel that may be worn rapidly.

Enamel infraction (T/FX/EI): Incomplete fracture (crack) of the enamel without loss of tooth substance

Enamel fracture (T/FX/EF): Fracture with loss of crown substance confined to the enamel

Tooth Formation Abnormalities

Persistent deciduous tooth (DT/P): A deciduous tooth that is present when it should have exfoliated

Supernumerary tooth (T/SN): Presence of an extra tooth (also called hyperdontia)

Hypodontia (HYP): Developmental absence of a few teeth

Oligodontia (OLI): Developmental absence of numerous teeth

Anodontia (ANO): Failure of all teeth to develop

Macrodontia (T/MAC): Tooth/teeth larger than normal

Microdontia (T/MIC): Tooth/teeth smaller than normal

Transposition (T/TRA): Two teeth that have exchanged position

Fusion (T/FUS): Combining of adjacent tooth germs and resulting in partial or complete union of the developing teeth; also called synodontia

Concrescence (T/CCR): Fusion of the roots of two or more teeth at the cementum level

Fused roots (T/FDR): Fusion of roots of the same tooth

Gemination (T/GEM): A single tooth bud's attempt to divide partially (cleft of the crown) or completely (presence of an identical supernumerary tooth); also called twinning

Supernumerary root (T/SR): Presence of an extra root

Dilaceration (T/DIL): Disturbance in tooth development, causing the crown or root to be abruptly bent or crooked

Dens invaginatus (T/DEN): Invagination of the outer surface of a tooth into the interior, occurring in either the crown (involving the pulp chamber) or the root (involving the root canal); also called dens in dente

Enamel pearl (E/P): Small, nodular growth on the root of a tooth made of enamel with or without a small dentin core and sometimes a covering of cementum

Unerupted tooth (T/U): Tooth that has not perforated the oral mucosa

Embedded tooth (T/E): Unerupted tooth covered in bone whose eruption is compromised by lack of eruptive force

Impacted tooth (T/I): Unerupted or partially erupted tooth whose eruption is prevented by contact with a physical barrier

Dentigerous cyst (DTC): Odontogenic cyst initially formed around the crown of a partially erupted or unerupted tooth; also called follicular cyst or tooth-containing cyst; removal is abbreviated **DTC/R**

Folliculitis (FOL): Inflammation of the follicle of a developing tooth

Pericoronitis (PEC): Inflammation of the soft tissues surrounding the crown of a partially erupted tooth

Tooth Resorption

Tooth resorption is classified based on the severity of the resorption (**Stages 1–5**) and on the location of the resorption (**Types 1–3**).

The AVDC classification of tooth resorption is based on the assumption that tooth resorption is a progressive condition.

Tooth resorption (TR): Resorption of dental hard tissue

Internal resorption (RR:) Tooth resorption originating within the pulp cavity

Stages of Tooth Resorption

Stage 1 (TR 1): Mild dental hard tissue loss (cementum or cementum and enamel).

Stage 2 (TR 2): Moderate dental hard tissue loss (cementum or cementum and enamel with loss of dentin that does not extend to the pulp cavity).

Stage 3 (TR 3): Deep dental hard tissue loss (cementum or cementum and enamel with loss of dentin that extends to the pulp cavity); most of the tooth retains its integrity.

Stage 4 (TR 4): Extensive dental hard tissue loss (cementum or cementum and enamel with loss of dentin that extends to the pulp cavity); most of the tooth has lost its integrity.

TR4a Crown and root are equally affected.

Stage 4 (TR 4): Extensive dental hard tissue loss (cementum or cementum and enamel with loss of dentin that extends to the pulp cavity); most of the tooth has lost its integrity.

TR4b: Crown is more severely affected than the root

Stage 4 (TR 4): Extensive dental hard tissue loss (cementum or cementum and enamel with loss of dentin that extends to the pulp cavity); most of the tooth has lost its integrity.

TR4c: Root is more severely affected than the crown.

Stage 5 (TR 5): Remnants of dental hard tissue are visible only as irregular radiopacities, and gingival covering is complete.

Types of Resorption Based on Radiographic Appearance

Type 1 (T1): On a radiograph of a tooth with type 1 (T1) appearance, a focal or multifocal radiolucency is present in the tooth with otherwise normal radiopacity and normal periodontal ligament space.

Type 2 (T2): On a radiograph of a tooth with type 2 (T2) appearance, there is narrowing or disappearance of the periodontal ligament space in at least some areas and decreased radiopacity of part of the tooth.

Type 3 (T3): On a radiograph of a tooth with type 3 (T3) appearance, features of both type 1 and type 2 are present in the same tooth. A tooth with this appearance has areas of normal and narrow or lost periodontal ligament space, and there is focal or multifocal radiolucency in the tooth and decreased radiopacity in other areas of the tooth.

Tooth Fracture Classification

The **Tooth fracture (T/FX)** classification shown below can be applied for brachyodont and hypsodont teeth, which covers domesticated species and many wild species.

Fractures of teeth in some wild species may not fit into this classification because of differences in the tissues present in the teeth.

When used in AVDC case log entries, the **tooth fracture abbreviations** noted below are to be stated as T/FX/ (specific abbreviation [e.g., **T/FX/CCF**]).

Enamel infraction (T/FX/EI): Incomplete fracture (crack) of the enamel without loss of tooth substance

Enamel fracture (T/FX/EF): Fracture with loss of crown substance confined to the enamel

Uncomplicated crown fracture (T/FX/UCF): Fracture of the crown that does not expose the pulp

Complicated crown fracture (T/FX/CCF): Fracture of the crown that exposes the pulp

Uncomplicated crown-root fracture (T/FX/UCRF): Fracture of the crown and root that does not expose the pulp

Complicated crown-root fracture (T/FX/CCRF): Fracture of the crown and root that exposes the pulp

Root fracture (T/FX/RF): Fracture involving the root

Retained root or reserve crown (RTR): Presence of a root remnant or reserve crown remnant

Retained crown-root or clinical crown-reserve crown or clinical crown-reserve crown and root (RCR): Presence of a crown-root remnant (in brachyodont teeth), clinical crown-reserve crown remnant (in aradicular hypsodont teeth) or clinical crown-reserve crown and root remnant (in radicular hypsodont teeth)

Enamel infraction (EI): An incomplete fracture (crack) of the enamel without loss of tooth substance. Example:

Enamel fracture (EF): A fracture with loss of crown substance confined to the enamel. Example:

Uncomplicated crown fracture (UCF): A fracture of the crown1 that does not expose the pulp. Example:

Complicated crown fracture (CCF): A fracture of the crown1 that exposes the pulp. Example:

Uncomplicated crown-root fracture (UCRF): A fracture of the crown and root that does not expose the pulp. Example:

Complicated crown-root fracture (CCRF): A fracture of the crown and root that exposes the pulp. Example:

Root fracture (RF): A fracture involving the root.

ENDODONTIC TERMINOLOGY

Endodontics is a specialty in dentistry and oral surgery that is concerned with the prevention, diagnosis, and treatment of diseases of the pulp–dentin complex and their impact on associated tissues.

Apexogenesis: Physiologic formation of the apex of a vital tooth

Pulp (PU): Soft tissue in the pulp cavity

Odontoblasts: Cells of mesenchymal origin that line the outer surface of the pulp and whose biological function is formation of dentin (dentinogenesis)

Predentin: Unmineralized dentin matrix produced by odontoblasts

Dentin: Mineralized tissue surrounding the pulp and containing dentinal tubules that radiate outward from the pulp to the periphery

Primary dentin: Dentin produced until root formation is completed (e.g., dogs, cats) or the tooth comes into occlusion (e.g., horses)

Secondary dentin: Dentin produced after root formation is completed

Tertiary dentin: Dentin produced as a result of a local insult; can be reactionary (produced by existing odontoblasts) or reparative (produced by odontoblast-like cells that differentiated from pulpal stem cells as a result of an insult)

Sclerotic dentin: Transparent dentin characterized by mineralization of the dentinal tubules as a result of an insult or normal aging

Periapical (PA): Pertaining to tissues around the apex of a tooth, including the periodontal ligament and the alveolar bone

Fracture (FX): Breaking of a bone or tooth

Vital tooth (T/V): Tooth with vital pulp

Nonvital tooth (T/NV): Tooth with nonvital pulp or from which the pulp has been removed

Pulp stones (PU/S): Intrapulpal mineralized structures

Mineralization of the pulp (PU/M): Pulpal mineralization resulting in regional narrowing or complete disappearance of the pulp cavity

Hypercementosis (HC): Excessive deposition of cementum around the root or reserve crown of a tooth

Near pulp exposure (T/NE): Thin layer of dentin separating the pulp from the outer tooth surface

Pulp exposure (T/PE): Tooth with an opening through the wall of the pulp cavity uncovering the pulp

Tooth luxation (T/LUX): Clinically or radiographically evident displacement of the tooth within its alveolus

Tooth avulsion (T/A): Complete extrusive luxation with the tooth out of its alveolus

Periapical pathology (PA/P): Pertaining to disease around the apex of a tooth

Periapical cyst (PA/C): Odontogenic cyst formed around the apex of a tooth after stimulation and proliferation of epithelial rests in the periodontal ligament (also known as a radicular cyst)

Periapical granuloma (PA/G): Chronic apical periodontitis with accumulation of mononuclear inflammatory cells and an encircling aggregation of fibroblasts and collagen that on diagnostic imaging appears as diffuse or circumscribed radiolucent lesion

Periapical abscess (PA/A): Acute or chronic inflammation of the periapical tissues characterized by localized accumulation of suppuration

Osteosclerosis (OSS): Excessive bone mineralization around the apex of a vital tooth caused by low-grade pulp irritation (asymptomatic; not requiring endodontic therapy)

Condensing osteitis (COO): Excessive bone mineralization around the apex of a nonvital tooth caused by long-standing and low-toxic exudation from an infected pulp (requiring endodontic therapy)

Alveolar osteitis (AOS): Inflammation of the alveolar bone considered to be a complication after tooth extraction

Osteomyelitis (OST): Localized or wide-spread infection of the bone and bone marrow

Osteonecrosis (OSN): Localized or wide-spread necrosis of the bone and bone marrow

Phoenix abscess: Acute exacerbation of chronic apical periodontitis

Intraoral fistula (IOF): Pathologic communication between tooth, bone, or soft tissue and the oral cavity; use **IOF/R** for its repair

Orofacial fistula (OFF): Pathologic communication between the oral cavity and face; use **OFD/R** for its repair

Indirect pulp capping (PCI): Procedure involving the placement of a medicated material over an area of near pulp exposure

Direct pulp capping (PCD): Procedure performed as part of vital pulp therapy and involving the placement of a medicated material over an area of pulp exposure

Vital pulp therapy (VPT): Procedure performed on a vital tooth with pulp exposure, involving partial pulpectomy, direct pulp capping, and access/fracture site restoration

Apexification (APN): Procedure to promote apical closure of a nonvital tooth

Standard (orthograde) root canal therapy (RCT): Procedure that involves accessing, debriding (including total pulpectomy), shaping, disinfecting, and obturating the root canal and restoring the access and/or fracture sites

Surgical (retrograde) root canal therapy (RCT/S): Procedure that involves accessing the bone surface (through mucosa or skin), fenestration of the bone over the root apex, apicoectomy, and retrograde filling

Apicoectomy (AP/X): Removal of the apex of a tooth; also called root end resection

Retrograde filling: Restoration placed in the apical portion of the root canal after apicoectomy

Tooth repositioning (T/RP): Repositioning of a displaced tooth

Interdental splinting (IDS): Fixation using intraoral splints between teeth within a dental arch (e.g., for avulsed or luxated teeth that underwent reimplantation or repositioning); if performed for jaw fracture repair, use FX/R/IDS

Operative Dentistry and Prosthodontic Terminology

Operative (or restorative) dentistry is a specialty in dentistry and oral surgery that is concerned with the art and science of the diagnosis, treatment, and prognosis of defects of teeth that do not require prosthodontic crowns for correction.

Prosthodontics (or dental prosthetics or prosthetic dentistry) is a specialty in dentistry and oral surgery that is concerned with the provision of suitable substitutes for the clinical crown of teeth or for one or more missing or lost teeth and their associated parts. Maxillofacial prosthetics is considered a subspecialty of prosthodontics, involving palatal obturators and maxillofacial prostheses to replace resected or lost tissues.

Odontoplasty (ODY): Surgical contouring of the tooth surface

Defect preparation (DP): Removal of dental hard tissue to establish in a tooth the biomechanically acceptable form necessary to receive and retain a defect restoration

Restoration (R): Anything that replaces lost tooth structure, teeth, or oral tissues, including fillings, inlays, onlays, veneers, crowns, bridges, implants, dentures, and obturators

Defect restoration: Filling made of amalgam (R/A), glass ionomer (R/I), composite (R/C), or compomer (R/CP) within a prepared defect

Bridge (BRI): Fixed partial denture used to replace a missing or lost tooth by joining permanently to adjacent teeth or implants

Crown preparation (CR/P): Removal of enamel or enamel and dentin to establish on a tooth the biomechanically acceptable form necessary to receive and retain a prosthodontic crown

Temporary crown (CR/T): Provisional, short-term cap made of resin to protect a prepared crown until cementation of a prosthodontic crown

Full crown: Prosthodontic crown made of metal (CR/M), resin (CR/R), ceramic (CR/C), or porcelain fused to metal (CR/PFM) that covers the tip and all sides of a prepared crown

Partial crown: Prosthodontic crown (e.g., three-quarter crown) made of metal (CR/M/P), resin (CR/R/P), ceramic (CR/C/P), or porcelain fused to metal (CR/PFM/P) that covers part of a prepared crown

Implant (IMP): Titanium rod-shaped endosseous device to support intraoral prosthetics that resemble a tooth or group of teeth to replace one or more missing or lost teeth

Crown reduction (CR/XP): Partial removal of tooth substance to reduce the height or an abnormal extension of the clinical crown

Crown amputation (CR/A): Total removal of clinical crown substance

Post and core (PCB): Placing a post into the root canal of a tooth that had root canal therapy and build-up of a core made of filling material around the portion of post that extends out from the pulp cavity

JAW AND TMJ ABNORMALITIES

Jaw and TMJ Anatomy

All mammals have two maxillas (or maxillae) and two mandibles. The adjective "maxillary" is often used in a wider sense (e.g., "maxillary fractures") to include other facial bones, in addition to the maxillary bone proper.

Reference(s): Anonymous: *Nomina anatomica veterinaria* ed. 4, Zurich and Ithaca, 1994, World Association of Veterinary Anatomists.

Evans HE: The skull. In: Evans HE, ed: *Miller's anatomy of the dog*, ed 4, Philadelphia, 1993, W.B. Saunders, 128–166.

Hildebrand M: *Analysis of vertebrate structure*, ed 4, New York, 1995, John Wiley & Sons.

Nickel R, Schummer A, Seiferle E, et al: Teeth, general and comparative. In: *The viscera of domestic mammals*, ed 1, Berlin, 1973, Verlag Paul Parey, 75–99.

Verstraete FJM: Maxillofacial fractures. In: Slatter DH, ed: *Textbook of small animal surgery*, ed 3, Philadelphia, 2003, WB Saunders Co, 2190–2207.

Incisive Bones

In domestic animals, the correct name for the paired bones that carry the maxillary incisors, located rostral to the maxillary bones, is the incisive bones, not the premaxilla.

Reference(s): Anonymous. *Nomina anatomica veterinaria*, ed 4, Zurich and Ithaca, 1994, World Association of Veterinary Anatomists.

CLINICALLY RELEVANT TERMS RELATED TO THE MANDIBLE AND TEMPOROMANDIBULAR JOINT: ANATOMIC STRUCTURE COMMENTS

Mandible: All animals have two mandibles, not one; removing one entire mandible is a total mandibulectomy not a hemimandibulectomy

Body of the mandible: The part that carries the teeth; often incorrectly referred to as horizontal ramus

Incisive part: The part that carries the incisors

Molar part: The part that carries the premolars and molars; premolar-molar part would probably have been more accurate

Alveolar margin: Often incorrectly referred to as alveolar crest

Ventral margin: Free ventral border

Mandibular canal: Contains a neurovascular bundle; often incorrectly referred to as the medullary cavity of the mandible

Mental foramens or foramina: Rostral, middle, or caudal mental foramina in the dog and cat

Ramus of the mandible: The part that carries the three processes; often incorrectly referred to as the vertical ramus

Angular process: Caudoventral process (in *carnivora*)

Coronoid process: Process for the attachment of the temporal muscle

Condylar process: Consisting of mandibular head and mandibular neck; often incorrectly referred to as condyloid process

Mandibular head: Articular head of the condylar process

Mandibular neck: Neck of the condylar process

Mandibular notch: The notch on the caudal aspect, between the coronoid and condylar processes; not to be confused with the facial vascular notch

Mandibular angle: Angle between the body and ramus of the mandible.

Facial vascular notch: Shallow indentation on the ventral aspect of the mandible, rostral to the angular process (absent in carnivores)

Mandibular foramen: The entrance to the mandibular canal

Intermandibular joint (mandibular symphysis): Median connection of the bodies of the right and left mandibles (in adult Sus and Equus replaced by a synostosis), consisting of intermandibular synchondrosis and intermandibular suture

Intermandibular synchondrosis: The smaller part of the intermandibular joint formed by cartilage

Intermandibular suture: The larger part of the intermandibular joint formed by connective tissue

Temporomandibular joint (TMJ): The area where the condylar process of the mandible articulates with the mandibular fossa of the temporal bone

Articular disk: A flat structure composed of fibrocartilagenous tissue and positioned between the articular surfaces of the condylar process of the mandible and mandibular fossa of the temporal bone, separating the joint capsule in dorsal and ventral compartments; often incorrectly referred to as meniscus.

Mandibular fossa: Concave depression in the temporal bone that articulates with the mandibular head

Retroarticular process: A projection of the temporal bone that protrudes ventrally from the caudal end of the zygomatic arch and carries part of the mandibular fossa

Reference(s): Anonymous: *Nomina anatomica veterinaria,* ed 4, Zurich and Ithaca, 1994, World Association of Veterinary Anatomists.

Scapino RP: The third joint of the canine jaw, *J Morphol* 116:23–50, 1965.

OTHER TERMS RELATING TO THE JAWS AND TMJ

Alveolar jugum (plural: alveolar juga): The palpable convexity of the buccal alveolar bone overlying a large tooth root.

Reference(s): Anonymous: *Nomina anatomica veterinaria,* ed 4, Zurich and Ithaca, 1994, World Association of Veterinary Anatomists. Evans HE: *Miller's anatomy of the dog,* ed 3, Philadelphia: 1993, WB Saunders Co.

Dental arch: Referring to the curving structure formed by the teeth in their normal position; upper dental arch formed by the maxillary teeth, lower dental arch formed by the mandibular teeth

Jaw quadrant: Referring to the left or right upper or lower jaw

Interarch: Referring to the area between the upper and lower dental arches

Interquadrant: Referring to the area between the left and right upper or lower jaw quadrants

Jaw and Related Abbreviations

Mandible/mandibular (MN): Referring to the lower jaw

Maxilla/maxillary (MX): Referring to the upper jaw

Mandibular symphysis (SYM): Joint between the left and right mandibles (intermandibular joint)

Zygomatic arch (ZYG): Consisting of the zygomatic process of the temporal bone and the temporal process of the zygomatic bone; also called zygoma

PERIODONTAL ANATOMY AND DISEASE

Definitions of Stage, Grade and Index

Stage: The assessment of the extent of pathologic lesions in the course of a disease that is likely to be progressive (e.g., stages of periodontal disease, staging of oral tumors)

Grade: The quantitative assessment of the degree of severity of a disease or abnormal condition at the time of diagnosis, irrespective of whether the disease is progressive (e.g., a grade 2 mast cell tumor based on mitotic figures)

Index: A quantitative expression of predefined diagnostic criteria whereby the presence and/or severity of pathologic conditions are recorded by assessing a numerical value (e.g., gingival index, plaque index)

STAGES OF PERIODONTAL DISEASE

The degree of severity of periodontal disease (PD) relates to a single tooth; a patient may have teeth that have different stages of periodontal disease.

Normal (PD0): Clinically normal; gingival inflammation or periodontitis is not clinically evident.

Stage 1 (PD1): Gingivitis only without attachment loss; the height and architecture of the alveolar margin are normal.

Stage 2 (PD2): Early periodontitis; less than 25% of attachment loss or, at most, there is a stage 1 furcation involvement in multirooted teeth. There are early radiologic signs of periodontitis. The loss of periodontal attachment is less than 25% as measured either by probing of the clinical attachment level, or radiographic determination of the distance of the alveolar margin from the cementoenamel junction relative to the length of the root.

Stage 3 (PD3): Moderate periodontitis; 25% to 50% of attachment loss as measured either by probing of the clinical attachment level, radiographic determination of the distance of the alveolar margin from the cementoenamel junction relative to the length of the root, or there is a stage 2 furcation involvement in multirooted teeth.

Stage 4 (PD4): Advanced periodontitis; more than 50% of attachment loss as measured either by probing of the clinical attachment level, or radiographic determination of the distance of the alveolar margin from the cementoenamel junction relative to the length of the root, or there is a stage 3 furcation involvement in multirooted teeth.

Reference(s): Wolf HF, Rateitschak EM, Rateitschak KH, et al: *Color atlas of dental medicine: periodontology,* ed 3, Stuttgart, 2005, Georg Thieme Verlag.

Furcation Involvement and Mobility Index

Furcation Index

Stage 1 (F1): Furcation 1 involvement exists when a periodontal probe extends less than half way under the crown in any direction of a multirooted tooth with attachment loss.

Stage 2 (F2): Furcation 2 involvement exists when a periodontal probe extends greater than half way under the crown of a multirooted tooth with attachment loss but not through and through.

Stage 3 (F3): Furcation exposure exists when a periodontal probe extends under the crown of a multirooted tooth, through and through from one side of the furcation out the other.

Tooth Mobility Index

Stage 0 (M0): Physiologic mobility up to 0.2 mm.

Stage 1 (M1): The mobility is increased in any direction other than axial over a distance of more than 0.2 mm and up to 0.5 mm.

Stage 2 (M2): The mobility is increased in any direction other than axial over a distance of more than 0.5 mm and up to 1.0 mm.

Stage 3 (M3): The mobility is increased in any direction other than axial over a distance exceeding 1.0 mm or any axial movement.

Gingival and Periodontal Pathology

Gingivitis: Inflammation of gingiva

Periodontitis: Inflammation of nongingival periodontal tissues (i.e., the periodontal ligament and alveolar bone)

Gingival recession (GR): Root surface exposure caused by apical migration of the gingival margin or loss of gingiva.

Gingival enlargement (GE): Clinical term, referring to overgrowth or thickening of gingiva in the absence of a histologic diagnosis

Gingival hyperplasia (GH): Histologic term, referring to an abnormal increase in the number of normal cells in a normal arrangement and resulting clinically in gingival enlargement

Abnormal tooth extrusion (ATE): Increase in clinical crown length not related to gingival recession or lack of tooth wear

Alveolar bone expansion (ABE): Thickening of alveolar bone at labial and buccal aspects of teeth

Periodontal Treatment

Professional oral care includes mechanical procedures performed in the oral cavity.

Professional dental cleaning (PRO) refers to scaling (supragingival and subgingival plaque and calculus removal) and polishing of the teeth with power/hand instrumentation performed by a trained veterinary health care provider under general anesthesia. See also AVDC Position Statements on Dental Health Care Providers and on Non-Professional Dental Scaling.

Periodontal therapy refers to treatment of diseased periodontal tissues that includes professional dental cleaning as defined above and one or more of the following: root planing, gingival curettage, periodontal flaps, regenerative surgery, gingivectomy/gingivoplasty, and local administration of antiseptics/antibiotics.

Home oral hygiene refers to measures taken by pet owners that are aimed at controlling or preventing plaque and calculus accumulation.

Gingival curettage (GC): Removal of damaged or diseased tissue from the soft tissue lining of a periodontal pocket.

Root planing (RP): Removal of dental deposits from and smoothing of the root surface of a tooth; it is closed (**RP/C**) when performed without a flap or open (**RP/O**) when performed after creation of a flap.

Gingivectomy (GV): Removal of some or all gingiva surrounding a tooth

Gingivoplasty (GV): A form of gingivectomy performed to restore physiological contours of the gingiva

Guided tissue regeneration (GTR): Regeneration of tissue directed by the physical presence and/or chemical activities of a biomaterial; often involves placement of barriers to exclude one or more cell types during healing of tissue

Crown lengthening (CR/L): Increasing clinical crown height by means of gingivectomy/gingivoplasty, apically positioned flaps, post and core build-up, or orthodontic movement

Frenuloplasty (frenulotomy, frenulectomy) (FRE): Reconstructive surgery or excision of a frenulum

Hemisection (HS): Splitting of a tooth into two separate portions

Trisection (TS): Splitting of a tooth into three separate portions.

Partial tooth resection (T/XP): Removal of a crown-root segment with endodontic treatment of the remainder of the tooth

Root resection/amputation (RO/X): Removal of a root with maintenance of the entire crown and endodontic treatment of the remainder of the tooth

Flap Surgery

Flap (F): A sheet of tissue partially or totally detached to gain access to structures underneath or to be used in repairing defects; can be classified based on the location of the donor site (local or distant), attachment to donor site (pedicle, island, or free), tissue to be transferred (e.g., mucosal, mucoperiosteal, cutaneous, myocutaneous), tissue thickness (partial-thickness or full-thickness), blood supply (random pattern or axial pattern), and direction and orientation of transfer (envelope, advancement, rotation, transposition, and hinged).

Location of Donor Site:

Local flap: Harvested from an adjacent site
Distant flap: Harvested from a remote site

Attachment to Donor Site:

Pedicle flap: Attached by tissue through which it receives its blood supply
Island flap (F/IS): Attached by a pedicle made up of only the nutrient vessels
Free flap: Completely detached from the body; it has also been suggested that a free flap be termed a graft

Tissue to be Transferred

Mucosal flap: Containing mucosa
Mucoperiosteal flap: Containing mucosa and underlying periosteum
Cutaneous (or skin) flap: Containing epidermis, dermis, and subcutaneous tissue
Myocutaneous flap: Containing skin and muscle
Gingival flap: Containing gingiva
Alveolar mucosa flap: Containing alveolar mucosa
Periodontal flap: Containing gingiva and alveolar mucosa
Labial flap: Containing lip mucosa
Buccal flap: Containing cheek mucosa
Sublingual flap: Containing sublingual mucosa
Palatal flap: Containing palatal mucosa
Pharyngeal flap: Containing pharyngeal mucosa

Tissue Thickness

Partial-thickness (or split-thickness) flap: Consisting of a portion of the original tissue thickness

Full-thickness flap: Having the original tissue thickness

Blood Supply

Random pattern flap: Randomly supplied by nonspecific arteries
Axial pattern flap: Supplied by a specific artery

Direction and Orientation of Transfer

Envelope flap (F/EN): Retracted away from a horizontal incision; there is no vertical incision
Advancement (or sliding) flap (F/AD): Carried to its new position by a sliding technique in a direction away from its base
Rotation flap (F/RO): A pedicle flap that is rotated into a defect on a fulcrum point
Transposition flap (F/TR): Flap that combines the features of an advancement flap and a rotation flap
Hinged flap (F/HI): Folded on its pedicle as though the pedicle was a hinge; also called a turnover or overlapping flap
Apically positioned flap (F/AP): Moved apical to its original location
Coronally positioned flap (F/CO): Moved coronal to its original location
Mesiodistally or distomesially positioned flap: Moved distal or mesial to its original location along the dental arch; also called a laterally positioned flap (**F/LA**)

ORAL PATHOLOGY: INFLAMMATORY DISEASES, TUMORS, OTHER ABNORMALITIES

Oral Inflammation

Note that a definitive diagnosis of inflammation often cannot be made based on physical examination findings alone.

Oral and oropharyngeal inflammation is classified by location:

Gingivitis: Inflammation of gingiva
Periodontitis: Inflammation of nongingival periodontal tissues (i.e., the periodontal ligament and alveolar bone)
Alveolar mucositis: Inflammation of alveolar mucosa (i.e., mucosa overlying the alveolar process and extending from the mucogingival junction without obvious demarcation to the vestibular sulcus and to the floor of the mouth)

Sublingial mucositis: Inflammation of mucosa on the floor of the mouth

Labial/buccal mucositis: Inflammation of lip/cheek mucosa

Caudal mucositis: Inflammation of mucosa of the caudal oral cavity, bordered medially by the palatoglossal folds and fauces, dorsally by the hard and soft palate, and rostrally by alveolar and buccal mucosa

Stomatitis (ST): Inflammation of the mucous lining of any of the structures in the mouth; in clinical use the term should be reserved to describe wide-spread oral inflammation (beyond gingivitis and periodontitis) that may also extend into submucosal tissues (e.g., marked caudal mucositis extending into submucosal tissues may be termed caudal stomatitis (ST/CS). Note: The fauces are defined as the lateral walls of the oropharynx that are located medial to the palatoglossal folds. The areas lateral to the palatoglossal fold, commonly involved in feline stomatitis, are not the fauces.

Contact mucositis and contact mucosal ulceration (CU): Lesions in susceptible individuals that are secondary to mucosal contact with a tooth surface bearing the responsible irritant, allergen, or antigen. They have also been called "contact ulcers" and "kissing ulcers."

Palatitis: Inflammation of mucosa covering the hard and/or soft palate

Glossitis: Inflammation of mucosa of the dorsal and/or ventral tongue surface

Osteomyelitis (OST): Inflammation of the bone and bone marrow

Cheilitis: Inflammation of the lip (including the mucocutaneous junction area and skin of the lip)

Tonsillitis (TON/IN): Inflammation of the palatine tonsil

Pharyngitis (PHA/IN): Inflammation of the pharynx

AUTOIMMUNE CONDITIONS AFFECTING THE MOUTH

Pemphigus vulgaris (PV): Autoimmune disease characterized histologically by intraepithelial blister formation (after breakdown or loss of intercellular adhesion), biochemically by evidence of circulating autoantibodies against components of the epithelial desmosome–tonofilament complexes, and clinically by the presence of vesiculobullous and/or ulcerative oral and mucocutaneous lesions

Bullous pemphigoid (BUP): Autoimmune disease characterized histologically by subepithelial clefting (separation at the epithelium–connective tissue interface), biochemically by evidence of circulating autoantibodies against components of the basement membrane, and clinically by the presence of erythematous, erosive, vesiculobullous and/or ulcerative oral lesions

Lupus erythematosis (LE): Autoimmune disease characterized histologically by basal cell destruction, hyperkeratosis, epithelial atrophy, subepithelial and perivascular lymphocytic infiltration, and vascular dilation with submucosal edema; biochemically by the evidence of circulating autoantibodies against various cellular antigens in both the nucleus and cytoplasm; and clinically by the presence of acute lesions (systemic **LE**) to skin, mucosa and multiple organs or chronic lesions (discoid **LE**) mostly confined to the skin of the face and mucosa of the oral cavity

Masticatory muscle myositis (MMM): Autoimmune disease affecting the temporal, masseter, and medial and lateral pterygoid muscles of the dog. The term masticatory myositis is an acceptable alternative

ORAL TUMORS

The AVDC Nomenclature Committee is working with human oral pathologists, veterinary pathologists, and veterinary oncologists to develop a set of names for specific tumor types that will be acceptable for standard use in veterinary dental patients.

Abbreviations to be used in AVDC case logs are shown in (blue in brackets).

The term "epulis" (plural = "epulides") is a general term referring to a gingival mass lesion of any type. Examples of epulides include the following: focal fibrous hyperplasia, peripheral odotogenic fibroma, acanthomatous ameloblastoma, nonodontogenic tumors, pyogenic granulomas, and reactive exostosis.

Types of Neoplasms Occurring in Oral Tissues (Listed in Alphabetical Order)

Acanthomatous ameloblastoma (OM/AA): A typically benign, but aggressive, histologic variant of a group of epithelial odontogenic tumors known collectively as ameloblastomas which have a basic structure resembling the enamel organ (suggesting derivation from ameloblasts); the acanthomatous histologic designation refers to the central cells within nests of odontogenic epithelium that are squamous and may be keratinized rather than stellate

Adenoma (OM/AD): Benign epithelial tumor in which the cells form recognizable glandular structures or in which the cells are derived from glandular epithelium

Adenocarcinoma (OM/ADC): An invasive, malignant epithelial neoplasm derived from glandular tissue of either the oral cavity, nasal cavity, or salivary tissue (major or accessory)

Amyloid producing odontogenic tumor (OM/APO): A benign epithelial odontogenic tumor characterized by the presence of odontogenic epithelium and extracellular amyloid

Anaplastic neoplasm (OM/APN): A malignant neoplasm whose cells are generally undifferentiated and pleomorphic (displaying variability in size, shape, and pattern of cells and/or their nuclei)

Cementoma (OM/CE): A benign odontogenic neoplasm of mesenchymal origin, consisting of cementum-like tissue deposited by cells resembling cementoblasts

Feline inductive odontogenic tumor (OM/FIO): A benign tumor unique to adolescent and young adult cats that originates multifocally within the supporting connective tissue as characteristic, spherical condensations of fibroblastic connective tissue associated with islands of odontogenic epithelium; has also been incorrectly called inductive fibroameloblastoma

Fibrosarcoma (OM/FS): An invasive, malignant mesenchymal neoplasm of fibroblasts; a distinct histologically low-grade, biologically high-grade variant is often found in the oral cavity

Giant cell granuloma (OM/GCG): A benign, tumor-like growth consisting of multi-nucleated giant cells within a background stroma on the gingiva (peripheral giant cell granuloma) or within bone (central giant cell granuloma); also called giant cell epulis

Granular cell tumor (OM/GCT): A benign tumor of the skin or mucosa with uncertain histogenesis, most commonly occurring on the tongue; also called myoblastoma

Hemangiosarcoma (OM/HS): A malignant neoplasm of vascular endothelial origin characterized by extensive metastasis; it has been reported in the gingiva, tongue, and hard palate

Lipoma (OM/LI): A benign mesenchymal neoplasm of lipocytes

Lymphosarcoma (OM/LS): A malignant neoplasm defined by a proliferation of lymphocytes within solid organs such as the lymph nodes, tonsils, bone marrow, liver, and spleen; the disease also may occur in the eye, skin, nasal cavity, oral cavity, and gastrointestinal tract; also known as lymphoma

Malignant melanoma (OM/MM): An invasive, malignant neoplasm of melanocytes or melanocyte precursors that may or may not be pigmented (amelanotic); also called melanosarcoma

Mast cell tumor (OM/MCT): A local aggregation of mast cells forming a nodular tumor, having the potential to become malignant; also called mastocytoma

Multilobular tumor of bone (OM/MTB): A potentially malignant and locally invasive neoplasm of bone that more commonly affects the mandible, hard palate, and flat bones of the cranium with a multilobular histologic pattern of bony or cartilaginous matrix surrounded by a thin layer of spindle cells that gives it a near pathognomonic radiographic "popcorn ball" appearance; also called multilobular osteochondrosarcoma, multilobular osteoma, multilobular chondroma, chondroma rodens, and multilobular osteosarcoma

Osteoma (OM/OO): A benign neoplasm of bone consisting of mature, compact, or cancellous bone

Osteosarcoma (OM/OS): A locally aggressive malignant mesenchymal neoplasm of primitive bone cells that have the ability to produce osteoid or immature bone

Papilloma (OM/PAP): An exophytic, pedunculated, cauliflower-like benign neoplasm of epithelium; canine papillomatosis is thought to be caused by infection with canine papillomavirus in typically young dogs; severe papillomatosis may be recognized in older immunocompromised dogs

Peripheral nerve sheath tumor (OM/PNT): A group of neural tumors arising from Schwann cells or perineural fibroblasts (or a combination of both cell types) of the cranial nerves, spinal nerve roots, or peripheral nerves; they may be classified as histologically benign or malignant

Peripheral odontogenic fibroma (OM/POF): A benign mesenchymal odontogenic tumor associated with the gingiva and believed to originate from the periodontal ligament; characterized by varying amounts of inactive-looking odontogenic epithelium embedded in a mature, fibrous stroma, which may undergo osseous metaplasia; historically has been referred to as fibromatous epulis or—when bone or tooth-like hard tissue present within the lesion—ossifying epulis

Plasma cell tumor (OM/PCT): A proliferation of plasma cells, commonly occurring on the gingiva or dorsum of the tongue; also called plasmacytoma

Rhabdomyosarcoma (OM/RBM): A malignant neoplasm of skeletal muscle or embryonic mesenchymal cells

Squamous cell carcinoma (OM/SCC): An invasive, malignant epithelial neoplasm of the oral epithelium with varying degrees of squamous differentiation

Undifferentiated neoplasm (OM/UDN): A malignant neoplasm whose cells are generally immature and lack distinctive features of a particular tissue type

Diagnostic and Nonsurgical Treatment Procedures

Biopsy (B): Removal of tissue from a living body for diagnostic purposes. The term has also been used to describe the tissue being submitted for evaluation

Guided biopsy: Using computed tomography or ultrasonography to guide an instrument to the selected area for tissue removal

Surface biopsy (B/S): Removal of tissue brushed, scraped, or obtained by an impression smear from the intact or cut surface of a tissue in question

Needle aspiration (B/NA): Removal of tissue by application of suction through a hollow needle attached to a syringe

Needle biopsy (B/NB): Removal of tissue by puncture with a hollow needle

Core needle biopsy (B/CN): Removal of tissue with a large hollow needle that extracts a core of tissue

Bite biopsy (B/B): Removal of tissue by closing the opposing ends of an instrument

Punch biopsy (B/P): Removal of tissue by a punch-type instrument

Incisional biopsy (B/I): Removal of a selected portion of tissue by means of surgical cutting

Excisional biopsy (B/E): Removal of the entire tissue in question by means of surgical cutting **Guided biopsy:** Using computed tomography or ultrasonography to guide an instrument to the selected area for tissue removal

Radiotherapy (RTH): Use of ionizing radiation to control or kill tumor cells; also called radiation therapy

Chemotherapy (CTH): Use of cytotoxic anti-neoplastic drugs (chemotherapeutic agents) to control or kill tumor cells

Immunotherapy (ITH): Use of the immune system to control or kill tumor cells

Radiography (RAD): Two-dimensional imaging of dental, periodontal, oral, and maxillofacial structures using an x-ray machine and radiographic films, sensor pads, or phosphor plates

Computed tomography (CT): A method of medical imaging that uses computer-processed x-rays to produce tomographic images or "slices" of specific areas of the body; digital geometry processing is used to generate three-dimensional images of an object of interest from a large series of two-dimensional x-ray images taken around a single axis of rotation

Cone-beam CT (CT/CB): Variation of traditional CT that rotates around the patient, capturing data using a cone-shaped x-ray beam

Magnetic resonance imaging (MRI): A method of medical imaging that uses the property of nuclear magnetic resonance to image nuclei of atoms inside the body

Ultrasonography (US): A method of medical imaging of deep structures of the body by recording the echoes of pulses of ultrasonic waves directed into the tissues and reflected by tissue planes where there is a change in density

Scintigraphy (SCI): A method of medical imaging that uses radioisotopes taken internally (e.g., by mouth, injection, inhalation); the emitted radiation is captured by external detectors (gamma cameras) to form two-dimensional images

Surgical Treatment Procedures for Oral Tumors

Surgery (S): Branch of medicine that treats diseases, injuries, and deformities by manual or operative methods

Buccotomy (BUC): Incision through the cheek (e.g., to gain access to an intraoral procedure)

Cheiloplasty/commissuroplasty (CPL): Reconstructive surgery of the lip/lip commissure

Commissurotomy (COM): Incision through the lip commissure (e.g., to gain access to an intraoral procedure)

Partial mandibulectomy (S/M): Surgical removal (en block) of part of the mandible and surrounding soft tissues

Dorsal marginal mandibulectomy (S/MD): A form of partial mandibulectomy in which the ventral border of the mandible is maintained, also called marginal mandibulectomy or mandibular rim excision

Segmental mandibulectomy (S/MS): A form of partial mandibulectomy in which a full dorsoventral segment of the mandible is removed

Bilateral partial mandibulectomy (S/MB): Surgical removal of parts of the left and right mandibles and surrounding soft tissues

Total mandibulectomy (S/MT): Surgical removal of one mandible and surrounding soft tissues

Partial maxillectomy (S/X): Surgical removal (en block) of part of the maxilla and/or other facial bones and surrounding soft tissues

Bilateral partial maxillectomy (S/XB): Surgical removal of parts of the left and right maxillae and/or other facial bones and surrounding soft tissues

Partial palatectomy (S/P): Partial resection of the palate

OTHER ORAL PATHOLOGY

Chewing lesion (CL): Mucosal lesion resulting from self-induced bite trauma on the cheek (**CL/B**), lip (**CL/L**), palate (**CL/P**), or tongue/sublingual region (**CL/T**)

Eosinophilic granuloma (EOG): Referring to conditions affecting the lip/labial mucosa (**EOG/L**), hard/soft palate (**EOG/P**), tongue/sublingual mucosa (**EOG/T**), and skin that are characterized histopathologically by the presence of an eosinophilic infiltrate

Pyogenic granuloma (PYO): Inflammatory proliferation at the vestibular mucogingival tissues of the mandibular first molar tooth (in the cat probably owing to malocclusion and secondary traumatic contact of these tissues by the ipsilateral maxillary fourth premolar tooth)

Erythema multiforme (EM): Typically drug-induced hypersensitivity reaction characterized by erythematous, vesiculobullous, and/or ulcerative oral and skin lesions

Calcinosis circumscripta (CC): Circumscribed areas of mineralization characterized by deposition of calcium salts (e.g., in the tip of the tongue)

Retrobulbar abscess (RBA): Abscess behind the globe of the eye

Retropharyngeal abscess (RPA): Abscess behind the pharynx

Craniomandibular osteopathy (CMO): Disease characterized by cyclical resorption of normal bone and excessive replacement by immature bone along mandibular, temporal, and other bone surfaces in immature and adolescent dogs

Calvarial hyperostosis (CHO): Disease characterized by irregular, progressive proliferation, and thickening of the cortex of the bones forming the calvarium in adolescent dogs

Fibrous osteodystrophy (FOD): Disease characterized by the formation of hyperostotic bone lesions, in which deposition of unmineralized osteoid by hyperplastic osteoblasts and production of fibrous connective tissue exceed the rate of bone resorption; usually caused by primary or secondary hyperparathyroidism; resulting in softened, pliable, and distorted bones of the face ("rubber jaw," "bighead," or "bran disease")

Periostitis ossificans (PEO): Periosteal new bone formation in immature dogs, manifesting clinically as (usually) unilateral swelling of the mid to caudal body of the mandible and radiographically as two-layered (double) ventral mandibular cortex

TONGUE, LIPS, PALATE, PHARYNX, NOSE, FACE, SALIVARY GLANDS AND LYMPH NODES

Anatomy of the Tongue, Lips, Cheek and Palate

Tongue (LIN): Fleshy muscular organ in the mouth used for tasting, licking, swallowing, articulating, and thermoregulation; use **LIN/X** for tongue resection

Lip/cheek (LIP): Fleshy parts that form the upper and lower edges of the opening of the mouth/side of the face below the eye; use **LIP/X** for lip/cheek resection

Hard palate: The part of the palate supported by bone

The **midline of the hard palate** is not a symphysis but is formed by the interincisive suture, the median palatine suture of the palatine processes of the maxillary bones, and the median suture of the palatine bones.

Reference(s): Anonymous: *Nomina anatomica veterinaria,* ed 4, Zurich and Ithaca, 1994, World Association of Veterinary Anatomists. Evans HE: *Miller's anatomy of the dog,* ed 3, Philadelphia, 1993, WB Saunders Co.

Palatine rugae: Transverse ridges of mucosa on the hard palate

Incisive papilla: Elevation of mucosa at the rostral end of the median line of junction of the halves of the palate, concealing the orifices of the incisive ducts

Soft palate: The caudal part of palate that is not supported by bone

Abnormalities of the Palate

Palate defect (PDE): Acquired communication between the oral and nasal cavities along the hard or soft palate; surgical repair is abbreviated **PDE/R**

Cleft lip (CFL): Congenital longitudinal defect of the upper lip or upper lip and most rostral hard palate (regardless of location); surgical repair is abbreviated **CFL/R**

Cleft palate (CFP): Congenital longitudinal defect in the midline of the hard and soft palate; surgical repair is abbreviated **CFP/R**

Cleft soft palate (CFS): Congenital longitudinal defect in the midline of the soft palate only; surgical repair is abbreviated **CFS/R**

Unilateral soft palate defect (CFSU): Congenital longitudinal defect of the soft palate on one side only; surgical repair is abbreviated **CFSU/R**

Soft palate hypoplasia (CFSH): Congenital decrease in length of the soft palate; surgical lengthening of the soft palate is abbreviated **CFSH/R**

Traumatic cleft palate (CFT): Acquired longitudinal defect in the midline of the hard and/or soft palate resulting from trauma; surgical repair is abbreviated **CFT/R**

Oronasal fistula (ONF): Acquired communication between the oral and nasal cavities along the upper dental arch; surgical repair is abbreviated **ONF/R**

Oroantral fistula (OAF): Acquired communication between the oral cavity and maxillary sinus in pigs, ruminants, and equines (also called oromaxillary fistula in equines); surgical repair is abbreviated **OAF/R**

Elongated soft palate (ESP): Congenital increase in length of the soft palate; surgical reduction of the soft palate is abbreviated **ESP/R**

Palatal obturator (POB): Prosthetic device for temporary or permanent closure of palate defects

ANATOMY OF THE NOSE, PHARYNX, TONSIL, AND FACE

Palatine tonsil (TON): Tonsil related to the lateral attachment of the soft palate

Tonsillar fossa: Depression containing the palatine tonsil

Semilunar fold: Mucosal fold from the ventrolateral aspect of the soft palate, forming the medial wall of the tonsillar fossa

Pharynx (PHA): Throat caudal to the oral cavity and divided into nasopharynx and oropharynx

Fauces: The fauces are defined as the lateral walls of the oropharynx that are located medial to the palatoglossal folds. The areas lateral to the palatoglossal fold, commonly involved in feline stomatitis, are not the fauces.

Reference(s): Anonymous: *Nomina anatomica veterinaria,* ed 4, Zurich and Ithaca, 1994, World Association of Veterinary Anatomists. Evans HE: *Miller's anatomy of the dog,* ed 3, Philadelphia, 1993, WB Saunders Co.

Nose/nasal (N): Referring to the part of the face or facial region that contains the nostrils and nasal cavity

SALIVARY GLAND ABNORMALITIES AND DIAGNOSTIC PROCEDURES

Ptyalism (PTY): Excessive flow of saliva; also called hypersalivation

Sublingual sialocele (SG/MUC/S): Mucus extravasation phenomenon manifesting in the sublingual region; also called **ranula**

Pharyngeal sialocele (SG/MUC/P): Mucus extravasation phenomenon manifesting in the pharyngeal region

Cervical sialocele (SG/MUC/C): Mucus extravasation phenomenon manifesting in the intermandibular or cervical region

Mucus retention cyst (SG/RC): Intraductal mucus accumulation with duct dilation resulting from obstruction of salivary flow (e.g., owing to a sialolith)

Sialadenitis (SG/IN): Inflammation of a salivary gland

Sialadenosis (SG/ADS): Noninflammatory, nonneoplastic enlargement of a salivary gland; also called **sialosis**

Necrotizing sialometaplasia (SG/NEC): Squamous metaplasia of the salivary gland ducts and lobules with ischemic necrosis of the salivary gland lobules; also called **salivary gland infarction**

Salivary gland adencarcinoma (SG/ADC): Adenocarcinoma arising from salivary glandular or ductal tissue; use abbreviations under **OM** for other salivary gland tumors.

Sialocele (or salivary mucocele): Clinical term indicating a swelling that contains saliva and including mucus extravasation phenomenon and mucus retention cyst

Mucus extravasation phenomenon: Accumulation of saliva that leaked from a salivary duct into subcutaneous or submucosal tissue and consequent tissue reaction to saliva

Sialolithiasis (SG/SI): Condition characterized by the presence of one or more sialoliths, a calcareous concretion or calculus (stone) in the salivary duct or gland

Sialography (RAD/SG): Radiographic technique where a radiopaque contrast agent is infused into the ductal system of a salivary gland before imaging is performed.

Salivary gland resection (SG/X): Surgical removal of a salivary gland

Marsupialization (MAR): Exteriorization of an enclosed cavity by resecting a portion of the cutaneous or mucosal wall and suturing the cut edges of the remaining wall to adjacent edges of the skin or mucosa, thereby creating a pouch; use **SG/MAR** for marsupialization of a sublingual or pharyngeal sialocele.

LYMPH NODES

Lymph node (LN): Lymphoid tissue that produces lymphocytes and has a capsule; filters lymph fluid, as afferent lymph vessels enter the node and efferent lymph vessels leave the node

Tonsil (TON): Lymphoid tissue that produces lymphocytes, but lacks a capsule; not filtering lymph fluid, as there are no afferent lymph vessels

Lymph node enlargement (LN/E): Palpable or visual enlargement of a lymph node

Regional metastasis (MET/R): Neoplastic spread to regional lymph node(s) confirmed by biopsy

Distant metastasis (MET/D): Neoplastic spread to distant sites confirmed by biopsy or diagnostic imaging

Lymph node resection (LN/X): Surgical removal of a lymph node

OCCLUSAL ABNORMALITIES
Normal Occlusion

Ideal occlusion can be described as perfect interdigitation of the upper and lower teeth. In the dog, the ideal tooth positions in the arches are defined by the occlusal, interarch and interdental relationships of the teeth of the archetypal dog (i.e., wolf). This ideal relationship with the mouth closed can be defined by the following:

Maxillary incisor teeth are all positioned rostral to the corresponding mandibular incisor teeth.

The crown cusps of the mandibular incisor teeth contact the cingulum of the maxillary incisor teeth.

The mandibular canine tooth is inclined labially and bisects the interproximal (interdental) space between the opposing maxillary third incisor tooth and canine tooth.

The maxillary premolar teeth do not contact the mandibular premolar teeth.

The crown cusps of the mandibular premolar teeth are positioned lingual to the arch of the maxillary premolar teeth.

The crown cusps of the mandibular premolar teeth bisect the interproximal (interdental) spaces rostral to the corresponding maxillary premolar teeth.

The mesial crown cusp of the maxillary fourth premolar tooth is positioned lateral to the space between the mandibular fourth premolar tooth and the mandibular first molar tooth.

Normal Occlusion in a Dog

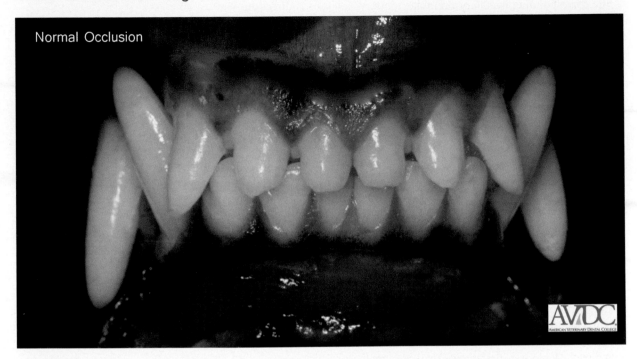

Normal Occlusion

Normal Occlusion in a Cat

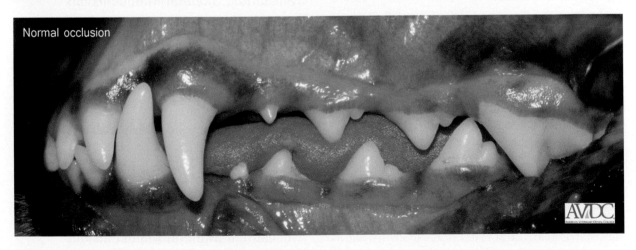

Normal occlusion

Normal occlusion in cats is similar to dogs.

Maxillary incisor teeth are labial to the mandibular incisor teeth, with the incisal tips of the mandibular incisors contacting the cingula of the maxillary incisors or occluding just palatal to the maxillary incisors.

Mandibular canine teeth fit equidistant in the diastema between the maxillary third incisor teeth and the maxillary canine teeth, touching neither.

The incisor bite and canine interdigitation form the dental interlock.

Each mandibular premolar tooth is positioned mesial to the corresponding maxillary premolar tooth.

The maxillary second premolar tooth points in a space between the mandibular canine tooth and third premolar tooth.

The subsequent teeth interdigitate, with the mandibular premolars and first molar being situated lingual to the maxillary teeth.

The buccal surface of the mandibular first molar tooth occludes with the palatal surface of the maxillary fourth premolar tooth.

The maxillary first molar tooth is located distopalatal to the maxillary fourth premolar tooth.

Malocclusion

Malocclusion (MAL) is any deviation from normal occlusion described above.

Malocclusion may be caused by abnormal positioning of a tooth or teeth (dental malocclusion) or by asymmetry or other deviation of bones that support the dentition (skeletal malocclusion).

The diagnosis for a patient with malocclusion is abbreviated as: MAL (malocclusion) 1 or 2 or 3 or 4 (= malocclusion class designation)/specific malocclusion abbreviation and tooth or teeth number(s).

Example: MAL1/CB/R202 for a dog with class 1 malocclusion and a rostral crossbite of the left maxillary second incisor.

If multiple teeth have the same malocclusion, include the tooth numbers with a comma in between (e.g., MAL1/CB/R202,302).

Dental Malocclusions

Neutroclusion: Class 1 Malocclusion (MAL1)

A normal rostrocaudal relationship of the maxillary and mandibular dental arches with malposition of one or more individual teeth

Distoversion (MAL1/DV) describes a tooth that is in its anatomically correct position in the dental arch, but which is abnormally angled in a distal direction.

Mesioversion (MAL1/MV) describes a tooth that is in its anatomically correct position in the dental arch, but which is abnormally angled in a mesial direction.

Linguoversion (MAL1/LV) describes a tooth that is in its anatomically correct position in the dental arch, but which is abnormally angled in a lingual direction.

Palatoversion (MAL1/PV) describes a tooth that is in its anatomically correct position in the dental

arch, but which is abnormally angled in a palatal direction.

Labioversion (MAL1/LABV) describes an incisor or canine tooth that is in its anatomically correct position in the dental arch, but which is abnormally angled in a labial direction.

Buccoversion (MAL1/BV) describes a premolar or molar tooth that is in its anatomically correct position in the dental arch, but which is abnormally angled in a buccal direction.

Crossbite (CB) describes a malocclusion in which a mandibular tooth or teeth have a more buccal or labial position than the antagonist maxillary tooth. It can be classified as rostral or caudal:

In rostral crossbite (CB/R), one or more of the mandibular incisor teeth is labial to the opposing maxillary incisor teeth when the mouth is closed; similar to posterior crossbite in human terminology.

In caudal crossbite (CB/C), one or more of the mandibular cheek teeth is buccal to the opposing maxillary cheek teeth when the mouth is closed; similar to posterior crossbite in human terminology.

SKELETAL MALOCCLUSIONS

Symmetrical Skeletal Malocclusions

Mandibular Distoclusion: Class 2 Malocclusion (MAL2)

An abnormal rostrocaudal relationship between the dental arches in which the mandibular arch occludes caudal to its normal position relative to the maxillary arch.

Mandibular mesioclusion: Class 3 Malocclusion: (MAL3)

An abnormal rostralcaudal relationship between the dental arches in which the mandibular arch occludes rostral to its normal position relative to the maxillary arch. Example:

Aymmetrical Skeletal Malocclusions

Maxillomandibular Asymmetry: Class 4 Malocclusion (MAL4)

Asymmetry in a rostrocaudal, side-to-side, or dorsoventral direction:

Maxillomandibular asymmetry in a rostrocaudal direction (MAL4/RC) occurs when mandibular mesioclusion or distoclusion is present on one side of the face while the contralateral side retains normal dental alignment.

Maxillomandibular asymmetry in a side-to-side direction (**MAL4/STS**) occurs when there is loss of the midline alignment of the maxilla and mandible.

Maxillomandibular asymmetry in a dorsoventral direction (**MAL4/DV**) results in an open bite, which is defined as an abnormal vertical space between opposing dental arches when the mouth is closed.

The expression "wry bite" is a layman term that has been used to describe a wide variety of unilateral occlusal abnormalities. Because "wry bite" is nonspecific, its use is not recommended.

Management of Malocclusion

Orthodontics is a specialty in dentistry and oral surgery that is concerned with the prevention, interception, and correction of malocclusion.

Preventive orthodontics is concerned with the client's education, the development of the dentition and maxillofacial structures, the diagnostic procedures undertaken to predict malocclusion, and the therapeutic procedures instituted to prevent the onset of malocclusion. Preventive procedures are undertaken in anticipation of development of a problem. Examples of preventive procedures include:

- Client education about time tables on exfoliation of deciduous teeth and eruption of permanent teeth
- Fiberotomy (severing of gingival fibers around a permanent tooth to prevent its relapse after corrective orthodontics)
- Operculectomy (surgical removal of an operculum to enable eruption of a permanent tooth)
- Extraction of a tooth that could pose a risk to development of malocclusion

Interceptive orthodontics is concerned with the elimination of a developing or established malocclusion. Interceptive procedures are typically undertaken in the growing patient. Examples of interceptive procedures include:

- Crown reduction of a permanent tooth in malocclusion
- Extraction of a tooth in malocclusion

Corrective orthodontics is concerned with the correction of malocclusion without loss of the maloccluded tooth or part of its crown. This is accomplished by means of tooth movement. Examples of corrective procedures include:

- Surgical repositioning of a tooth
- Orthognathic surgery to treat skeletal malocclusion
- Passive movement of a tooth using an inclined plane
- Active movement of a tooth using an elastic chain

Treatment plan (TP): Written document that outlines the progression of therapy (advantages, disadvantages, costs, alternatives, outcome, and duration of treatment)

Impression (IM): Detailed imprint of hard and/or soft tissues that is formed with specific types of impression materials

Full-mouth impression (IM/F): Imprints of the dentition and/or surrounding soft tissues of the upper and lower dental arches

Diagnostic cast (DC): Positive replica created by pouring a liquid material into an impression or placing an impression into a liquid material; once the material has hardened, the cast is removed and used to study and to plan treatment; also called die (**DC/D**) when made from an impression of a particular tooth/area of interest or stone model (**DC/SM**) when made from a full-mouth impression

Bite registration (BR): Impression used to record a patient's occlusion, which is then used to articulate diagnostic casts

Fiberotomy (FT): Severing gingival fibers around a permanent tooth to prevent its relapse after corrective orthodontics

Operculectomy (OP): Surgical removal of an operculum to enable eruption of a permanent tooth

Surgical repositioning (SR): Repositioning of a developmentally displaced tooth

Orthognathic surgery (OS): Surgical procedure to alter relationships of dental arches; typically performed to correct skeletal malocclusion

Bracket/button/hook (OA/BKT): Device made of metal or plastic that is bonded to the tooth surface and aids in the attachment of wires or elastics; use **OA/CMB** if custom-made

Elastic chain/tube/thread (OA/EC): Orthodontic elastics used to move teeth

Orthodontic wire (OA/WIR): Metal wire with "memory" used to move teeth

Arch bar (OA/AR): Device attached to one dental arch to move individual teeth in between the device's attachments

Orthodontic appliance (OA): Device attached to a tooth or teeth to move a tooth or teeth

Orthodontic appliance adjustment (OA/A): Abbreviation used at the time of adjustment of the orthodontic appliance

Orthodontic appliance installation (OA/I): Abbreviation used at the time of installation of the orthodontic appliance

Orthodontic appliance removal (OA/R): Abbreviation used at the time of removal of the orthodontic appliance

Orthodontic counseling (OC): Client communication on the genetic basis, diagnosis, and treatment of malocclusion and the legal and ethical implications of orthodontics

Ball therapy (BTH): Removable orthodontic device in the form of a ball or cone-shaped rubber toy (e.g., to passively move linguoverted mandibular canine teeth)

Inclined plane (IP): Fixed orthodontic device made of acrylic (**IP/A**), composite (**IP/C**), or metal (**IP/M**) with sloping planes (for example to passively move linguoverted mandibular canine teeth)

Orthodontic recheck (OR): Examination of a patient treated with an orthodontic appliance.

Oral Surgery

Tooth Extraction-Related Terminology

Closed extraction (X or XS): Extraction of teeth without flap creation; **X** is used when closed extraction is performed without tooth sectioning; **XS** is used when closed extraction is performed with tooth sectioning or removal of interproximal crown tissue

Open extraction (XSS): Extraction of teeth after flap creation and alveolectomy

Alveolectomy (ALV): Removal of some or all of the alveolar bone

Alveoloplasty (ALV): A form of alveolectomy performed to restore physiologic contours or achieve smooth contours of the alveolar bone

Palate, Pharynx and Nasal Surgery
Palate Surgery: Click the link

Naroplasty (NAS/R): Surgical correction of stenotic nares

Tonsillectomy (TON/X): Surgical resection of the palatine tonsil

Grafts and Related Terminology

Transplantation: Act or process of transferring something from one part or individual to another

Transplant: Something transferred from one part or individual to another

Graft (GF): Nonliving material or living tissue used for implantation or transplantation to replace a diseased part or compensate for a defect

Gingival graft (GF/G): Gingiva or gingiva-like tissue (e.g., from the hard palate) used to replace gingiva in a gingival defect

Connective tissue graft (GF/CT): Connective tissue from a keratinized mucosa (e.g., from the hard palate) placed in a gingival defect and which is partially or completely covered with gingiva and/or alveolar mucosa in the recipient bed

Mucosal graft (GF/M) Mucosa used to take place of a removed piece of mucosa or cover a mucosal defect

Bone graft (GF/B): A surgical procedure by which bone or a bone substitute is used to take the place of a removed piece of bone or bony defect

Cartilage graft (GF/C): Cartilage used to take the place of a removed piece of bone or fill a bony defect

Skin graft (GF/S): Skin used to take place of a removed piece of skin/mucosa or skin/mucosa defect

Venous graft (GF/V): A vein used to take place of a removed segment of artery/vein or arterial/venous defect

Nerve graft (GF/N): A nerve used to take place of a removed segment of nerve or nerve defect

Fat graft (GF/F): Adipose tissue used to provide volume to a defect or to prevent ingrowth of other tissues into the defect

Autograft: Tissue transferred from one area to another area of the animal's own body

Isograft: Tissue transferred between genetically identical animals

Allograft: Tissue transferred between genetically dissimilar animals of the same species

Xenograft: Tissue transferred between animals of different species

Particulate graft: A graft containing equally or variably sized particles

Full-thickness graft: A graft consisting of the full thickness of a tissue

Partial-thickness (split-thickness) graft: A graft consisting of a portion of the thickness of a tissue

Mesh graft: A type of partial-thickness graft in which multiple small incisions have been made to increase stretching and flexibility of the graft

Composite graft: A graft composed of at least two different tissues (e.g., skin-muscle-and-bone graft)

Implant (IMP): Something inserted into or applied onto living tissue

Implantation: The act or process of inserting something into or applying something onto living tissue

American Veterinary Dental College Position Statement

VETERINARY DENTAL HEALTHCARE PROVIDERS

The American Veterinary Dental College (AVDC) has developed this position statement as a means to safeguard the veterinary dental patient and to ensure the qualifications of persons performing veterinary dental procedures.

Primary Responsibility for Veterinary Dental Care

The AVDC defines veterinary dentistry as the art and practice of oral health care in animals other than man. It is a discipline of veterinary medicine and surgery. The diagnosis, treatment, and management of veterinary oral health care is to be provided and supervised by licensed veterinarians or by veterinarians working within a university or industry.

Who May Provide Veterinarian-Supervised Dental Care

The AVDC accepts that the following health care workers may assist the responsible veterinarian in dental procedures or actually perform dental prophylactic services while under direct, in-the-room supervision by a veterinarian if permitted by local law: licensed, certified, or registered veterinary technician or a veterinary assistant with advanced dental training, dentist, or registered dental hygienist.

Operative Dentistry and Oral Surgery

The AVDC considers operative dentistry to be any dental procedure that invades the hard or soft oral tissue including, but not limited to, a procedure that alters the structure of one or more teeth or repairs damaged and diseased teeth. A veterinarian should perform operative dentistry and oral surgery.

Extraction of Teeth

The AVDC considers the extraction of teeth to be included in the practice of veterinary dentistry. Decision-making is the responsibility of the veterinarian, with the consent of the pet owner, when electing to extract teeth. Only veterinarians shall determine which teeth are to be extracted and to perform extraction procedures.

Dental Tasks Performed by Veterinary Technicians

The AVDC considers it appropriate for a veterinarian to delegate maintenance dental care and certain dental tasks to a veterinary technician. Tasks appropriately performed by a technician include dental prophylaxis and certain procedures that do not result in altering the shape, structure, or positional location of teeth in the dental arch. The veterinarian may direct an appropriately trained technician to perform these tasks providing that the veterinarian is physically present and supervising the treatment.

Veterinary Technician Dental Training

The AVDC supports the advanced training of veterinary technicians to perform additional ancillary dental services: taking impressions, making models, charting veterinary dental pathology, taking and developing dental radiographs, performing nonsurgical, subgingival root scaling and debridement, providing that they do not alter the structure of the tooth.

Tasks That May Be Performed By Veterinary Assistants (Not Registered, Certified, or Licensed)

The AVDC supports the appropriate training of veterinary assistants to perform the following dental services: supragingival scaling and polishing, taking and developing dental radiographs, taking impressions, and making models.

Tasks That May Be Performed By Dentists, Registered Dental Hygienists, and Other Dental Health Care Providers

The AVDC recognizes that dentists, registered dental hygienists, and other dental health care providers in good standing may perform those procedures for which they have been qualified under the direct supervision of the veterinarian. The supervising veterinarian will be responsible for the welfare of the patient and any treatment performed on the patient.

The AVDC understands that individual states have regulations that govern the practice of veterinary medicine. This position statement is intended to be a model for veterinary dental practice and does not replace existing law.

Adopted by the Board of Directors April 1998, revised October 1999, revised September 2006.

BIBLIOGRAPHY

Allen DG, Dowling PM, Smith DA, et al: *Handbook of veterinary drugs,* ed 3, Philadelphia, 2005, Lippincott Williams & Wilkins.

Bellows J: *The practice of veterinary dentistry: a team effort,* Ames, IA, 1999, Iowa State University Press.

Bellows J: *Feline dentistry: oral assessment, treatment, and preventative care,* Hoboken, NJ, 2010, Wiley-Blackwell.

Capello V, Gracis M, Lennox A: *Rabbit and rodent dentistry handbook,* Hoboken, NJ, 2005, Wiley-Blackwell.

Capello V, Gracis M: *Rabbit and rodent dentistry handbook,* Lake Worth, FL, 2005, Zoological Education Network.

Colgin LMA, Schulman FY, Dubiezig RR, Multiple epulides in 13 cats. *Vet Pathol* 38:227–229, 2001.

Conlon KC, Corbally MT, Bading JR, et al: Atraumatic endotracheal intubation in small rabbits. *Lab Anim Sci* 40:221–222, 1990.

Crossley DA: Dental disease in ferrets. In Quesenberry K, Carpenter JW, eds: *Ferrets, rabbits and rodents: clinical medicine and surgery,* Philadelphia, 2003, WB Saunders.

Crossley DA: Oral biology and disorders of lagomorphs, *Vet Clin North Am Exot Anim Pract* 6:629–659, 2003.

Davis EM: How I treat refractory feline chronic gingivostomatitis. *Clinicians Brief,* January, 2015 19–22.

Dental abstracts: Elsevier Science International (last 5 years).

Dental clinics of North America: Philadelphia, WB Saunders (last 5 years).

DuPont GA, DeBowes LJ: *Atlas of dental radiography in dogs and cats,* St. Louis, 2009, Saunders Elsevier.

Emily P, Penman S: *Handbook of small animal dentistry,* Oxford, 1990, Pergamon Press.

Erne JB, Mann FA: Surgical hemostasis compendium. VetLearn.com 25:10, 2003.

Eroshin VV, Reiter AM, Rosenthal K, et al: Oral examination results in rescued ferrets: clinical findings, *J Vet Dent* 2011;8:8–15.

Fossum TW: *Small animal surgery,* ed 3, St. Louis, 2007, Mosby.

Hargreaves KM, Cohen MA: *Cohen's pathways of the pulp,* ed 10. St. Louis, 2010, Mosby.

Harvey CE: *Veterinary dentistry,* Philadelphia, 1985, WB Saunders.

Holmstrom SE (guest ed): *Dentistry: the veterinary clinics of North America: small animal practice,* Philadelphia, 2005, WB Saunders.

Holmstrom SE (guest ed): *Clinical veterinary dentistry: the veterinary clinics of North America: small animal practice,* Philadelphia, 2013, Elsevier.

Holmstrom SE, Frost P, Eisner ER: *Veterinary dental techniques,* ed 3, Philadelphia, 2004, WB Saunders.

Holmstrom SE, Frost P, Gammon RG: *Veterinary dental techniques for the small animal practitioner,* Philadelphia, 1992, WB Saunders.

Holmstrom SE (guest ed): *Canine dentistry: the veterinary clinics of North America: small animal practice,* Philadelphia, 1998, WB Saunders.

Hoyer NK, Bannon KM: Diagnostic imaging in veterinary dental practice, *J Am Vet Med Assoc* June 2014;244(12).

Jennings MW, Lewis JR: Effect of tooth extraction on stomatitis in cats: 95 cases (2000–2013), *J Am Vet Med Assoc* March 15, 2015;246(6).

Johnson D: *Intubation of rabbits and rodents,* Davis, CA, 2006, Veterinary Information Network, Inc.

Journal of Veterinary Dentistry: Volume 7(no.1): January 1990 to present.

Lappin MR, Management of stomatitis in cats, Wild West Veterinary Conference, 2015.

Lobprise HB, Wiggs RB: Dental and oral disease in lagomorphs, *J Vet Dent* 1991;8(2):11–17.

Lommer M: Feline chronic gingivostomatitis: what we know and what we can do about it. In: Proceedings, Veterinary Dental Forum, Nashville, September 2017.

Manfra Marretta S, Leesman M, Burgess-Cassler A, et al: Pilot evaluation of a novel test strip for the assessment of dissolved thiol levels, as an indicator of canine gingival health and periodontal status. *CVJ* 53:1260–1265, 2012.

Muir WW, Hubbell JAE, Bednarski RM, et al: *Handbook of veterinary anesthesia,* ed 4, St. Louis, 2007, Mosby Elsevier.

Mulligan TW, Aller MS, Williams CA: *Atlas of canine and feline dental radiography,* Trenton, NJ, 1998, Veterinary Learning Systems.

Newman MG, Takei H, Klokkevold PR, et al: *Carranza's clinical periodontology,* ed 11. Philadelphia, 2011, Saunders.

Niemiec B: *Veterinary periodontology,* Ames, 2013, Wiley-Blackwell.

Page RC, Schroeder HE: *Periodontitis in man and other animals,* New York, 1982, Karger.

Shipp AD, Fahrenkrug P: *Practitioners' guide to veterinary dentistry,* Beverly Hills, CA, 1992, Dr. Shipp's Labs Publishing.

Snyder LBC, Snyder CJ, Hetzel, S: Effects of buprenorphine added to bupivacaine infraorbital nerve blocks on isoflurane minimum alveolar concentration using a model for acute dental/oral surgical pain in dogs. *J Vet Dent* June 33(2):90–96, 2016.

Tholen MA: *Concepts in veterinary dentistry,* Edwardsville, KS, 1983, Veterinary Medicine Publishing.

Thomas S, Lappin D, Spears, J, et al: Prevalence of feline calicivirus in cats with odontoclastic resorptive lesions and chronic gingivostomatitis. *Res Vet Sci* 111:124–126, 2017.

Verstraete FJM, ed: *Self-assessment color review of veterinary dentistry,* Ames, IA, 1999, Iowa State University Press.

Verstraete FJM, Lommer MJ: *Oral and maxillofacial surgery in dogs and cats,* Philadelphia, 2012, Saunders.

Winer JN, Arzi B, Verstraete FJM: Feline chronic gingivostomatitis: a systematic review of the literature. *Front Vet Sci* 3:Article 54, 2016.

White SC, Pharoah MJ: *Oral radiology: principles and interpretation,* ed 6, St. Louis, 2008, Mosby.

Wiggs RB, Lobprise HB: Dental and oral disease in rodents, *J Vet Dent* 7(3):6–8, 1990.

Wiggs RB, Lobprise HB: *Veterinary dentistry principles and practice,* Philadelphia, 1997, Lippincott-Raven.

Wilkins EM: *Clinical practice of the dental hygienist,* Baltimore, 1994, Williams & Wilkins.

Year book of dentistry, St. Louis, Mosby-Year Book (last 5 years).

Winer JN, Arizi B, Verstraete JM: Therapeutic management of feline chronic gingivostomatitis: a systematic review of the literature. *Front Vet Sci* 3:Article 54, 2016.

Zwarych PD: Does the intermediate plexus of periodontal ligament exist? *Penn Dent J* 69:60–67, 1996.

GLOSSARY

Absorbent points Tightly rolled, tapered paper used for drying a pulp canal after it has been prepared (debrided) and irrigated.

Acanthomatous ameloblastoma Proliferating epithelial cells of dental origin. Although classified as benign, these epulides tend to invade bone, which makes dental radiographic evaluation and aggressive surgery important.

Acepromazine An injectable medication used as a form of tranquilization.

Alginate An irreversible hydrocolloid impression material in dentistry for making impressions of jaws in the preparation for orthodontic appliances.

Alternating current (AC) The usual waveform of an AC power circuit is a sine wave.

Alveolar mucosa The less densely keratinized gingival tissue covering the bone.

Alveolar mucositis Inflammation of alveolar mucosa (i.e., mucosa overlying the alveolar process and extending from the mucogingival junction without obvious demarcation to the vestibular sulcus and to the floor of the mouth).

Alveolus The tooth socket.

Ameloblasts Cells that take part in forming dental enamel.

Amelogenesis imperfecta An abnormality of enamel formation, including genetic and/or developmental enamel formation and maturation abnormalities such as enamel hypoplasia and enamel hypomineralization.

Anaerobic bacteria Bacteria that do not require oxygen to survive.

Anatomic numbering system A numbering system used for medical record annotation in which the correct anatomic names of teeth are written out in full or abbreviated.

Anionic detergent A class of detergents (soap) having a negatively charged surface-active ion such as sodium alkylbenzene sulfonate. The detergent work by destroying the cell walls of bacteria.

Anisognathic jaw relationship Naturally unequal jaw relationship in which the upper dental arch is slightly wider than the lower.

Ankylosis Fusion of dental root to the bone.

Anodontia The absence of teeth.

Antiseptic Any substance that inhibits the growth of bacteria.

Apex The pointed end of a cone-shaped part, or the end of a tooth root where blood vessels and nerves enter the tooth.

Apical Toward the apex of the tooth.

Apicoectomy Excision of the apical portion of the root of a tooth through an opening in overlying tissues of the jaw.

Aradicular hypsodont A tooth that grows continuously throughout life.

Arkansas stone A sharpening stone used for final sharpening of an instrument that is already close to sharpness.

Association of American Feed Control Officials (AAF-CO) AAFCO is a voluntary membership association of local, state, and federal agencies charged by law to regulate the sale and distribution of animal feeds and animal drug remedies.

Atraumatic malocclusion Malposition of the teeth caused by hereditary factors or by nutritional or other atraumatic changes in teeth, temporomandibular joints, mandibular symphysis, or bone that result in improper tooth alignment.

Attrition The wearing away of a tooth, resulting from the friction of teeth against each other.

Autoclaving An equipment sterilization technique using a combination of pressure and steam heat.

American Veterinary Dental College (AVDC) Certifying organization authorized by the American Veterinary Association to board certify veterinary dentists.

Avulsion Complete displacement of the tooth from the socket.

Barbed broach Instrument useful in the removal of intact pulp. It can also be used to remove from the root canal absorbent points, cotton pellets, separated file tips, and other foreign material, such as dirt, gravel, and grass.

Biofilm An aggregate of bacterial colonies protected by a polysaccharide complex.

Bisecting-angle technique A radiographic technique obtained by visualizing an imaginary line that bisects the angle formed by the x-ray film and the structure being radiographed.

Blind intubation Placing an endotracheal tube into the trachea without being able to visualize the epiglottis. Usually performed in rabbits and other small mammals.

Bone augmentation A procedure in which bone is "built" using a synthetic material.

Bone graft substitute Materials placed into areas where periodontal or endodontic disease has resulted in bone loss.

Bone necrosis Cellular death of the bone.

Brachycephalic Having a short wide head. Characteristic of some breeds (e.g., Boxers, Pugs, Bulldogs, and Persian cats).

Brachyodont A tooth with true distinction between crown and root structure, with a root that does not grow once the tooth erupted.

Bradycardia Slowness of the heartbeat, in dogs and cats to less than 60 beats per minutes.

Buccal The direction toward the outside of the teeth, usually toward the cheeks.

Buccotomy A full-thickness incision through the skin, mucosa, and subcutaneous tissue to allow for direct visualization and the ability to treat cheek teeth.

Buccoversion A premolar or molar tooth that is in its anatomically correct position in the dental arch but which is abnormally angled in a buccal direction.

Bupivacaine A local anesthetic. It is the drug of choice at a 0.5% solution or 5 mg/mL.

Bur A type of cutter used in a dental handpiece.

Calcium hydroxide A compound used topically in solution or lotions; in dentistry used to encourage deposition of secondary dentin.

Calicivirus A virus that causes disease in cats. It is one of the two important viral causes of respiratory infection in cats, and may be a trigger leading to feline chronic ulcerative gingivostomatitis.

Calculus Mineralized deposits of calcium phosphate and carbonate, with organic matter, deposited on tooth surfaces. May initiate caries and periodontal disease.

Calculus removal forceps A dental instrument that allows for quick removal of large pieces of calculus.

Canine oral viral oral papillomatosis Warts on the oral mucous membrane (and sometimes on the lips) caused by a virus. They will generally go away with time.

Canine tooth The long, pointed tooth in the interdental space between incisors and cheek teeth; there is one in each jaw on both sides.

Caries Cavities.

Carious erosion The wasting away or loss of tooth substance.

Carnassial tooth Shearing tooth that is the upper P4 and lower M1 in the dog and cat.

Carnivore Any animal, particularly mammals of the order Carnivora, that eats primarily flesh. Includes cats, dogs, bears, etc.

Caudal crossbite A malocclusion in which one or more of the mandibular cheek teeth is buccal to the opposing maxillary cheek teeth when the mouth is closed.

Caudal mandibular block A regional nerve block in which all of the teeth of the mandible on the side of infiltration as well as adjacent bone and soft tissue are blocked.

Caudal maxillary block A regional nerve block in which both the maxillary nerve (rostrally becomes the infraorbital nerve) and the sphenopalatine nerve or ganglia is anesthetized.

Caudal mucositis Inflammation of mucosa of the caudal oral cavity, bordered medially by the palatoglossal folds and fauces, dorsally by the hard and soft palate, and rostrally by alveolar and buccal mucosa.

Caudal stomatitis The painful inflammation and ulceration extending into the tissues of the lateral palatine folds.

Cementoenamel junction The tooth location where the enamel and the cementum meet.

Cementum The bonelike connective tissue that attaches the periodontal ligament to the tooth.

Cheek pouch impaction A condition in which food is impacted in the cheek pouches, causing mild buccal irritation or stomatitis. Treatment consists of removal of the impacted material, and in severe cases, antibiotic therapy may be warranted.

Cheek retractors Single-bladed instruments that retract the cheek on a single-side or double-bladed instruments with a spring wire that spreads both buccal folds at the same time.

Cheilitis Inflammation of the lip (including the mucocutaneous junction area and skin of the lip).

Chemical plaque control Removal of plaque with a chemical agent.

Chlorhexidine An antiseptic with antibacterial, antifungal, and some antiviral activity.

Chronic ulcerative gingivostomatitis (CUGS) Widespread oral inflammation beyond gingivitis and periodontitis.

Cingulum A ledge on the palatal side of the maxillary incisors.

Class I malocclusion Overall normal occlusion except that one or more teeth are out of alignment.

Class II occlusion A malocclusion occurring when the mandible is shorter than normal. This may cause the adult canines and incisors to penetrate the hard palate, and irritation and ulceration of the hard palate may result.

Class III occlusion A malocclusion that has several forms, and may be caused by the mandible being too long (mandibular prognathism). As a result, the mandibular incisors occlude labial to the maxillary incisors.

Clip art Premade images used to illustrate any medium.

Closed periodontal debridement Procedure performed with hand instruments and an ultrasonic device to remove plaque, calculus, and debris from a periodontal pocket.

Closed position The position obtained when the face of the curette is facing the foot surface when inserted into the pocket.

Composite restoration materials Supplies used for restoring decay or for cosmetic improvements. Most cosmetic restoration materials require an acid etch for maximal adhesion.

Composites A variety of resins used in restorative dentistry.

Conical stone A sharpening stone that is used to provide a final sharpening to the instrument by working on its face.

Consent form A form used to obtain permission before a procedure is performed.

Contact mucositis (also contact mucosal ulceration) Lesions in susceptible individuals that are secondary to mucosal contact with a tooth surface bearing the responsible irritant, allergen, or antigen. They have also been called "contact ulcers" and "kissing ulcers."

Coronal The direction toward the crown.

Coronal direction Away from the gumline.

Cranial mandibular osteodystrophy An inherited condition in which nonneoplastic bone forms in the region of the temporomandibular joint and occasionally extends into the mandible. It occurs primarily in West Highland white terriers and occasionally in other breeds.

Crossbite A malocclusion in which a mandibular tooth or teeth have a more buccal or labial position than the antagonist maxillary tooth. It can be classified as rostral or caudal.

Curettage The cleansing of a diseased surface.

Curette A dental instrument used for the removal of calculus both supragingivally and subgingivally.

Dental elevator An exodontic instrument used to engage teeth and raise them from the root socket.

Dental models A manufactured copy of dentition made for orthodontic evaluation and treatment as well as for the manufacture of restorative crowns.

Dental radiographic film X-ray film used in the dental office.

Dental x-ray system Digital radiology equipment consisting of a control unit, a tube head that produces radiation, a collimator that aims and confines the radiation, and a timer that turns the unit on.

Dentigerous cyst A cyst in which all or part of a tooth is in the cyst. It causes a local swelling of the jaw which may be visible externally.

Dentin One of the hard tissues of the teeth that constitutes most of its bulk. It lies between the pulp cavity and the enamel; where it is not covered by enamel, it is covered by cementum, the third hard substance of the tooth.

Dentinal tubules Minute channels in the dentin of a tooth that extend from the pulp cavity to the cement or the enamel.

Dermatitis Inflammation of the skin. Dermatitis can result from various animal, vegetable, and chemical substances; from heat or cold; from mechanical irritation; from certain forms of malnutrition; or from infectious disease.

Diastema A space or cleft (e.g., the space in the dental arch between the incisors and canines and cheek teeth).

Digital veterinary dental radiology (DVDR) The two basic components to DVDR are the dental x-ray machine and the digital x-ray system; these x-rays require no film.

Digital x-ray system   Digital or direct radiology (DR) system can include a sensor or phosphorous plate; also known as indirect or computerized radiology (CR).

Dilacerated root   An abnormally formed root

Dilaceration   An abnormally shaped root resulting from trauma during tooth development.

Direct current (DC)   DC is the unidirectional flow of electric charge.

Direct pulp-capping   A procedure, similar to vital pulpectomy, performed aseptically after purposeful or accidental iatrogenic pulpal exposure.

Disclosing solution   A solution that selectively stains all soft debris, pellicle, and bacterial plaque on teeth.

Distal   The portion farthest from the center of the dental arch.

Distoversion   A type of Class I malocclusion in which a tooth is in its anatomically correct position in the dental arch but which is abnormally angled in a distal direction.

Dolichocephalic   Having a narrow, long head. Characteristic of some breeds (e.g., Collie, Borzoi, Greyhound, and Siamese cats).

Double palatal flap   A flap to repair oronasal fistulas that inverts a palatal graft, which is covered by tissues from the gingiva and mucous membrane.

Edentulous   The absence of teeth.

Embedded tooth   A tooth that is usually covered in bone, has not erupted into the oral cavity, and is not likely to erupt.

Enamel hypomineralization   Inadequate mineralization of enamel matrix.

Enamel hypoplasia   A defect in tooth enamel production.

Endodontic abscess   A localized collection of pus in a cavity formed by the disintegration of tissue. They frequently result from some form of trauma that has exposed the pulp and resulted in devitalization of the tooth.

Endodontic therapy   Treatment of the dental pulp, including saving vital pulp, removing live or dead pulp, and preventing or treating infection.

Endodontics   Dental specialty dealing with the treatment of conditions inside the tooth.

Endoscopic intubation   Intubation using an otoscope with an endotracheal tube or intravenous (IV) catheter. This form of intubation calls for the use of an ear cone in a size appropriate for the size and depth of the animal's oral cavity. This form of intubation is primarily used with rats, hamsters, gerbils, chinchillas, and smaller rodents and lagomorphs.

Endotoxins   A heat-stable toxin present in the intact bacterial cell but not in cell-free filtrates of cultures of intact bacteria.

Endotracheal intubation   The insertion of a tube into the trachea. The purpose of intubation varies with the location and type of tube inserted; generally, the procedure is performed to maintain an open airway and for the administration of anesthetics or oxygen.

Endo-ring   A metal or plastic instrument that fits around the finger. An attached disposable sponge in which the files can be placed in ascending order of size helps organize the files during the dental procedure.

Epithelial attachment   The epithelium attaching the gingiva to the tooth.

Ergonomics   The science of designing the workplace so that operators remain in the most neutral positions possible.

Estimate   An approximate calculation.

Exodontics   The branch of dentistry dealing with extraction of teeth.

Explorer   A hand instrument used to detect plaque and calculus. It is also used to explore for cavities and check for exposed pulp chambers.

Extraction forceps   An exodontic instrument used to grasp the tooth and remove it from the socket.

Eye shield   A shield worn over the eyes that protects the wearer from either bacterial spray or, if filtered, intense light from light-curing units that may cause permanent retinal damage.

Feline orofacial pain syndrome (FOPS)   A pain disorder of cats with behavioral signs of oral discomfort and tongue mutilation. It occurs mainly in Burmese cats, and is thought to be caused by damage to the nerves of the peripheral nervous system possibly involving central and/or ganglion processing of sensory trigeminal information.

Ferret   A member of the order Carnivora and the family Mustelidae.

Fibrosarcoma   A sarcoma occurring in the mandible or maxilla that may create fleshy, protruding, firm masses that are sometimes friable.

File   Instrument used to clean the root canal and remove dead or infected tissues.

Fistula   Any abnormal, tubelike passage within body tissue.

Flat stone   A stone used for sharpening dental equipment.

Floating   Creating a level occlusal surface.

Force technique   An exodontic technique that breaks bone and tooth root and causes more trauma than necessary. This technique is discouraged.

Free gingiva   Portion of the gingiva not directly attached to the tooth that forms the gingival wall of the sulcus.

Frenectomy   Excision of a frenum.

Frenula   Small folds of integument or mucous membrane that limit the movements of an organ or part.

Full-coverage metal crowns   A metal crown used to protect the surface of the endodontically treated tooth from further injury and to provide renewed height, shape, and function of severely deformed, fractured teeth.

Furcation   The area in which the roots join the crown.

Fusion   The joining of two developing teeth that have different tooth buds.

Gemini tooth   A tooth in which a tooth bud has partially divided in the attempt to form two teeth.

Gingiva   The gums, which consists of the mucosal tissue that lies over the alveolar bone.

Gingival hyperplasia   The proliferation of gingival cells.

Gingivectomy   Surgical excision of all loose, infected, and diseased gingival tissue to eradicate periodontal infection and reduce the depth of the gingival sulcus.

Gingivitis   Inflammation of the gingiva most often caused by bacterial plaque.

Gingivoplasty   Surgical remodeling of the gingiva.

Glass ionomers   A dental restorative material used for a base layer with composites to fill teeth.

Glossitis   Inflammation of mucosa of the dorsal and/or ventral tongue surface.

Glucose oxidase   A chemical that, when combined with lactoperoxidase, produces the hypothiocyanite ion, which is the same ion produced naturally in saliva to help inhibit bacterial growth.

Gram-positive aerobic bacteria Bacteria that resist decolorization by alcohol in Gram's method of staining. They require oxygen to survive.

Granuloma A tumor-like mass or nodule of granulation tissue.

Gutta-percha The coagulated latex used as a dental cement and in splints. It is the most popular core material used by veterinary practitioners.

Halitosis Bad breath.

Handle The part of the hand instrument that is grasped. Handles come in a variety of round, tapered, and hexagonal shapes.

Handouts Printed copies of information that give the client additional information on the procedure or procedures being performed.

HAZCOM The Federal Hazard Communication Standard (also known as HCS). Enforced by the Occupational Safety and Health Administration (OSHA) of the United States Department of Labor, HAZCOM is based on employees' rights and their "need to know" identities of hazardous substances to which they may be exposed in the work environment.

Herbivore Animals that subsist in their natural state entirely by eating plants and plant products.

Heterodont dentition Having teeth of different shapes, as molars, incisors, etc.

High-speed handpiece A handpiece used for cutting teeth in extractions and making access holes into the teeth in root canal therapy.

Hyperglobulinemia Elevated globulin.

Hyperproteinemia Elevated blood protein.

Hypotension Diminished tension; lowered blood pressure. In animals, almost the only occurrence is in severe peripheral circulatory failure, especially traumatic, toxemic, or anaphylactic shock.

Hypoventilation Reduction in the amount of air entering the pulmonary alveoli.

Iatrogenic Resulting from the activity of a medical professional.

Iatrogenic pulpal exposure The exposure of pulp induced by a medical professional.

Iatrogenic slab fracture The breaking of the enamel layer on a tooth induced inadvertently by a medical professional.

iM3 42-12 unit A veterinary ultrasonic tooth scaler.

Impacted tooth A nonerupted or partially erupted tooth that is prevented from erupting further by any structure.

Impression tray A receptacle or device that is used to carry impression material to the mouth, confine the material in apposition to the surfaces to be recorded, and to control the impression material while it sets to form the impression.

Incisors The front teeth of either jaw.

India stone A sharpening stone used for "coarse" sharpening of an overly dull instrument or for changing the plane of one or more of the sides of the instrument.

Indirect pulp-capping A restorative procedure performed when the preparation of a carious lesion does not penetrate the pulp but is perilously close (0.5 mm) to it.

Infiltration blocks A method of local anesthesia. Rather than blocking an entire quadrant, infiltration blocks block only the area where the infiltration has been administered.

Inflammatory resorption The dissolving of a tooth's root caused by injury of the periodontal ligament leading to necrotic pulp.

Interceptive orthodontics The process of extracting primary teeth to prevent orthodontic malocclusions.

Intermediate plexus A middle zone of the periodontal membrane situated between the cemental group of fibers attached to the root of the tooth and the alveolar group of fibers attached to the alveolar bone.

Internet marketing A form of marketing involving e-mail, websites, and social forums such as Facebook, Twitter, and LinkedIn.

Interproximal The area between adjacent surfaces of adjoining teeth.

Interproximal area The area between the teeth.

Intraoral film Nonscreen radiographic film that fits neatly into the oral cavity. It can be processed in 1 to 2 minutes with minimal loss of detail.

Intubation The insertion of a tube, as into the larynx. The purpose of intubation varies with the location and type of tube inserted; generally, the procedure is done to allow for drainage, to maintain an open airway, or for the administration of anesthetics or oxygen.

Irrigation The washing of a wound by a stream of water or other fluid.

Isoflurane An inhalant form of anesthesia.

Junctional epithelium The epithelium which lies at the base of the gingival sulcus.

Ketamine An injectable medication used as a form of anesthesia.

Kilovoltage peak (kVp) The highest kilovoltage used in producing a radiograph.

Labial The direction toward the outside of the teeth, usually toward the lips.

Labial/buccal mucositis Inflammation of lip/cheek mucosa.

Labioversion An incisor or canine tooth that is in its anatomically correct position in the dental arch, but which is abnormally angled in a labial direction.

Lactoperoxidase A chemical that, when combined with glucose oxidase, produces the hypothiocyanite ion, which is the same ion produced naturally in saliva to help inhibit bacterial growth.

Lagomorph A member of the order Lagomorpha. Includes the domestic rabbit, hare, and cottontail.

LaGrange scissors A type of small scissors, helpful in trimming periodontal tissue.

Lamina dura A radiographic term referring to the dense cortical bone forming the wall of the alveolus. It appears radiographically as a bony white line next to the dark line of the periodontal space.

Lamina lucida A radiographic term referring to the periodontal space between the lamina dura and tooth. It is occupied by the periodontal ligament.

Laryngoscope An instrument used for endotracheal intubation.

Lateral palatine fold The area where the two jaws join in the back of the oral cavity.

Lateral recumbency A clinical term used to describe an animal that is positioned on its side.

Linguoversion A tooth that is in its anatomically correct position in the dental arch, but which is abnormally angled in a lingual direction.

Locking cotton pliers A tool used to pick up paper points or gutta-percha without contaminating the container or points. Also known as college pliers.

Low-speed handpiece A handpiece used for polishing with prophy angles and for performing other dental procedures with contra angles.

Lucency An area of an x-ray image that represents the absorption of less radioactive energy than the surrounding tissue. Lucent areas appear dark compared with the surrounding area.

Luxation   Partial displacement of the tooth from the socket.

Malignant melanoma   A tumor occurring on any site in the oral cavity: gingiva, buccal mucosa, hard and soft palates, and tongue. The tumor is locally invasive and highly metastatic to the lungs, regional lymph nodes, and bone.

Mandible   The lower jaw.

Mandibular periostitis ossificans   A benign lesion seen in young breed dogs that will spontaneously resolve with age.

Mandibular prognathism   A condition in which the mandible is too long.

Manipulation   Skillful or dextrous treatment by the hands.

Marketing   A system of activities designed to identify and satisfy consumer needs and desires.

Material safety data sheet (MSDS)   A form with data regarding the properties of a particular substance. The MSDS provides workers with procedures for handling or working with a particular substance in a safe manner.

Maxilla   The upper jaw.

Maxillary brachygnathism   A malocclusion in which the maxilla is too short and the mandible appears to be normal length.

Maxillary-mandibular asymmetry   Skeletal malocclusions that can occur in a rostrocaudal, side-to-side, or dorsoventral direction.

Mechanical plaque control   Removal of plaque with a device such as a toothbrush, fingerbrush, or cotton-tipped applicator.

Mesaticephalic   A skull with the cranium and nasal cavity about equal lengths. Seen in a majority of dog breeds.

Mesial   Situated in the middle; median; nearer the center of the dental arch.

Mesioversion   A type of Class I malocclusion in which a tooth that is in its anatomically correct position in the dental arch is abnormally angled in a mesial direction.

Milliamperage (mA)   Measurement of x-ray current.

Modified pen grasp   The preferred method for holding hand instruments in which the instrument is held with the thumb and index finger. The instrument rests on the index finger, and the middle, ring, and little fingers are extended. The middle ring and little fingers are then placed alongside the index finger.

Molars   The permanent, primary cheek teeth that are not preceded by premolars.

Monofluorophosphate (MFP) fluoride   MFP fluoride is the form of fluoride most commonly found in over-the-counter products.

Mouth gag   Instruments that keep the mouth open during inspection and treatment. Most are spring activated or may expand with a screw device.

Mucogingival junction   The line of demarcation where the attached gingiva and alveolar mucosa meet.

Mucogingival line   The junction between gingiva attached to underlying bone and the flap overlying the tooth.

Mucositis   The painful inflammation and ulceration of the mucosal tissues lining the digestive tract.

Neutral position   Sitting with the knees slightly below the hips, the back straight, the elbows at a 90-degree angle, and the thumbs relaxed at the top of the hand.

Nonneoplastic bone   Proliferative bone that does not contain cancer cells.

Normograde   Direction from the crown to the apex.

Occlusal equilibration   Creating a level occlusal surface.

Occlusion   The way the teeth fit together. Dogs and cats have sectorial occlusion, which means chewing occurs on the sides of the teeth.

Odontoblastic cells   Connective tissue cells that deposit dentine and form the outer surface of the dental pulp adjacent to the dentine.

Odontoblasts   Cells that line the pulp chamber and produce dentine.

Odontoma   A mass of cells that have enamel, dentin, cementum, and small tooth-like structures.

Odontoplasty   The process of recontouring a tooth surface, which is not limited to leveling an occlusal surface.

Omnivore   Animals that eat both plant and animal foods.

Opacity   An area on a radiograph that indicates absorption of more radioactive energy than the surrounding tissue and will appear as lighter spots.

Open position   The position obtained when the curette is moved over the calculus and repositioned so that the cutting surface is under the calculus ledge.

Oral medicine   Dental specialty dealing with the effects of cancer and other medical conditions on the mouth.

Oral neoplasia   Tumors in the mouth.

Oronasal fistula   An abnormal opening between the oral and nasal cavities.

Orthodontics   The correction of dental malocclusions.

OSHA   Occupational Safety and Health Administration.

Osteomyelitis   Inflammation of the bone and bone marrow.

Otoscope   An instrument for inspecting the ear.

Palatal   The direction toward the inside of the maxillary tooth.

Palatitis   Inflammation of mucosa covering the hard and/or soft palate.

Palpation   The technique of examining parts of the body by touching and feeling them.

Parallel technique   A radiographic technique indicated to evaluate the caudal mandibular teeth and nasal cavity.

***Pasteurella* species**   A genus of gram-negative facultatively anaerobic, rod-shaped bacteria. Pasteurella species are most likely an antigenic trigger leading to feline chronic ulcerative gingivostomatitis (CUGS).

Patency   The condition of being open.

Pathogenesis   The development of morbid conditions or of disease; more specifically, the cellular events and reactions and other pathologic mechanisms occurring in the development of disease.

Pedodontics   Dental specialty dealing with the treatment of dental disease in the puppy and kitten.

Peg teeth   Abnormally formed supernumerary teeth.

Perioceutic therapy   The application of antibiotics directly into the periodontal pockets after root planing or periodontal debridement. In addition to the antibacterial action, there can also be anticollagenase activity.

Periodontal abscess   A localized collection of pus in a cavity formed by the disintegration of tissue.

Periodontal debridement   The treatment of gingival and periodontal inflammation. Its goal is the mechanical removal of surface irritants while maintaining soft tissue and allowing it to return to a healthy, noninflamed state.

Periodontal disease   An inflammation and infection of the tissues surrounding the tooth, collectively called the periodontium.

Periodontal pockets   An area of diseased gingival attachment, characterized by loss of attachment and eventual damage to the tooth's supporting bone.

Periodontal probe   An instrument in dentistry primarily used to measure pocket depths around the tooth in order to establish the state of health of the periodontium.

Periodontal-endodontic abscess   A localized collection of pus in a cavity formed by the disintegration of tissue. These abscesses are some of the most commonly detected facial or jaw abscesses. They occur owing to extension of periodontal disease apically to enter the pulp of the tooth.

Periodontics   Dental specialty dealing with the treatment of conditions in the surrounding tooth structure (perio means around, and dontics means tooth).

Periodontitis   Inflammation of nongingival periodontal tissues (i.e., the periodontal ligament and alveolar bone).

Periosteal elevator   An instrument used to lift the gingiva away from the bone during periodontal surgery.

Peripheral odontogenic fibroma   Fibroma characterized by the presence of a tumor in the tissues of the gingiva, it contains primarily fibrous tissues, and is also known as fibromatous epulis.

Persistent primary teeth   Baby teeth that may cause orthodontic and periodontic abnormalities by possibly displacing the adult teeth.

Pharyngitis   Inflammation of the pharynx.

Piezoelectric   An ultrasonic scaler that uses crystals in the handpiece to pick up the vibration. These units have a wide, back-and-forth tip motion.

Pigtail explorer   A curved explorer that allows the operator to easily avoid touching the parts of the tooth that are not being explored.

Plaque   A mass adhering to the enamel surface of a tooth, composed of a mixed colony of bacteria.

Plugger   An instrument with blunted tips used to obtain vertical (apical) condensation.

Pocket   A space resulting from the gingiva separating from the tooth owing to inflammation.

Porcelain-fused-to-metal crowns   A cosmetically pleasing crown with a metal shell on which is fused a veneer of porcelain. It is used to protect the surface of the endodontically treated tooth from further injury and to provide renewed height, shape, and function of severely deformed, fractured teeth.

Power scaler   A scaler that converts electric or pneumatic energy into a mechanical vibration. When the power scaler is placed against the calculus, the vibration shatters it, freeing it from the tooth surface.

Premolars   Cheek teeth present in both generations found between the molars and canines.

Prophy   A shortened version of the word prophylaxis.

Prophy angles   Attachments on slow-speed or electric motor handpiece that are used to polish teeth.

Prophy cup   The rubber cup used on the prophy angle for polishing teeth.

Prophy paste   The paste used for polishing teeth.

Prophylaxis   Prevention of or protective treatment for disease.

Prosthodontics   Dental specialty dealing with the process of restoring the tooth to normal health.

Pseudopocket   A pocket, adjacent to a tooth, resulting from gingival hyperplasia or swelling, and the periodontal membrane and alveolar bone are normal.

Pull stroke   A hand instrument technique for the removal of calculus.

Pulp   Blood vessels, nerves, and connective tissues that support the odontoblastic cells lining the pulp chamber and root canal.

Pulpectomy   Removal of dental pulp.

Pulse   Measurement of setting certain dental x-ray machine timers (one-sixtieth of a second).

Rasps   Instruments used to level an abnormally uneven occlusive table of the teeth.

Reamer   Instrument used to clean the root canal and remove dead or infected tissues. Reamers are used in a twisting, auger-like motion that delivers filings from the depth of the canal to the access site.

Recall system   System of reminding the client to return for repeat visits.

Regional anesthesia   A method of local anesthesia in which an entire quadrant is blocked.

Repetitive motion disorder   A family of muscular conditions that result from repeated motions performed in the course of normal work or daily activities.

Restorative dentistry   Restoring the form and function of damaged teeth.

Retrograde intubation   Intubation in which a needle is inserted through the midventral neck region between two of the tracheal rings and directed toward the head. The needle is stopped as soon as it penetrates the trachea. This type of intubation can be used on all sizes of rodents and lagomorphs, but it can be traumatic and irritating to the trachea.

Rodent   A member of the order Rodentia. Includes rats and mice and allied species, the squirrels and beavers, the porcupines and their related species, and the African mole rat in four separate suborders.

Root canal sealant   Cements or pastes used to seal the apical one-third of the root, dentinal tubules that radiate from the walls of the canal, and apical delta.

Root planing   The traditional method of periodontal therapy. The objective of root planing is the removal of calculus and cementum from the root surface and the creation of a clean, smooth, glasslike root surface. In this treatment, everything, including cementum, is removed from the root surface.

Rostral crossbite   A malocclusion in which one or more of the mandibular incisor teeth is labial to the opposing maxillary incisor teeth when the mouth is closed.

Rostral mandibular block   A regional nerve block in which the inferior alveolar nerve within the mandibular canal via the middle mental foramen is anesthetized.

Rostral maxillary block   A regional nerve block in which the infraorbital nerve is infiltrated as it exits the infraorbital canal.

Rotary scaler   A type of scaler that is discouraged because it can easily damage the tooth. Also, the burs must be replaced often because they become dull very quickly.

Rugae palatinae   Irregular ridges on hard palate mucosa shaped to facilitate the movement of food back toward the pharynx.

Scaler   A dental instrument used for scaling calculus from the crown surface. These instruments are particularly useful in removing calculus from narrow but deep fissures such as that located on the buccal surface of the fourth premolar.

Scissors bite   Normal occlusion in dogs and cats, in which the mandibular (lower) teeth come into contact with the palatal side (inside) of the maxillary (upper) teeth.

Scurvy   Disease caused by a nutritional deficiency of ascorbic acid (vitamin C).

Sealer   A product applied to a clean tooth surface with a sponge applicator or gloved finger that reduces plaque and tartar formation by repelling water and preventing bacteria from attaching to the teeth.

Sevoflurane   An inhalant form of anesthesia.

Shank   The part of the hand instrument that joins the working end with the handle.

Sharps   Needles, scalpel blades, broken ampoules; anything in a hospital or clinic that has been used on patients and that may be contaminated with infectious material; to be discarded into special containers for disposal without any risk to disposal personnel.

Shepherd's hook   The most commonly found explorer.

Simple buccal sliding flap   A gingival flap using gingiva and mucous membrane to cover extraction sites or oronasal fistulas.

Slab fracture   The most common fracture of the fourth premolar, resulting from the force placed on a very small area of tooth (cusp) when the patient bites down. The shear force fractures enamel and dentin, exposing the pulp.

SLOB rule   Same lingual opposite buccal (SLOB) rule used to identify roots that are laying side by side.

Slobbers   A condition in which excess salivation results in a moist dermatitis.

Smile book   A pictorial description of procedures performed in the practice. One effective strategy is to include "before and after" photographs of dental procedures.

Social media site   The use of web-based and mobile technology to turn communication into an interactive dialogue.

Sodium hypochlorite   An irrigating solution that helps break down and remove organic material.

Sonic scaler   An ultrasonic scaler that operates at 6000 cycles per second with a 0.5-mm amplitude and an elliptic, figure-of-eight motion.

Spearing canines   A Class I orthodontic condition in which the maxillary canines are tipped in a rostral position and trapped by the mandibular canines; also known as mesioversion.

Spreader   An instrument with a tapered, round shaft and pointed tip used to compress gutta-percha laterally and force sealant into dentinal tubules.

Squamous cell carcinoma   A histologically distinct form of cancer arising in a variety of locations in the mouth. The cell's type is from the epithelium, and the appearance varies, but generally it is a nodular, gray-to-pink, irregular mas that invades the bone and cause tooth mobility.

Stannous fluoride   The most bactericidal fluoride. It is stable at a pH of 6.5.

Stethoscope-aided intubation   Intubation in which an endotracheal tube is attached to a standard clinical stethoscope using an appropriate adapter.

Stomatitis   Inflammation of the mucous lining of any of the structures in the mouth; in clinical use the term should be reserved to describe widespread oral inflammation (beyond gingivitis and periodontitis) that may also extend into submucosal tissues (e.g., marked caudal mucositis extending into submucosal tissues may be termed caudal stomatitis).

Subgingival scaling   Removal of tartar from the teeth beneath the free margin of gingival tissue.

Sublingual   The structures and surfaces beneath the tongue.

Sublingual mucositis   Inflammation of mucosa on the floor of the mouth.

Substantivity   The ability of chlorhexidine, parachlorometaxylenol, and triclosan to stick to surfaces.

Sulcus   The groove between the surface of the tooth and the epithelium lining the free gingiva.

Supernumerary teeth   Teeth in excess of the regular number; extra teeth.

Supragingival gross calculus   Gross calculus formed adjacent to the opening of the submandibular salivary gland duct.

Supragingival scaling   Removal of tartar from the teeth on the side of the gingival margin toward the dental crown.

Surgical flaps   A mass of tissue used for grafting, usually including skin, only partially removed from one part of the body so that it retains its own blood supply during transfer to another site.

Suturing   Application of stitches to secure apposition of the edges of a surgical or traumatic wound.

Tartar   A yellowish film formed of calcium phosphate and carbonate, food particles, and other organic matter that is deposited on the teeth by the saliva.

Temporomandibular joint (TMJ)   The hinge joint of the jaw that connects the mandible to the maxilla.

Terminal shank   The part of the shank that is closest to the working end of the hand instrument.

Three-way syringe   Part of the dental unit that creates a water spray and an air spray. The water spray is used for irrigating a tooth surface and clearing away prophy paste, tooth shavings, and other debris. The air spray can be used to dry the field.

Tongue entrapment   A condition in which the tongue is "pinned" in the intermandibular space because of mandibular cheek teeth growing to meet at the midline.

Tongue retractors   Instruments with a single, flat blade used to move the tongue away from the area to be inspected or treated.

Tonsillitis   Inflammation of the palatine tonsil.

Tooth abrasion   Wear of teeth not associated with normal tooth-to-tooth contact.

Tooth extrusion   A pushing out (e.g., an orthodontic procedure that makes a tooth emerge further from its alveolus).

Tooth resorption   A process by which all or part of a tooth structure is lost.

Torque   The ability to overcome resistance to movement.

Toxicity   The characteristic or quality of being poisonous, especially the degree of virulence of a toxic microbe or of a poison.

Tracheotomy intubation   Intubation in which a tracheotomy is performed by making a longitudinal skin incision over the trachea midway between the larynx and thoracic inlet. A stab incision is made between two of the tracheal rings, and the endotracheal tube is passed into the trachea and then anchored with umbilical tape, which is tied to the tube and then around the animal's neck to prevent accidental extubation.

Traumatic malocclusion   Malposition of the teeth resulting from injury to the teeth resulting in broken crowns, which may cause overgrowth of the opposing tooth because of the lack of normal attrition.

Triadan numbering system   A numbering system used for medical record annotation in which three numbers are used to identify each tooth. The first number identifies the quadrant (remember that there are four) of the mouth. The second and third numbers identify the tooth, which is always represented by two numbers.

Turbine   The internal portion of the high-speed handpiece that spins at an extremely high speed.

Ulcerative eosinophilic stomatitis   A disease of the King Charles Spaniel characterized by focal raised areas on the palate. Histologically, they do not have granuloma formation. The cause is unknown.

Ultrasonic ferroceramic rod   An ultrasonic device that vibrates at 42,000 cycles per second. All sides of the tip are equally active.

Ultrasonic instrument   Dental instrument that converts energy from a power source into a sound wave.

Ultrasonic metal strips/stacks   Ultrasonic devices that vibrate at 18,000, 25,000, and 30,000 cycles per second. The amplitude of tip movement is between 0.01 and 0.05 mm, which is extremely narrow.

Ultrasonic scaler   A type of scaler used to quickly remove smaller deposits of supragingival calculus.

Uremic ulceration   Ulcerations on the tip of the tongue.

Veterinary Oral Health Council (VOHC)   Established by the AVDC in 1997, the VOHC sets testing protocol for products. If product testing is approved, the product is awarded the VOHC seal of approval.

Vital pulp therapy   A procedure performed to maintain tooth vitality. It may be required when injury or iatrogenic action causes exposure of the pulp.

Vital pulpotomy   Removal of exposed, contaminated pulp and disinfection of remaining pulp and access site. This procedure is indicated for recent fractures to preserve healthy dental pulp.

Working end   The part of the hand instrument that comes in contact with the tooth.

Xylitol   An ingredient commonly used in chewing gum and water additives for plaque control. Properly formulated, it can be safe to use; however, it can be toxic in high doses.

Zinc ascorbate   A product (also known as MaxiGuard) that is effective in the elimination of plaque and the stimulation of healing. It contains vitamin C and zinc sulfate, which are reported to clean the mouth and help decrease inflammation.

ANSWERS TO WORKSHEETS

ANSWERS TO CHAPTER 1 WORKSHEET

1. oral disease
2. mouth
3. roots
4. lateral palatine folds
5. 28; 42
6. Enamel
7. odontoblasts
8. sulcus; pocket
9. periodontal ligament
10. $2 \times (3/3I, 1/1C, 4/4P, 2/3M) = 42$
11. $2 \times (3/3I, 1/1C, 3/2P, 1/1M) = 30$
12. $^{123}I^{123}$, $^1C^1$, $^1P^1$ or 101, 102, 103, 104, 105, 201, 202, 203, 204, 205
13. $_{234}P_{234}$, $_{12}M_{12}$, or 306, 307, 308, 406, 407, 408, 309, 310, 409, 410
14. $^4P^4$, $^{12}M^{12}$, or 108, 109, 110, 208, 209, 210
15. $^4P^4$, $^1M^1$, or 108, 109, 208, 209
16. lower case
17. 1; 2; 3; 4
18. 01; 02; 03; 04; 05
19. canine; first molar
20. 205; 407

ANSWERS TO CHAPTER 2 WORKSHEET

1. deciduous; baby
2. Interceptive
3. West Highland White Terriers
4. II
5. shortened
6. wry
7. Gingivitis
8. Periodontal
9. Enamel; dentin
10. Abrasion
11. Attrition
12. Enamel hypoplasia
13. Endodontics
14. endodontic (root canal) therapy; extraction
15. slab
16. hemorrhage
17. avulsion
18. feline odontoclastic resorptive lesions; resorptive lesions; cervical line lesions
19. Benign
20. bad breath (or oral bleeding)

ANSWERS TO CHAPTER 3 WORKSHEET

1. explorers; periodontal probes; curettes; scalers (and calculus removal forceps)
2. working end
3. 3
4. 15 mm; 18 mm
5. three
6. supragingival
7. mirror imaged
8. cutting edge
9. universal
10. dull; sharp
11. 75; 80
12. flashing
13. electric; pneumatic
14. magnetostrictive; piezoelectric.
15. crystals
16. compressed air
17. 30; 40
18. Water
19. higher; less
20. sharps

ANSWERS TO CHAPTER 4 WORKSHEET

1. law or OSHA
2. their own safety
3. chemical; physical; biologic; ergonomic
4. bacteria
5. handwashing
6. cold
7. immediately
8. material safety data sheets
9. sterile
10. life

ANSWERS TO CHAPTER 5 WORKSHEET

1. supervising veterinarian
2. 0.5; 5
3. decrease the chance of toxicity
4. toxicity to skeletal muscle; anaphylactic reactions; permanent nerve damage
5. 0.1; 0.2; 0.3
6. 2.0
7. increase
8. entire
9. rostral maxillary; caudal maxillary; rostral mandibular; caudal mandibular
10. distal; third; infraorbital
11. caudally; infraorbital
12. frenulum
13. notch; condylar process
14. third; first
15. aspirate

ANSWERS TO CHAPTER 6 WORKSHEET

1. inflammation; infection
2. acquired pellicle
3. gram-negative
4. Supragingival; free-floating subgingival; attached to tooth or gingival; invasive into gingiva
5. "Doggy breath"
6. plaque; calculus
7. bone (or attachment) loss
8. attachment loss
9. early periodontitis
10. 4 (advanced periodontitis)

ANSWERS TO CHAPTER 7 WORKSHEET

1. Prophy or prophylaxis; periodontal therapy
2. gross
3. calculus removal forceps
4. mechanical etching; thermal heating
5. lightly; tightly
6. Water flow
7. light
8. modified
9. oxygenates
10. Dental radiographs

ANSWERS TO CHAPTER 8 WORKSHEET

1. before
2. "demonstrator"
3. coronal
4. Visual aids; client handouts
5. plaque control
6. Veterinary Oral Health Council
7. chlorhexidine
8. parental guidance (proper supervision)
9. Daily
10. 6; 8

ANSWERS TO CHAPTER 9 WORKSHEET

1. treat periodontal disease
2. 2; 3; 4
3. Scaling
4. root planing
5. horizontal; vertical; oblique
6. Periodontal debridement
7. cementum
8. disrupting
9. doxycycline
10. 100

ANSWERS TO CHAPTER 10 WORKSHEET

1. chronic ulcerative gingivostomatitis; tooth resorption; feline oral pain syndrome
2. Stomatitis
3. Plasma
4. Feline orofacial pain syndrome
5. antibiotics; steroids; NSAIDs; pain medications
6. 50 to 75
7. resorption
8. 1
9. extraction
10. Dental radiographs

ANSWERS TO CHAPTER 11 WORKSHEET

1. plastic or paper
2. layer of paper
3. lead safety aprons; screens; distance.

4. root
5. mandibular posterior teeth; nasal cavity
6. bisecting-angle technique
7. elongation
8. foreshortening
9. parallel
10. 45
11. 6
12. 45; 45
13. movement
14. Black
15. developer
16. sink
17. pulses; pulses
18. subject; sensor, or film
19. air
20. Sensor, or film
21. subject

ANSWERS TO CHAPTER 12 WORKSHEET

1. home care
2. authorization
3. laws
4. extraction
5. surgery
6. Dental elevators
7. Extraction forceps
8. 301; 301s; 301ss
9. Heidbrink
10. small (cat) extraction
11. sterile instruments
12. force
13. discouraged
14. rotational
15. Single
16. vertical
17. multirooted
18. "T"
19. Dental radiographs
20. flap

ANSWERS TO CHAPTER 13 WORKSHEET

1. subgingival; tissues
2. dental x-ray; periodontal probe
3. 3
4. Gingivectomy

5. lip
6. Endodontic therapy
7. fractured tooth
8. pulpal hemorrhage (or pulpal death)
9. black
10. less
11. 48
12. Root canal (or endodontic)
13. K; Hedstrom
14. length; diameter
15. Pluggers
16. level bite
17. base narrowed
18. wry bite
19. Dental impressions
20. Rubber mixing bowls

ANSWERS TO CHAPTER 14 WORKSHEET

1. aradicular; aradicular; brachyodont
2. incisors; premolars; molars; canine
3. intermediate plexus
4. traumatic; atraumatic
5. mandibular canine
6. 4
7. slobbers, or wet dewlap
8. Anisognathic jaw relationship
9. enamel
10. No restriction is required

ANSWERS TO CHAPTER 15 WORKSHEET

1. identify; satisfy; needs; desires
2. "doctoring"
3. "smile book"
4. handouts
5. Treatment plans
6. handouts
7. Recall cards (or e-mails)
8. February
9. occlusion
10. better service
11. Facebook; Twitter; LinkedIn
12. design; structure; content
13. blog
14. e-mail; permission; e-mail
15. dental recalls; newsletters

Note: Page numbers followed by "*f*" indicate figures, "*t*" indicate tables, and "*b*" indicate boxes.